Everyone's Guide to CANCER SURVIVORSHIP

RELATED BOOKS

Everyone's Guide to Cancer Therapy

Everyone's Guide to Cancer Supportive Care

Everyone's Guide to

CANCER SURVIVORSHIP

A Road Map for Better Health

Ernest H. Rosenbaum, M.D., F.A.C.P.
David Spiegel, M.D.
Patricia Fobair, L.C.S.W., M.P.H
Holly Gautier, R.N.

With Louise Maffitt, B.F.A.

Foreword by Sandra Horning, M.D.,
Immediate Past President, American Society of Clinical Oncology

Andrews McMeel Publishing, LLC
Kansas City

07 08 09 10 11 RR4 10 9 8 7 6 5 4 3 2 1

Library of Congress Cataloging-in-Publication Data

Everyone's guide to cancer survivorship : a road map for better health / Ernest H. Rosenbaum . . . [et al.].
p. cm.
Includes bibliographical references and index.
ISBN-13: 978-0-7407-6870-5
ISBN-10: 0-7407-6870-0
1. Cancer—Popular works. 2. Cancer—Patients—Rehabilitation. 3. Cancer—Patients—Life skills guides. I. Rosenbaum, Ernest H.

RC263.E93 2007
616.99'406—dc22

2007019862

Although they do not appear with the "TM" symbol in this book, the brand names of drugs listed are the trademarks of the pharmaceutical companies that produce them.

Parts of *Everyone's Guide to Cancer Survivorship* have been adapted from:

"American Cancer Society Guidelines on Nutrition and Physical Activity for Cancer Prevention: Reducing the Risk of Cancer with Healthy Food Choices and Physical Activity," Lawrence H. Kushi, Tim Byers, Colleen Doyle, Elisa V. Bandera, Marji McCullough, Ted Gansler, Kimberly S. Andrews, Michael J. Thun, and the American Cancer Society 2006 Nutrition and Physical Activity Guidelines Advisory Committee. *CA Cancer J Clin* 2006;56(5):254–81. http://caonline.amcancersoc.org/cgi/content/full/56/5/254.

From Cancer Patient to Cancer Survivor, Lost in Transition, Committee on Cancer Survivorship: Improving Care and Quality of Life, National Cancer Policy Board; Maria Hewitt, Sheldon Greenfield, and Ellen Stovall, editors. Washington, D.C.: Institute of Medicine, National Research Council, The National Academies Press, 2005.

A Cancer Survivor's Almanac, Barbara Hoffman, J.D., National Coalition for Cancer Survivorship, Hoboken, NJ: John Wiley & Sons, 2004.

"Nutrition and Physical Activity During and After Cancer Treatment: An American Cancer Society Guide for Informed Choices," Colleen Doyle, Lawrence H. Kushi, Tim Byers, Kerry S. Courneya, Wendy Demark-Wahnefried, Barbara Grant, Anne McTiernan, Cheryl L. Rock, Cyndi Thompson, Ted Gansler, Kimberly S. Andrews, and the 2006 Nutrition, Physical Activity, and Cancer Survivorship Committee. *CA Cancer J Clin* 2006;56(6):323–53.http://caonline.amcancersoc.org/cgi/content/full/56/6/323.

"Riding the Crest of the Teachable Moment: Promoting Long-Term Health After the Diagnosis of Cancer," Wendy Denark-Wahnefried et al., *J Clin Oncol* 2006; 23(24):12585-1530.

Design and composition by Kelly & Company, Lee's Summit, Missouri

www.andrewsmcmeel.com

This book is dedicated to the survivors of cancer who have struggled with great difficulty to achieve a satisfying and productive quality of life after their diagnosis and treatment, and whose courage and perseverance have inspired others to live their lives to the fullest.

All royalties will be donated to the Stanford Cancer Survivorship Program in the Stanford Center for Integrative Medicine.

Contents

Foreword

Sandra J. Horning, M.D.,
Immediate Past President,
American Society of
Clinical Oncology

Cancer survivors have increased in number more than threefold over the last thirty years to the current level of 10 million and growing. Among patients diagnosed in 2006, nearly two thirds are expected to survive five or more years. With these burgeoning survivor numbers, a growing body of data on the side effects of treatment, and increased professional and public awareness, a guide to cancer survivorship is a welcome and timely resource. Using the latest data from multiple sources, including a recent Institute of Medicine report on adult survivorship, Dr. Rosenbaum and the co-editors of *Everyone's Guide to Cancer Survivorship* have combined their expertise to empower survivors with the knowledge and self-determination to promote health and quality of life after a cancer diagnosis.

Current success in cancer treatment may be attributed to the expertise of multidisciplinary healthcare providers precisely executing a complex plan based on clinical research. Yet after a period of orchestrated and frequent interaction with healthcare professionals, the end of treatment may be marked by patient anxiety and uncertainty because of the lack of an ongoing plan for cancer survivorship. Appropriately, this significant volume begins with a program to help physicians coordinate and provide comprehensive survivor care and continues with a wealth of resources for patients, covering the major areas for optimal survivorship. The topics include a road map to health and longevity, ways to improve lifestyle, disease prevention and control, side effect control, and improved survival through creative expression. With this guide, cancer survivors can take proactive steps to promote their total well-being with practical advice on diet, exercise, and further prevention.

As a cancer survivor and an oncologist, I deeply appreciate the supportive and positive tone in this guide and its comprehensiveness. This volume for survivors complements efforts of professional societies such as the American Society of Clinical Oncology to include survivorship issues in training curricula, provide ongoing education to practicing healthcare providers, and encourage scientific inquiry in the health and social outcomes of survivors.

An entire generation of cancer survivors has unmet needs that are addressed in *Everyone's Guide to Cancer Survivorship*. Dr. Rosenbaum, his co-editors, and the distinguished contributors are to be congratulated for this valued resource.

Preface

Ernest H. Rosenbaum, David Spiegel, Patricia Fobair, and Holly Gautier

Over the last twenty-five years, a large series of papers with evidence-based research have shown that by adopting a healthier lifestyle, including a prudent diet, exercise, smoking cessation, and limited alcohol intake, and by following a disease surveillance and preventive program, cancer survivors can live longer, reduce the risk of recurrence of breast, prostate, and colon cancers, and help prevent the occurrence of a new cancer.

This book, *Everyone's Guide to Cancer Survivorship,* is written for both survivors and health professionals, some of whom are cancer survivors, too. Our goal is to provide you with a survivor's road map so you will meet the fewest possible obstacles while going through diagnosis, therapy, and posttherapy survivorship. The ideas, strategies, and solutions offered here are intended to help prevent or reduce many of the toxic side effects of treatment, and offer a survivor plan for follow-up care. With this practical cancer healthcare guide, your journey through cancer care can be easier and safer.

We also imagine this book as a guide to preventive and surveillance care to help reduce the risk of second cancers and recurrent cancers. Thus, the book can be a companion guide, pointing the direction for a healthier future.

Finally, we hope that cancer survivors everywhere will adopt preventive lifestyle programs to help them live longer, fuller lives with the fewest possible treatment-related problems.

Acknowledgments

We wish to acknowledge that this book is the result of the writings and ideas of many authors (credited in the text) compiled to create a comprehensive guide to help cancer survivors find optimal ways of coping with the challenges they face and live better lives by addressing their problems and adopting coping techniques.

We appreciate the efforts of the American Society of Clinical Oncology (ASCO), the National Institutes of Health (NIH), the Institute of Medicine (IOM), the National Coalition for Cancer Survivors (NCCS), the Oncology Nursing Society (ONS), the American Cancer Society (ACS), and the Office of Cancer Survivorship (at the NIH) for their leadership efforts to promote survivorship programs to improve the quality of life for cancer patients and survivors and their families.

The IOM Committee on Cancer Survivorship: Improving Care and Quality of Life (who wrote *From Cancer Patient to Cancer Survivor, Lost in Transition,* 2005) National Cancer Policy Board:

Sheldon Greenfield *(Chair)*, director, Center for Health Policy Research, University of California at Irvine, Irvine, CA

Ellen Stovall *(Vice Chair)*, president and CEO, National Coalition for Cancer Survivorship, Silver Spring, MD

John Z. Ayanian, associate professor of medicine and healthcare policy, Harvard Medical School and Brigham and Women's Hospital, Boston, MA

Regina M. Benjamin, founder and CEO, Bayou La Batre Rural Health Clinic, Inc., Bayou La Batre, AL

Harris A. Berman, dean of public health and professional degree programs and chair, Department of Public Health and Family Medicine, Tufts University School of Medicine, Boston, MA

Sarah S. Donaldson, Catharine and Howard Avery Professor, Stanford University School of Medicine, Stanford, CA

Craig Earle, assistant professor, Dana-Farber Cancer Institute, Department of Health Policy and Management, Harvard University, Boston, MA

Betty R. Ferrell, research scientist, Department of Nursing Research and Education, City of Hope National Medical Center, Duarte, CA

Patricia A. Ganz, professor, UCLA Schools of Medicine and Public Health, director, Division of Cancer Prevention and Control Research, Jonsson Comprehensive Cancer Center at UCLA, Los Angeles, CA

Frank E. Johnson, professor of surgery, Saint Louis University Health Sciences Center, St. Louis, MO

Mark S. Litwin, professor of health services and urology, UCLA School of Medicine, Los Angeles, CA

Karen Pollitz, project director, Georgetown University Health Policy Institute, Washington, DC

Pamela Farley Short, professor of health policy and administration, director of the Center for Health Care and Policy Research, Pennsylvania State University, University Park, PA

Bonnie Teschendorf, director, Quality of Life Sciences, American Cancer Society, Atlanta, GA

Mary M. Vargo, associate professor, Department of Physical Medicine and Rehabilitation, Case Western Reserve University at MetroHealth Medical Center, Cleveland, OH

Rodger J. Winn, clinical consultant, National Quality Forum, Washington, DC

Steven H. Woolf, professor of family practice, preventive medicine and community health, Virginia Commonwealth University, Richmond, VA

Staff

Maria Hewitt, study director

Roger Herdman, director, National Cancer Policy Board

Elizabeth J. Brown, research associate

Jaehee Yi, intern

Anike Johnson, administrative assistant

We also want to thank Louise Maffitt, B.F.A., Lane Butler, Michelle Daniel, and Carol Anne Peschke, for their superb editing; Paula Chung for her transcription skill and total support through the book-writing process; and Gail Sorrough, Gloria Won, and Laura Olson for library support, which helped make this book possible.

Contributors

Alexandra Andrews, Webmaster, cancersupportivecare.com

David G. Bullard, Ph.D., private psychology practice, UCSF Medical Center

Jean Chan, B.A., M.A., S.Ed., consultant for computer art graphics

David Claman, M.D., director, Sleep Center, UCSF Medical Center

John P. Cooke, M.D., Ph.D., cardiovascular medicine, Stanford University School of Medicine

J. Ben Davoren, M.D., Ph.D., director, Clinical Informatics, San Francisco VA Medical Center

Christine M. Derzko, M.D., F.R.C.S.C., associate professor, obstetrics & gynecology and internal medicine (endocrinology), University of Toronto

Charles M. Dollbaum, M.D., Ph.D., clinical professor of medicine, UCSF Comprehensive Cancer Center

Malin Dollinger, M.D., medical oncologist, University of Southern California

Patricia Fobair, L.C.S.W., M.P.H., group therapy, supportive care, integrative medicine, Stanford University School of Medicine

John Fox, C.P.T., Stanford University Hospital and Clinics

Holly Gautier, R.N., director, Stanford Cancer Center Concierge Services

Bernard Gordon, M.D., dermatologist, private practice, UCSF Medical Center

Jack D. Gordon, M.D. (deceased), internal medicine, UCSF Medical Center

Robert Ignoffo, Pharm.D., clinical professor of pharmacology, UCSF School of Pharmacy

Felix O. Kolb (retired), endocrinologist, professor of medicine, UCSF Medical Center

Jack LaLanne, physical fitness expert, television personality, author, and entrepreneur

Natalie Ledesma, M.S., R.D., dietitian, Resource Center, UCSF Comprehensive Cancer Center

Jay S. Luxenberg, M.D., private practice, internal medicine, UCSF Medical Center

Gerd Mairandries, wig master for the San Francisco Opera

Louise Maffitt, B.F.A., senior research associate, New Mexico Institute of Mining and Technology

Francine Manuel, R.P.T., private practice, physical therapist

Gary F. Milechman, M.D., F.A.C.C., cardiologist, California Pacific Medical Center

Lawrence Mintz, M.D., F.I.D.S.A., associate professor of medicine, infectious disease, UCSF

Jim Murdoch, musician, Art for Recovery, UCSF Comprehensive Cancer Center

Laura Olson, M.F.A., M.L.I.S., Web librarian, H. M. Fishbon Memorial Library, UCSF Medical Center at Mount Zion

Cynthia D. Perlis, B.S., director, Art for Recovery Program, UCSF Medical Center

John Phillips, medical librarian, H. M. Fishbon Memorial Library, UCSF Medical Center at Mount Zion

Wendye Robbins, M.D., clinical assistant professor, Stanford University School of Medicine, Department of Anesthesiology; president and CEO, Limerick NeuroSciences, Inc.

Mitchell Rosen, M.D., assistant professor, Department of Obstetrics and Gynecology, Division of Reproductive Endocrinology and Infertility, UCSF Medical Center

E rnest H. Rosenbaum, M.D., F.A.C.P., Cancer Supportive Care Program, Integrative Medicine, Stanford University School of Medicine and Clinical Professor of Medicine, UCSF Comprehensive Cancer Center

Isadora R. Rosenbaum, M.A. (retired), medical assistant, UCSF Comprehensive Cancer Center

Robert J. Rushakoff, M.D., F.A.C.P., endocrinologist, UCSF Medical Center

Richard Shapiro, M.D., chief of anesthesiology, Union Memorial Hospital, Baltimore, MD

Sol Silverman, Jr., M.A., D.D.S., professor emeritus of oral medicine, Department of Orofacial Sciences, UCSF

Gail Sorrough, M.L.I.S., director, Medical Li-b r a rySe rvices, H. M. Fishbon Memorial Library, UCSF Medical Center at Mount Zion

David Spiegel, M.D., Wilson Professor and Associate Chair of Psychiatry and Behavioral Sciences and director, Center for Integrative Medicine, Stanford University School of Medicine

Andrzej Szuba, M.D., cardiovascular medicine, Stanford University School of Medicine

Robert A. Wascher, M.D., F.A.C.S., director, Division of Surgical Oncology, Department of Surgery, Newark Beth Israel Medical Center

Chris Wilhite, manager, Friend to Friend Specialty Gift Shop, UCSF Medical Center at Mount Zion

Gloria Won, M.L.I.S., medical librarian, H. M. Fishbon Memorial Library, UCSF Medical Center at Mount Zion

Introduction

A cancer survivor is generally defined as one living from the time of diagnosis through the remainder of his or her life with or beyond cancer. The definition of the National Coalition for Cancer Survivorship is "living with, through, and beyond cancer." The U.S. Centers for Disease Control and Prevention and the Lance Armstrong Foundation define survivors as "anybody who has ever been diagnosed with cancer."

One of today's greatest medical challenges is to control and hopefully cure cancer through newer and better therapies that will prevent or stop the disease quickly so that survivors, no matter how you define them, can minimize medical problems and improve their social activities and quality of life.

Cancer Survival Rates Are Generally Increasing

Currently, more than 1.4 million new cases of cancer are diagnosed each year in the United States. The survival rate has risen from 3 million survivors thirty-five years ago to more than 10 million survivors in 2006. This survival rate will continue to increase as screening, early detection, diagnosis, treatment, and care advance. It is estimated that by 2030 there will be more than 20 million survivors. The National Cancer Institute and American Cancer Society currently project that about one-third of women and one-half of men will have cancer in their lifetime. One in four people are expected to die from the disease.

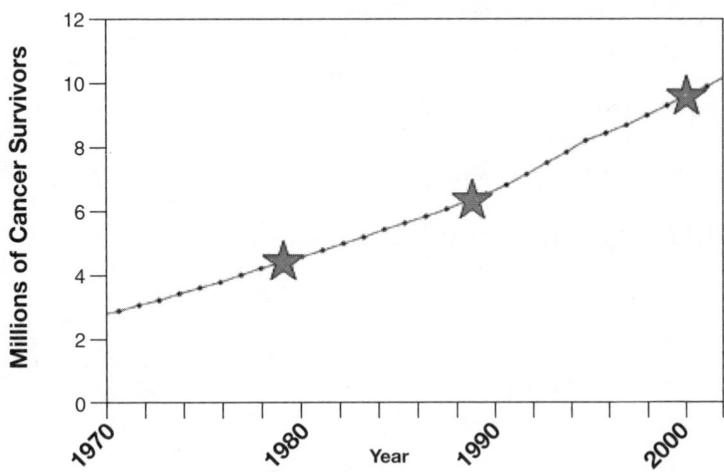

Cancer Has Become a Chronic Disease

Unfortunately, many cancer survivors may experience lasting adverse side effects of treatment. Although the current five-year survival rate is 64 percent (compared to 50 percent twenty-five years ago), the estimated follow-up needed for surveillance for other new diseases or the diagnosis of a secondary or new cancer is at least twenty years, the remainder of the survivor's life. With a good follow-up program, many cancer survivors can improve their overall health and longevity. Writer and activist Susan Sontag's cancer experience provides a good example of the potential for productivity, wellness, and longevity in survivorship. Diagnosed and treated for metastatic breast cancer at age forty-five, she died at age seventy-one of a new cancer.

Despite advances and innovations in cancer diagnosis and treatment, the long-term consequences for survivors remain serious. More than 50 percent of cancer survivors have residual side effects; approximately 15 percent experience recurrence or develop new cancers. It is estimated that 75 percent of survivors can have some health deficits related to their treatment.[1]

There is also overwhelming evidence that cancer survivors have higher death rates from other causes than do those who have not had cancer. Added to known cancer-specific vulnerabilities, the increased risk of additional illnesses (also called comorbid conditions), such as cardiovascular disease, diabetes, and osteoporosis, makes the need for follow-up programs for cancer survivors even more urgent.[2]

Age is a major risk factor, which has recently been shown to correlate with functional decline; 61 percent of cancer survivors are over age sixty-five. In the United States, 35 million people (12.4 percent of the population) are over sixty-five, and this figure will double by 2030 to 70 million (20 percent). As people experience greater longevity, there will also be more medical comorbidities and cancer cases.

This book is for both survivors and the medical teams responsible for their care. It is divided into sections for easy reference:

The first section explains the history of survivorship care programs, the development of the Institute of Medicine's report by the Committee on Survivorship Care, recommended guidelines, and essential elements of survivorship care programs.

The second section presents strategies and solutions for survivors and a basic outline of what survivors need to know after anticancer therapy.

The third section defines the elements of healthy lifestyles to improve survivorship and help prevent or reduce many of the toxic side effects of treatment. These chapters also include information from current research on the benefits of lifestyle improvements for survivors of specific cancers.

The fourth section provides descriptions and prevention measures for controlling potential comorbid conditions, or diseases that can be caused or exacerbated by the use of anticancer therapies.

The fifth section provides strategies for coping with and controlling the side effects of cancer and its therapies.

The sixth section describes ways to improve survival through creative expression.

A final section provides advice on ways to plan for the future and get your affairs in order.

PART I

A Physician Guidance Program

1 The Need for Survivorship Care

Physicians have the primary responsibility for directing the survivorship program, office or clinic program, nursing staff, and supportive care patient programs. The goal of survivorship care is to provide tools for patients and their medical team to chart the course forward to healthy survivorship.

The greatest of the many barriers to effective long-term survivorship care is a lack of awareness. Cancer survivors need to be made aware of the potential medical conditions and risks that follow cancer and its treatments and strategies they can use to reduce their risks. In order to provide this information, physicians need access to the most current standards in care and clinical guidelines. Often, after achieving a good healthy state five years after completing cancer treatments, patients are not in an optimal twenty-plus-year follow-up program, which should include surveillance for potential late toxic side effects of cancer therapy and screening for comorbid conditions, the possibility of a late recurrence of cancer, or the development of a new cancer. The American Society of Clinical Oncology (ASCO), the Institute of Medicine (IOM), the National Coalition for Cancer Survivorship (NCCS), the Office of Cancer Survivorship (at the National Institutes of Health [NIH]), the Oncology Nursing Society (ONS), and the American Cancer Society (ACS) have been working together on task forces to provide specific follow-up guidelines and templates for early and late side effects of therapy and follow-up surveillance programs. Web links to these resources are included in Appendix B.

One challenge in survivorship care programs is convincing patients of the need for follow-up care. After completing their therapy, some patients want to distance themselves from their cancer and their medical team. Another challenge is training physicians, nurses, and medical teams to provide patients with ways to make lifestyle changes for better health outcomes. A poll by the Lance Armstrong Foundation noted that the American healthcare system failed to meet cancer patients' medical needs: 70 percent of those polled reported that oncologists did not offer guidance for coping with these issues.

Oncologists and the medical team (including primary physicians or general practitioners and nurse specialists) can play a key role in cancer detection, treatment, surveillance, and prevention programs. Currently, only about 20 percent of oncologists actively guide survivors on better health practices and lifestyle changes that could improve physical and psychosocial well-being and promote better health, quality of life, and longevity.[1]

Specific Challenges of Survivorship Care

Comorbid Conditions

Comorbid conditions can threaten the lives of cancer survivors. Common problems include angina, congestive heart failure, osteoporosis, and diabetes. Unfortunately, with the growing obesity trend in the United States, comorbid problems will increase. African Americans, the poor, and older adults are less likely to receive necessary care, and if they are diagnosed with cancer, other comorbid conditions may not receive appropriate attention, resulting in 10 percent lower five-year survival rates for these groups because of poorer surveillance and an inability to afford optimal medical care.

Awareness of Both Physiological and Psychological Concerns

Survivors are also at risk for psychological and physiological changes, such as organ dysfunction (kidney, heart, nervous system, and lung), impairment of the immune response system, sexual dysfunction, cognitive changes, fatigue, depression, anxiety, family distress, and economic challenges related to insurance, job security, and financial survival.

Lack of Community-Based Education on Cancer and Survivorship

Community-based education programs are needed to raise awareness that cancer is a treatable chronic illness.

The Medical Approach to Long-Term Treatment

A multidisciplinary team approach and a variety of delivery systems are the best ways to address the medical, psychosocial, and lifestyle components of survivorship care. Physicians and other care providers need to change their approach to the wellness model, incorporating health promotion with surveillance and disease prevention rather than just treating problems when they arise. Better guidelines for evidence-based practices and advisory education are necessary and are now being addressed in cancer research programs.

Report on Essential Components of Survivorship Care

In 2005, an IOM Committee on Cancer Survivorship was formed with the NCCS, ACS, ONS, NIH, and others to investigate the conditions faced by cancer survivors. Composed of seventeen members representing many disciplines with special expertise, the committee extensively reviewed current patient care and condition data and posttreatment care strategies. Their report identifies the following essential components of survivorship care:

- Prevention of recurrent and new cancers and other late treatment side effects
- Surveillance for cancer spread, recurrence, or second cancers; assessment of medical and psychological late side effects
- Intervention for consequences of cancer and its treatment, including medical problems such as lymphedema, sexual dysfunction, pain, and fatigue; psychological distress of cancer survivors and their caregivers; and concerns related to employment, insurance, and disability
- Coordination between oncology specialists, primary care providers, and nurse specialists to ensure that all of the survivor's health needs are met

The IOM committee also identified the following survivor risk factor assessment variables:

- Age at diagnosis
- Current age (child or adult)
- Family genetic predisposition or immunodeficiency
- Current comorbidities
- Cancer therapies and latent toxicities
- Lifestyle factors

It is important that patients receive a cancer survivor care plan reviewing their medical history and treatments and a set of follow-up recommendations to help guide them over the next twenty or more years with appropriate surveillance and interventions to minimize or prevent further problems.[2] This includes information on their diagnosis and therapy, cancer warning signs, recommendations for screening, a list of potential side effects related to their cancer therapy, and clinical psychological advice and guidance for maintaining a healthy preventive lifestyle and coping with chronic recurrence-related anxiety.

The issues raised by long-lived survivors and their significant potential for comorbidities will be further exacerbated by the aging of the baby boomers, the first of whom will turn sixty-five in 2011. A concerted effort will be needed to reduce the impact of cancer on these millions of Americans.

Program Elements

Knowledge and awareness are the most important aspects of the services health providers give to their patients. To bolster their knowledge of ways to improve health and longevity, cancer survivors should be provided with medical team information, guideline forms, a discharge plan summary, medical records, and literature on supportive care that addresses the issues that will confront them. As patients focus on their mortality and vulnerabilities, they should be provided with guidelines and strategies for healthy survivorship.

A Proposed Framework for Survivorship Care Programs in Institutions, Medical Offices, and Clinics

A broad-spectrum approach covering the social and physical needs of cancer survivors is necessary. By facing these challenges with knowledge about how to overcome the obstacles, survivors gain confidence not only that life will go on but also that a good quality of life is attainable. Organized support from cancer centers, physician offices, the medical team, and community programs can provide psychosocial, physical, and preventive medicine programs. Information from literature, DVDs, videotapes, lectures, and various exercise programs is beneficial.

Information on implementing survivorship care programs can also be found on Web sites such as

www.cancersupportivecare.com
www.canceradvocacy.org
www.survivorshipguidelines.org
www.americancancersociety.org

As cancer patients live years and decades longer, the need for more educational follow-up clinics and supportive programs becomes vital.

The following flowchart by Ernest H. Rosenbaum and Rena Sellin of the M. D. Anderson Cancer Center outlines a potential structure for a shared-care survivorship care program.

The Structure of a Shared-Care Cancer Survivorship Program

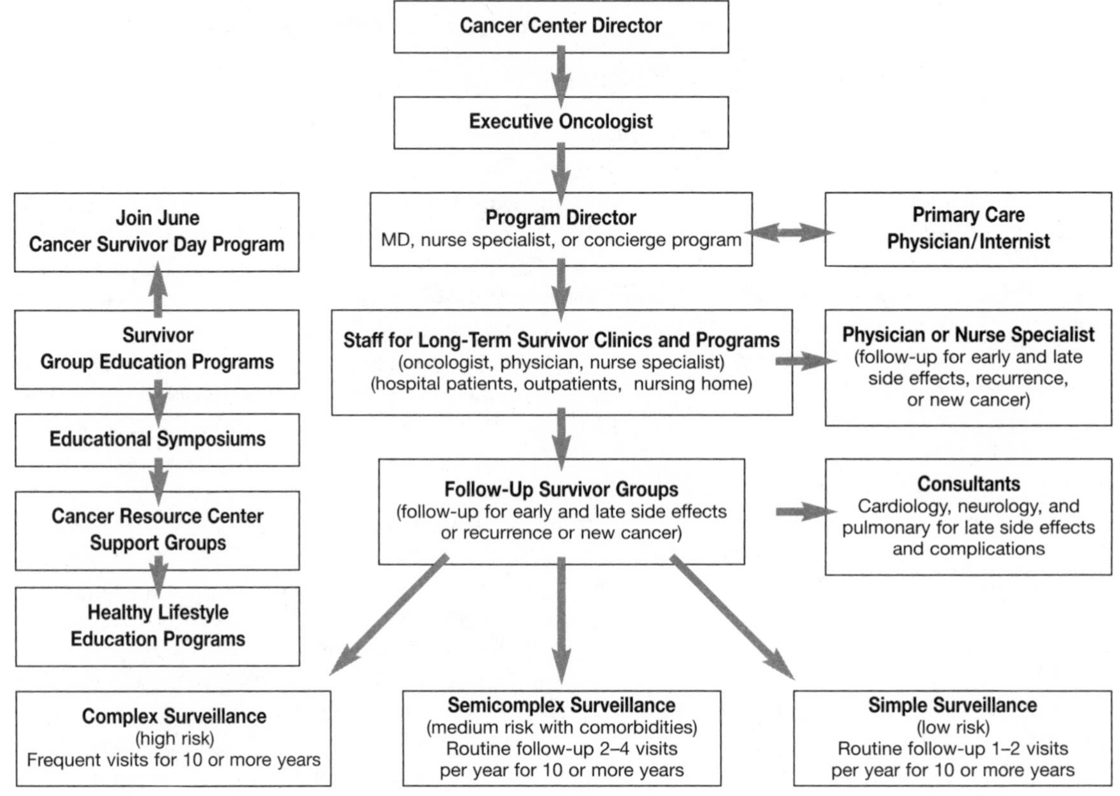

2 Guidelines for Survivorship Care

Ways for the Medical Community to Improve Health and Longevity

- Collect statistics on comorbid health problems and follow-up screening of survivors, assess treatment results and quality of life, and promulgate better lifestyle health practices.
- Collect and analyze data on disability and dysfunction caused by aging to identify ways to improve function and quality of life.[1]
- Promote better lifestyles (diet, exercise, psychological support, smoking cessation, alcohol moderation, bone health, sun exposure reduction) and screening for comorbid diseases, cancer recurrence, and new cancers.
- Reduce side effects of therapy and improve treatments of early comorbid problems (lymphedema, sexual dysfunction, fatigue, memory problems, and chemotherapy and radiation side effects such as mucositis) and late side effects (psychological, cardiac, renal effects, neurological deficits, osteoporosis, and pulmonary fibrosis [scarring]).
- Improve survival by reducing comorbidities and treatment side effects using improved treatments (e.g., sentinel node biopsies to avoid axillary dissections and lymphedema), adjuvant therapies, new drug treatments and immunotherapy to promote cures, longevity, quality of life, and survival.

The Objective

The goal is to improve the research on aging cancer survivors and to improve survival and quality of life with better treatments to ameliorate side effects and programs to provide coping mechanisms through patient and health team education. It is hoped that prevention programs and improved follow-up surveillance programs will enable survivors to have fewer preventable health problems and fewer premature deaths.

Prevention Measures

It is as important to make and implement positive recommendations for cancer prevention as it is to diagnose and treat cancer early. Preventing cancer spares patients the devastating psychological and physical morbidities, extreme expenses, and debility of a life-threatening illness.

The American Cancer Society proposes annual guidelines for cancer prevention and statistics that are published each year in their journal, *CA, A Cancer Journal for Clinicians*. Follow-up guidelines for primary, secondary, and tertiary prevention of cancers and surveillance include the following:

Primary Prevention

Prevention of cancer through healthful lifestyles, such as a healthy diet, smoking cessation, reduction of alcohol use, reduction of sun exposure, exercise to help decrease morbidity risks, and screening for precancerous lesions (such as colon polyps, cervical cell abnormalities, etc.).

Secondary Prevention

Screening and vaccination programs for prevention of cancer and comorbid diseases before and after cancer therapy, including cervix, breast, colon, melanoma, prostate, and lung cancer, osteoporosis, heart disease, diabetes, and other potential illnesses. Examples include the following:

- Screening for breast cancer many years after left chest mantle radiotherapy for Hodgkin's disease
- Screening for heart, kidney, and liver disease after radiotherapy and chemotherapy
- Screening for diabetes, pulmonary disease, and other comorbidities

Tertiary Prevention

Early detection, surveillance, and management of late cancer toxicities after radiotherapy, chemotherapy, or targeted immunotherapy (e.g., doxorubicin, epirubicin, bleomycin, and trastuzumab, which can have late toxic side effects). Examples include the following:

- Dexrazoxane and amifostine are drugs used to reduce doxorubicin or epirubicin cardiac toxicity or kidney toxicity from platinum drugs, respectively.
- Osteoporosis detection, evaluation, and prevention with diet, vitamin D, calcium, and/or bisphosphonate treatment and surveillance with a dual-energy x-ray absorptiometry (DEXA) bone density test for evaluation of bone density and treatment assessment as recommended.
- Dental preventive care is needed when one is using zoledronic acid, a bisphosphonate for bone pain or metastases to help prevent jaw bone necrosis.
- Dental care is needed before and after radiotherapy and chemotherapy for head and neck cancer.

Posttherapy Cancer Survivorship Measures

Survivors of cancer graduate to a new life but may face many consequences, both psychological and physical, related to their therapy. The challenges they face can best be overcome with a team approach, including their medical team, family, friends, community resources, and, most importantly, themselves.

The medical community needs to provide services that include the following:

- Knowledge about short- and long-term potential side effects and possible cancer recurrence or a new cancer
- A cancer care summary plan highlighting potential future problems and necessary follow-up observation programs
- Knowledge of lifestyle changes that can be implemented to help reduce the risk and severity of therapy side effects and comorbidities and promote better health
- Psychosocial and/or group therapy for support for anxiety, fear, isolation, and depression
- A list of community resources to aid in obtaining benefits, insurance, employment protection, and life support needs
- Ongoing communication of new advances in medicine and current research that could be of aid in reducing the aftereffects (sequelae) of both cancer and cancer therapy

Armed with this knowledge, survivors can be proactive, initiating necessary lifestyle changes to promote better health and longevity. With greater awareness of possible late side effects, survivors are alerted to potential problems and can take earlier action to prevent adverse outcomes. Awareness of risks also motivates survivor participation in surveillance programs. The goal is to promote wellness through health promotion and disease prevention.

New standards of care are being developed, and clinical guidelines are being developed to improve the quality of care. One of the challenges for the medical community is that the increasing number of survivors will present difficulties in busy oncological practices and ambulatory clinic practices. Informed survivors who adopt recommended lifestyle changes are less likely to need as much physician attention overall.

Recurrent and Second Tumors

Survivors need to be followed for twenty or more years to detect another cancer or a recurrence and to monitor late side effects of treatment. It's been estimated that up to 25 percent of patients face problems including bone marrow failure, myelodysplasia (dysfunctional bone marrow), or new cancers. A Stanford University Hospital study following a large number (2,498) of survivors treated for Hodgkin's disease found that the second cancers most likely to occur were leukemia, non-Hodgkin's lymphoma, lung cancer, breast cancer, salivary gland tumors, thyroid cancer, and pancreatic cancer. In an analysis by Donaldson et al. (1999) of 2,617 patients treated for Hodgkin's disease, the group estimated that 94 percent of patients were expected to survive.[2] Among those who do not survive, approximately half will die of Hodgkin's disease, 20 percent of new cancer, and 14 percent of cardiovascular complications.[3] Adopting healthful lifestyle practices can reduce the risk of comorbid conditions and possibly second cancers or delayed recurrences.

A British study called Second Malignancies Following Non-Hodgkin's Lymphoma Therapy found that although the therapy has improved over the last forty years with longer survivals and cures, there is still an elevated risk for second malignancy, mainly acute nonlymphocytic leukemia (ANLL), which is associated with alkylating chemotherapy or total nodal body irradiation.[4] Five percent of study participants (123 patients) developed a second malignancy. The majority of the malignancy risk was in the CHOP (cyclophosphamide, doxorubicin [hydroxydoxorubicin], vincristine [Oncovin], prednisone) chemotherapy group, for which the primary second malignancies were leukemia, lung, and colorectal cancers. Study participants had a 30 percent higher rate of second malignancies than the general population of England and Wales, primarily leukemia and lung cancer. Involved field of radiation treatments did not significantly increase the risk of leukemia, and the risk was believed to be related most to the alkylating cyclophosphamide chemotherapy. Of note, there was a higher risk of bladder cancer in the radiotherapy-only group. In some studies, lung cancer has been the most common second malignancy in patients with non-Hodgkin's lymphoma, and in this study there was a 60 percent increase of lung cancer, mainly related to chemotherapy (CHOP). It was noted that there was a lower risk of breast cancer but a higher risk of premature menopause and ovarian failure caused by the chemotherapy, mainly cyclophosphamide. The researchers concluded that the risk of second malignancy was elevated, with a fifteen-year cumulative probability 11.2 percent. There was also an elevated risk of leukemia, lung, and colorectal cancers. Therefore, long-term clinical follow-up is necessary after treatment for non-Hodgkin's lymphoma.

Recognizing Behavioral Challenges

Ernest H. Rosenbaum, M.D., F.A.C.P.

Three to four percent of the U.S. population has cancer, and a new case is diagnosed every twenty-three seconds. There are currently approximately 10 million survivors.

It is believed that lifestyles relate, in part, to the cause of cancer, and changing lifestyles can improve survival and longevity. Diet, exercise or other physical activity, smoking cessation, and alcohol reduction or abstinence are lifestyle changes that will improve functional and physical health and treatment outcomes.

Most cancer patients are aware of some of the changes needed, and those who have the courage and strength to initiate changes in diet, exercise, and lifestyle will see benefits from their efforts. These changes can help decrease the risk of progressive and possibly recurrent disease. Also, by reducing comorbid diseases such as cardiovascular disease, diabetes, obesity, and osteoporosis, these measures further reduce the risk of premature death.[5] Unfortunately, some recent studies show that many survivors make few changes in lifestyle, and in some cases they even increase smoking.[6] Physical activity, though recommended, often is not initiated, and many survivors do not meet the recommended intake of fruits, vegetables, fiber, and fat. Sedentary living and overeating habits often are difficult to change. It is hoped that with better understanding, better health practices will be initiated.

One study of prostate and colorectal cancer patients from the state of Washington found that overall, 66.3 percent of patients reported making lifestyle changes: 40.4 percent made one or more dietary changes, 20.8 percent added new physical activity, and 48.0 percent started taking new dietary supplements. Compared with men, women were 2.2 times more likely to take new dietary supplements. Compared with patients aged thirty-five to fifty-nine, those aged sixty to sixty-nine and seventy or older were statistically significantly less likely to make dietary changes or take new supplements. Compared with patients who received only one medical treatment, those receiving three or more treatments were more likely to make dietary changes or start new physical activity. Cancer survivors are likely to make lifestyle changes, and they could benefit from counseling on diet and physical activity.[7] In particular, some studies have shown that distance medicine–based interventions addressing multiple behaviors and targeting survivors (a high-risk group) can have a positive and broad public health impact.[7]

Diet

Many studies have been done on diet, but they are hard to compare, and the results have not been accepted by many researchers. The Women's Interventional Nutrition Study (WINS) recommended a diet consisting of less than 15 percent total calories from fat, but averaged approximately 20 percent total calories from fat. It involved 2,437 postmenopausal women and has been reported at several meetings with results suggesting that a low-fat diet has a protective effect, primarily among women with estrogen receptor–negative disease.[8] Another study, the Women's Healthy Eating and Living Study (WHELS), involving 3,088 premenopausal and postmenopausal women, tested the intake of five fruits and vegetables per day, vegetable juice, 30 grams of dietary fiber, and a 20 percent fat diet. The preliminary evaluation suggests that a low-fat diet can reduce the risk of recurrent breast cancer.[9] Obviously, more information is needed, and when further studies are completed it could give us the necessary guidelines for improved dietary lifestyle interventions. Therefore, a healthful diet is recommended.

Obesity

Almost 6 percent of the direct health costs in 1995 ($51.6 billion) were attributed to obesity, with an impact on coronary heart disease, stroke, diabetes, gallstones, osteoarthritis, and other conditions.[10] Obesity is a quickly growing health problem that healthcare professionals must discuss with their patients.

Scientists are now learning the mechanisms involved and are finding molecules called adipokines, which are secreted by fat tissue. One of the adipokines, adiponectin, has been implicated in regulating insulin sensitivity and lipid oxidation, and this might lower the risk of a myocardial infarction. Determining how it works in fighting obesity and heart disease is a high-priority research project.

Fat cells appear to be passive storage for fat but also generate signals and act as an endocrine organ in overall metabolism and hormone production, according to Robert Henry of the University of California, San Diego. Signaling agents include leptin, restin, tumor necrosis factor-alpha, interleukin-6, free radicals, and adiponectin. Although adiponectins increase the mass of adipose (fat) tissue, people who are obese have a low plasma adiponectin level because adiponectin production decreases with an increase in adipose (fat) mass. Therefore, adiponectin might have some therapeutic value in warding off weight gain or counteracting obesity.

Low adiponectin levels are associated with insulin resistance and type II diabetes and with premature vascular disease.[11] People who have a mutation in the adiponectin gene are at higher risk of cardiovascular disease and diabetes. There can also be a higher risk of myocardial infarction.[12]

People with high levels of adiponectin have high levels of high-density lipoproteins (good cholesterol), and studies are being conducted to develop and increase adiponectin levels and investigate the role of adiponectin in cancer development, cardiovascular disease, and diabetes. The reactions are very complex, involving many other molecules, so this is not an easy problem to solve.

As we learn more about the mechanisms of how adipokines and adiponectins work and interact in the targeted pathways, we will have better treatments for obesity, diabetes, and metabolic disorders. The discovery of leptin (an adipokine) in 1994 opened the door for chemical agents that could help melt away fat in obese people, and future learning on how to manipulate the complex nature of the metabolism and the action of these molecules could lead to effective antiobesity drugs.

Thus far, most studies on exercise, health, and obesity have been performed in the United States and Europe. A Korean study showed that obesity clearly increases the risk of many types of cancer and that obesity-related cancers appear to be rapidly increasing in Korea and other Asian countries.[13] Study authors recommend that controlling the obesity epidemic could be an effective tool for prevention of cancers in these areas. The following cancers all showed positive dose-dependent relationships with body mass index:

- Adenocarcinoma of the colon and rectosigmoid
- Renal cell carcinoma
- Hepatocellular carcinoma
- Cholangiocarcinoma
- Adenocarcinoma of the prostate
- Papillary carcinoma of the thyroid
- Small cell carcinoma of the lung
- Non-Hodgkin's lymphoma
- Melanoma

Although it is still a controversial subject, excess weight appears to promote the development of cancers; this study adds significant information about an Asian population.

Obesity interventions are common, especially commercial ones. Many of these methods have been tried and compared. The National Heart, Lung, and Blood Institute reviewed 236 randomized clinical trials, comparing their assessment of overweight and obesity, weight loss goals, and interventions to achieve weight loss. It was felt that reducing fat and dietary carbohydrates could facilitate caloric reduction, and an individualized diet planning program to reduce caloric intake by 500–2,000 kcal per day would be a good beginning to a weight loss program. Self-monitoring of eating habits, smaller portions, more physical activity, and stress management can also be very effective.[14]

Exercise Interventions

Exercise has been associated with improved quality of life, improved physical functioning, fitness, strength, flexibility, and weight control. Recent studies have shown that exercise can also improve a cancer patient's survival. Two Dana-Farber Cancer Institute studies demonstrated dramatic survival benefits for those who engaged in moderate physical activity. The Cancer and Leukemia Group B (CALGB) trial followed from a CALGB study presented at the 2005 American Society of Clinical Oncology meeting.[15]

- The CALGB treatment trial involved 832 Stage I to III colon cancer patients who had surgery and who then engaged in physical activity similar to those in the CALGB study. The results were a 61 percent lower chance of dying from any colorectal cancer compared with those who were inactive.
- In the CALGB study, patients who exercised at least 18 metabolic equivalent task (MET) hours per week (equivalent to six or more hours a week of moderate-paced walking at the rate of 2.0 to 2.9 miles per hour) had a 47 percent greater chance of disease-free survival six months after completion of therapy than those who did not exercise.

In a 2005 article, Jones and colleagues reported that although oncologists have a favorable attitude toward recommending exercise for patients with cancer, and actually recommended exercise to 28 percent of their patients, more encouragement is needed to help promote exercise.[16] Sixty-two percent of oncologists agree that exercise is beneficial, important, and safe. Sixty-three percent are in favor of exercise during treatment, and forty-three percent report recommending exercise to patients when appropriate. Of note is that younger oncologists are more apt to recommend exercise than older oncologists.

Current recommendations are three to five hours per week of walking or moderate physical exercise. Programs directed by physical therapy specialists are recommended for those with coronary artery disease, arthritis, and chronic obstructive pulmonary disease. Such programs are also valuable for those who have had anthracycline exposure, and they should include gradual increases in intensity.

Psychological Problems

The period after a diagnosis of cancer, which is generally considered life-threatening, is a psychologically taxing time for many survivors, necessitating counseling, psychiatric or psychosocial interventions, and often drug medication support. In the Nurses' Health Study of 48,892 women, 759 had breast cancer, and it was noted that many experienced an increase in pain and a decline in physical and social function, vitality, and ability to perform emotional and physical activities compared with the cancer-free women who were assessed as controls.[17,18]

In recent trials, few psychosocial interventions have been initiated for survivors beyond the early phases of diagnosis and treatment.[17] Unless active support programs were attached to the treating institution or physician's office, patients were more likely to learn about psychological support and specific cancer information *after* medical treatment. Therefore, there is a need to involve patients experiencing psychological distress in support groups or counseling and evaluate the potential need for antidepressant and anti-anxiety medications. It is of interest that survivors with fewer resources, less interpersonal support, and a lower level of education accept supportive care more readily than those who have such resources and often are better able to recover in their environment with a lower level of formal supportive intervention.[19]

Lifestyle studies show that personal behavior can exert a direct effect on cancer incidence. In their classic 1981 article, Doll and Peto compared site-specific cancer rates in the United States with the lowest incidence rates reported worldwide and concluded that 75–80 percent of cancers in the United States were the result of lifestyle factors such as tobacco and alcohol use, physical activity, and diet; biological factors such as birth weight, age at puberty, and reproductive history; and occupational and environmental exposure, and *could be avoided.*[20] Risk factors for many cancers can be controlled through behavior: Tobacco use, diet, physical activity, obesity and energy balance, and sun exposure are all linked to cancer. Intervention programs for prevention use various components of behavior modification. Clinical guidelines have already been established for smoking cessation, dietary compliance, physical activity, and obesity reduction, and new studies are helping to develop new tools for cancer prevention.

Behavior patterns can also influence the course of many cancers by affecting the patient's ability to tolerate chemotherapy, affecting the sensitivity of cancer screening, and reducing comorbid conditions.[21]

Tobacco use, physical activity levels, and weight have been shown to be important in the development of cancer. Interventions in these areas are available and are effective if used. It takes a lot of family and social support and personal perseverance to succeed in any exercise or weight loss program. Tobacco use and therefore lung cancer incidence and mortality rates are starting to decline and are leveling off for women after many decades of increase, suggesting that behavior changes are not only possible but also effective. Research, education, and public policy initiatives are beginning to be successful, but it is slow progress. One of the barriers is that it can be difficult to obtain information about effective interventions and how they can be applied in the community and the clinical setting. Clinical guidelines are being established for the behavioral aspects of smoking cessation treatment. The Cancer Information Service (1-800-4-Cancer) is available for information. Physicians and patients can obtain helpful information from cancercontrolplanet.cancer.gov and from the American Cancer Society, the U.S. Centers for Disease Control, and the National Cancer Institute.

Unfortunately, not everyone wants to change his or her lifestyle.The long latency period between exposure to risk factors and the development of cancer is one of the obstacles to motivating people to adopt healthy anticancer behaviors. Changing lifestyle behaviors entails an understanding of how these behaviors are learned and maintained. Each person has individualized differences and diverse social and environmental exposures. Therefore, different strategies must be created to promote better behavioral patterns. Social attitudes, values, and peer pressure play a role in lifestyle choices; family, friends, and social support can help people choose healthy habits. It is important to note that even after a cancer diagnosis there are still benefits to quitting smoking.

In the main, cancer survivors are more highly motivated to make changes to improve their survival and reduce the risk of recurrence or new cancer. Exercise and dietary intervention programs for survivors have been successful, but results have been difficult to maintain.

- Wing et al. (2006) studied 314 participants who lost an average of 42 pounds of body weight over a two-year period and received several interventions, including face-to-face contact, e-mails, and telephone calls to support their efforts to maintain weight loss.[22] They concluded that supportive care, including quarterly letters, a self-regulation program with daily weights, and face-to-face contact, was effective. All methods helped, but face-to-face contact appeared to be the optimal approach. Of note is that participants regained one-third of the weight in the first year, and by three to five years, they were back to their original baseline.

- The Fresh Start study, a ten-month, home-based program to study diet and exercise among cancer survivors to lower the risk of diabetes, cardiovascular disease, osteoporosis, and other cancers, found that the intervention was successful in changing the behavior of people with newly diagnosed cancers.[23] The study concluded that although many survivors made health-related lifestyle improvements, a substantial number did not. Therefore, intervention is needed, including dietary and exercise behavior programs to help control the multiple risk factors and late consequences of cancer and its treatment.[24]
- The U.S. surgeon general's 1996 report on physical activity and health concluded that it is very difficult to effect a change in physical activity over the long term.[25]

Although taking personal responsibility for healthy behavior patterns seems intuitive, compliance and adherence to programs may be difficult. There are many reasons why survivors may not comply with lifestyle modification guidance, including poor physician–patient communication, side effects of medication, impractical advice, and other problems, including job responsibilities, transportation problems, childcare costs, and communication and cultural barriers. Unfortunately, many programs are sketchy and difficult to follow, so promoting responsible behavior often is not easy.[26]

Supportive care is very important to the success of lifestyle interventions. Maintenance programs must be extensions of the original intervention program. Face-to-face contact and support over the Internet appear to be effective methods. Also, reinforcement from others, friend and family support, and automated telephone system contact can provide additional support.

Challenges for Childhood Cancer Survivors

Although the initial battle with cancer is often won, the subsequent battles with side effects and the fear of or occurrence of a recurrent or a new cancer can have devastating impacts on survivors, especially those who were diagnosed and treated in childhood. An estimated 20,000 children nationwide are diagnosed with cancer each year and are being treated in approximately twenty-six pediatric oncology research centers. The childhood cancer remission rate is now between 75 and 80 percent.[27] Although the treatments for both childhood and adult cancers have dramatically improved in both efficacy and safety, it is estimated that within five to twenty years after treatment, approximately three-quarters of childhood cancer survivors will have at least one comorbidity related to the cancer or its treatment. Pediatric cancer patients treated in the 1970s and 1980s are a high-risk population for subsequent health problems, often many years after treatment. Better solutions to short- and long-term side effects are needed and are being sought in ongoing research programs.[28]

A study by Kevin Oeffinger and colleagues (2006) elucidated many of the problems encountered by childhood survivors, who are at least eight times more likely than their cancer-free siblings to develop life-threatening chronic health conditions such as heart attacks, congestive heart failure, gonadal (ovary or testes) failure, second cancers, and cognitive dysfunction.[29] This diminished health status may cause survivors of pediatric cancers to die prematurely from the side effects of the cancer or its treatment. The study noted the extraordinarily high incidence of late and often permanent complications of intensive treatment with combination chemotherapy and ionizing radiation, showing that two-thirds of the pediatric cancer survivors studied reported at least one chronic health problem, and a quarter had three or more chronic health problems. As Dr. Oeffinger noted, "The impact of some of these health problems can be reduced with periodic survivor-focused follow up."

Vigorous long-term monitoring is essential. Surveillance and preventive programs are needed to detect recurrent or new cancers or deal with the late side effects of anthracycline-related cardiomyopathy, pulmonary fibrosis, and endocrinopathies (premature gonadal failure, thyroid disease, osteoporosis, and pituitary dysfunction). Preventive programs, such as control of hyperlipidemia (excess fat in the blood), hypertension, and diabetes, are vital to help reduce medical side effects.

The lifelong health of childhood cancer survivors depends largely on the treatments used and the length of exposure to drugs and radiation therapy. A significant increase in premature mortality and in serious morbidity and adverse health status has been noted.[30] Through preventive medicine technology (e.g., careful choice of the type of drug used, the amount administered, and the schedule of administration and modification dependent on observed side effects) and advances in patient care, some of the delayed side effects can be monitored, identified, and treated early and successfully. This approach has been successful in pediatric oncology and is now being applied to adult cancer care for survivors. The combination of risk-reducing technology, improved cancer surveillance, and increased efficiency and effectiveness of cancer treatments will spare many survivors the potentially fatal experience of late side effects.

There is a need to disseminate information about the side effects and comorbidities (those concurrent with the therapy and those emerging decades later), for both childhood cancer survivors and their attending physicians. More postgraduate programs are needed to review the treatments and potential solutions for the side effects and disseminate the conclusions and emerging recommendations.

Scientific evidence has shown the therapeutic value of a healthy diet, exercise, psychosocial health support from the medical team and clinics, weight control, and various lifestyle interventions for control and possible prevention of side effects. Lifestyle changes can help improve survival and reduce the short- and long-term side effects of therapy and cancer. Programs aimed at building better nutrition and physical activity habits are starting for our youth. These approaches have been most widely adopted for the leading three cancers (breast, colon, and prostate, which constitute about half of all cancers). Studies are ongoing to establish the effect of lifestyle changes on side effects and comorbidities caused by other types of cancer and their treatments, and programs are currently in development.

How to Plan a Patient's Trajectory After a Cancer Diagnosis

1. After reviewing a patient's records and diagnosis, a treatment plan is developed, usually in an oncologist's office or hospital. Patient, family, and physician usually discuss diagnosis, its meaning, and what therapy is recommended: surgery, radiation therapy, or chemotherapy.
2. Patients often join a support group to help introduce them into the "cancer system" and to promote, through discussions, supportive care necessary to help get them through treatments and the posttreatment period.

Cancer Life Trajectory

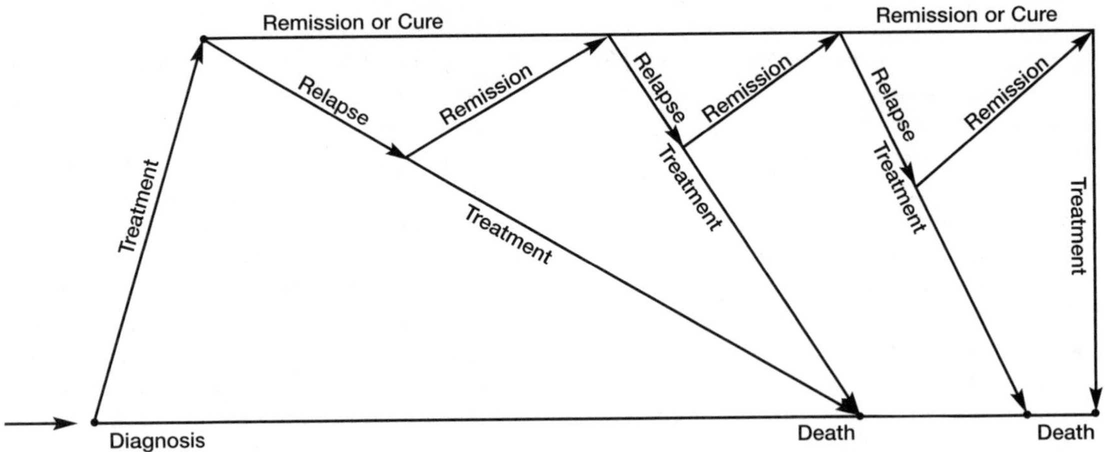

3. Each person has a different plan, but all follow a similar pathway. After treatment, they should receive a patient treatment care summary to give an overview of what they've gone through and plans for the future, including prevention, screening, and further follow-up visits and tests.
4. Many patients are followed by their oncologists or internists, and others are followed by a primary care physician or a survivorship clinic, with a nurse and medical staff.
5. This multidisciplinary approach follows survivors for ten to twenty more years.
6. Educational programs for survivors are promoted.
7. If cancer recurs or if there is a new cancer, oncologists reassess the patient. If there are long-term side effects, consults with cardiology, neurology, nephrology, and so on are arranged.
8. Postcancer problems such as pain, fatigue, distress, and psychosocial problems are continually reevaluated.
9. Programs that promote mental health and supportive care are involved and implemented.

Overall wellness is the goal, including exercise, nutrition, emotional support, spirituality support, sexual information, and other resources as well as medical treatment and surveillance. It is important to connect people and to foster relationships within the family, community, and circle of friends. Physicians and other care providers need to start thinking of cancer as a chronic illness. Knowledge of future problems and potential solutions can be very powerful to a patient's long-term wellness. It is as important to be living well as it is to be living—perhaps even more so.

Addressing insurance, work, and financial problems is also an important adjunct to cancer treatment, and being a cancer survivor advocate can play an important role for many patients, family, and friends. A cancer survivor begins a new lifelong battle that is best fought with a team approach. Because cancer has become a chronic illness, follow-up care emphasizing problems of age, comorbidities, and long-term follow-up is needed for the remainder of the patient's life.

Another important factor is the care of the caregivers, who are now devoting a part of their lives, unexpectedly, to helping their loved one or friend cope with any of the many problems of cancer and its treatments. The need for caregiver support is becoming better recognized. If caregivers burn out and become less functional, the cancer patient's recovery is hampered. As part of the team approach to cancer therapy, special support is now being given to cancer survivor caregivers to help keep them as functional as possible.

Often in follow-up care there is a large number of patients and a limited number of oncologists. Oncologists still need to provide guidance and leadership in how patients are being followed and be available to assess new problems, address side effects of the cancer or therapy, and provide screening and prevention recommendations. Additional support is provided by community action committees and organizations as well as from political sources.

Continued support is vital because when cancer treatments end, medical follow-ups may be at a distant time. Also, communication between the oncologist and the primary care physician or nurse team in a survivorship program is very important to promote optimal quality of care and quality of life. Fortunately, the American Society of Clinical Oncology (ASCO) is working to provide care and follow-up guidelines to assist oncologists and primary care physicians and nurses in follow-up care programs.

The ASCO is also adding survivorship as a key component of the ASCO Core Curriculum Outline for medical oncology training. This involves surveillance screening for second cancers, monitoring for short- and long-term side effects of cancer and therapy, prevention of secondary cancers, specialized follow-up for survivors with a predisposition to hereditary cancers, and assistance with psychosocial, insurance, employment, and other advocacy problems.

Cancer Survivorship Care Plan

By providing patients with a summary of their medical history and follow-up recommendations or a comprehensive letter with follow-up recommendations, oncologists make it possible for survivors to truly understand the lifelong scope of their condition and become partners in their medical care. Although many survivors want to forget their cancer experience at the end of therapy, many others need the reassurance of having a plan and knowing how to recognize what may be side effects of their disease or its treatment or a new or secondary cancer.

The essential elements of a posttherapy survival plan include the following:

- List of treating physicians and contact data.
- Periodic (to be specified) doctor visits for routine check-ups.
- Specific blood tests and x-rays, computed axial tomography (CAT) scans, and magnetic resonance imaging (MRI) scans as needed.
- Disease-specific follow-up screening guidelines.
- A review of short- and long-term potential side effects and discussion of signs and symptoms of a possible cancer recurrence or a new cancer.
- Recommendations for lifestyle changes to reduce the risk and severity of side effects and comorbidities.
- Preventive medical communication programs.
- Recommendations for psychosocial or group therapy for support for anxiety, fear, isolation, and depression.
- List of community resources to aid in obtaining benefits, insurance, employment protection, and life support as needed.
- Documents that provide hope. Relate ongoing communications of new advances in medicine and current research that

could be of aid in reducing the toxic side effects (sequelae) of both cancer and cancer therapy as needed.

Because each cancer and each patient are different, each survivor needs an individualized follow-up program, depending in part on the type of cancer, its risks, and its aggressiveness. Fortunately, the generalized cancer survivorship care plan guidelines in this book will aid physicians in patient follow-up planning, which can be organized for each specific cancer. Physicians should also check the *Journal of Clinical Oncology* for updated ASCO guidelines.

The following presents an outline of recommended elements for a survivor's follow-up guidance:

Cancer Survivor's Follow-Up Care Plan

Patient Name: ____________________

Telephone number: ____________________

Address: ____________________

City, state, zip code: ____________________

1. Hospitals where treated and medical record numbers: ____________________

   ____

2. Diagnosis: Type of cancer ____________________

   Pathology and grade: ____________________

3. Doctor involved in care: ____________________

   Name: ____________________

   Address: ____________________

   Telephone number: ____________________

   Name: ____________________

   Address: ____________________

   Telephone number: ____________________

4. Brief history: ____________________

   Clinical evaluation: ____________________

   X-ray: ____________________

   Lab tests: ____________________

5. Treatment: ____________________

   Surgery report: ____________________

   Radiation therapy report: ____________________

Type: ____________________

Dose: ____________________

X-ray field: ____________________

Where performed: ____________________

Chemotherapy or immunotherapy report: ____________________

Protocol: ____________________

Drugs: ____________________

Dosage: ____________________

Frequency: ____________________

6. Potential short- and long-term consequences of therapy (such as delayed cardiac toxicity or delayed physical impairment) and side effects: ____________________

____

____

7. Suggested posttreatment plan for potential second malignancies or recurrence: ____________________

____

____

____

8. Follow-up recommendations for the next ten or more years: ____________________

Intervals for follow-up doctor visits: ____________________

Tests needed (a plan): ____________________

9. Resources for supportive care for: ____________________
   - Group or family support
   - Occupational therapy or physical therapy
   - Home care
   - Psychosocial support for survivors
   - Physical care (pain, nutrition, fatigue, or sexual dysfunction)
10. Provide information on insurance, employment protection, and community resources.
11. Include medical reports from physician, x-ray, laboratory reports of vital information.
12. Give patient copies of cancer survivorship care plan, history, laboratory results, and x-rays and scans.

The Personal, Portable Survivorship Care Plan: Nothing to Carry?

J. Ben Davoren, M.D.

As previously noted, the elements of a cancer survivorship care plan are not particularly complex, but the information necessary to create a complete plan comes from many sources. In addition, the care plan must be shared with many sources and then updated again by many sources over time. The patient is the hub of all the activity. For decades, the idea of a personal, portable health record was romanticized as a way for the patient to keep the latest information, ensuring efficient and high-quality patient care, whether the patient was seeing his or her own doctor across town or an emergency room physician in another country. As magnetic strips on credit and other cards became more and more sophisticated, the natural desire was to incorporate medical information into a wallet-sized medical card that could be read and then updated at the local doctor's office, by a consultant across the country, or at any emergency room in the world.

Although there have been some basic successes in this matter, the sheer volume of information in a detailed medical record, especially one of a cancer survivor, has rapidly made this approach obsolete. In addition, with the large number of healthcare practitioners that an individual patient might see, it would be very cumbersome to keep the information up to date because each care provider would have to have physical access to the card to update it.

The advent of sophisticated Web technology has created the best place to store personal information: on the Internet. The ability to safely and securely access the Internet from almost anywhere in the world ensures that the information cannot be lost or stolen along with your wallet. Furthermore, new information can be posted at any time from anywhere so that one's health record can be as current as one's bank or credit card balance. The only thing that needs to be portable is the username and password information, with this important data locked away from prying eyes or ears until it becomes necessary.

What are the obstacles to creating Internet-based records, and why hasn't it already been widely adopted? One major obstacle is that as of 2006, more than three-quarters of physician groups in the United States were still using paper-based records to document and coordinate care. The good news is that there are multiple national and regional projects aiming to get medical care online instead. The dominant problem is that there is no standard format to make the process of moving clinical information from a clinician's office to the patient's Internet record site a smooth one. In contrast, if one uses a credit card at any store that takes one, automatic protocols route the information to the correct lender and the correct account and immediately establish whether the action is a credit or a debit and whether there are sufficient funds or credit available for the transaction, and confirmation of all this comes back to the merchant in seconds. In medicine, there's no standard format for your MRI results or for a dictated summary of care. Fortunately, such seemingly irrelevant Web phenomena as myspace.com and facebook.com have created examples in which trust relationships can be explicitly created with minimal effort.

On the positive side, almost every healthcare provider's office uses computers in some capacity. Dictated notes, laboratory or other diagnostic test results, hospital care summaries, and the actual computed tomography (CT) or MRI scans themselves usually are electronic, even if paper reports are still filed in doctors' offices. Secure e-mail of this information (except for actual radiology images, which are far too large to send as attachments) is now possible and being slowly adopted. Here, too, standards for security lag behind the need but are rapidly ramping up. Large medical groups, such as Kaiser Permanente, Partners Healthcare in Massachusetts, and the Veterans Healthcare Administration, are making more and more of their patients' information available to their patients online.

What can a cancer patient, survivor, or family do today? Even if your health plan does not yet have a personal health record Web site, there are a number of free or low-cost Web sites that facilitate the creation of a personal health record online, and these can be used to create the basics of your own cancer survivorship plan. For now, the work of posting that information is essentially all by the patient; after all, you are the hub of the plan. Encourage your healthcare providers to give you copies of your information, including CT scans and MRIs on CD or DVD to facilitate shared decision making. Although you might have to jump through hoops to get it, you are always entitled to the information.

There are other strategies to keep your information organized and accessible while medicine catches up with the Internet. Paper remains the most easily accessed medium, and at a minimum you should keep paper backup copies of critical information. Some people use a scanner attached to a personal computer to scan in important information and store that information on CD, DVD, or other portable media in a separate location away from home. One of the lessons of the Hurricane Katrina experience was that paper medical records are extremely vulnerable in a natural disaster. Enterprises that had their electronic information held remotely (such as Veterans Affairs) were able to resume business as usual after the disaster. A separate electronic strategy is to create a simple spreadsheet or word processing document that you can update on a home computer, and then create a free Internet mail account at google.com, yahoo.com, or another large, secure site. You can store your spreadsheet or document by starting an e-mail message to yourself, but instead of sending it, keep it as a draft message. That way, the content doesn't actually traverse the Internet, where prying eyes might find it, and it's in a spot you can always access as long as you have an Internet connection.

The Passport for Care: Development of a Novel Internet Resource for Managing Long-Term Health Risks

David G. Poplack, M.D., Michael Fordis, M.D., Marc E. Horowitz, M.D., Wendy Landier, R.N., M.S.N., C.P.N.P., C.P.O.N, Melissa M. Hudson, M.D., Smita Bhatia, M.D., Kevin C. Oeffinger, M.D., Ann C. Mertens, Ph.D.

Passport for Care (PFC) is an innovative project being developed at Baylor College of Medicine in collaboration with the Children's Oncology Group (COG) and the National Childhood Cancer Survivor Study. PFC addresses the need to provide survivors of cancer and chronic illnesses with access to their medical information and healthcare guidelines. The PFC is an interactive Internet resource that provides accurate, timely, and individualized healthcare information. The Passport for Care initially was developed for survivors of childhood cancer and will be extended to adult cancer survivors nationwide.

Survivors are often unfamiliar with the details of their treatment history and are unable to accurately share their medical information with their healthcare providers. Primary care providers, in turn, are often unfamiliar with cancer treatments or with recommendations for surveillance for long-term side effects or complications of cancer and cancer therapy.

An end-of-treatment Care Summary, completed by the treating institution with updates, would be available to the survivor, which can be securely shared with medical providers at the direction of the survivor. This Care

Summary will be used to generate recommendations for each survivor.

This will be readily accessible to the survivor and their healthcare provider (and hopefully transmitted via a secure Internet e-mail file). The information provided also helps empower the survivor. The survivor will have complete control over access to their medical follow-up in managing their long-term follow-up.

The goal is to produce an effective document that provides healthcare information for this growing population.

3 Posttherapy Screening Guidelines

Consensus guidelines for monitoring and management have been developed to promote wellness and quality of life from the time of diagnosis through the current standard of five years of posttreatment surveillance and even into long-term follow-up surveillance programs. Follow-up care is essential and usually is delivered by oncologists, primary care physicians, or specialty nurse teams. There is a need for experience in long-term follow-up for chronic conditions, even after a period of wellness, which may well be over ten to twenty years and for a lifetime. The recent Surveillance Epidemiology and End Results (SEER) study (2003) found that 16 percent of new cancer diagnoses were among people who had already been treated for cancer. This finding emphasizes the importance of long-term surveillance and screening follow-up for cancer survivors.[1] A recent study found that cancer survivors are at elevated risk for recurrence of their original malignancy or development of a second primary cancer.[2]

Suggested laboratory tests and ancillary procedures for postcancer, posttherapy surveillance include the following:

- *Breast cancer:* Perform a physical examination every six to twelve months and a mammogram of preserved breast tissue annually.
- *Colorectal cancer:* Periodic carcinoembryonic antigen level and colonoscopy, rectal exam, and stool occult blood test every three to six months for two years, then every six months for three to five years.
- *Prostate cancer:* Prostate-specific antigen (PSA) and rectal exam every six months for five years, and then annually.

Most follow-up programs should include recommended screening procedures for a span of twenty or more years.

Suggested Screening Guidelines for Specific Cancers and Associated Diseases

Breast Cancer

After age twenty-one, women should have their breasts examined by a physician as part of a physical examination every one to three years, with a review of any symptoms. A yearly examination is suggested if there are high-risk features (family history, genetic predisposition, prior history of breast cancer, or obesity). In a recent study, adiposity and a gain of 10 or more pounds increases the risk of breast cancer approximately three times. Height is an additional risk factor.[3]

Starting at age forty, a yearly mammogram is recommended unless clinically indicated to start earlier for high-risk women, in which case mammograms should coincide with clinical doctor visits.

In the last few years, digital mammogram imaging has become more available and offers additional information in detection of early breast cancer lesions. Digital mammography appears to be more sensitive and accurate, but computer-aided mammogram detection has reduced accuracy of interpretation, leading to increased biopsies (many of which are benign) and is not clearly associated with improved detection of invasive breast cancer.[4]

Women with a family history of breast cancer, women with a prior breast cancer diagnosis or assessment of the contralateral breast, or women who are otherwise at high risk of breast cancer may benefit from magnetic resonance imaging (MRI) screening, which is a more sensitive, accurate, and sometimes more cost-effective test. When there is a suspicious mass or when a woman is at high risk for breast cancer, a breast MRI should be done in a facility that also does guided breast needle biopsies to avoid the expense and time needed for a repeat MRI with a biopsy if needed.

The risk can be reduced with mastectomy, although many women prefer screening to surgery because MRI screening detects breast cancer earlier than mammography but is ten times more expensive.[5] Women who are at higher risk (family history, genetic tendencies, prior breast cancer, or obesity) should talk to their doctors about the benefits and limitations of starting screening earlier and having additional tests or more frequent examinations.

Recent studies have shown that breast cancer survivors who have been treated with doxorubicin (Adriamycin) and/or trastuzumab (Herceptin) may experience cardiac toxicity as a side effect, with the potential for congestive heart failure. A number of the study subjects had recurrent toxicity. Most cardiac toxicity is reversible. There is a need for cooperative follow-up with oncologist and primary care physician or survivorship clinic nurse.[6]

Of note, a recent research study concluded that exercise training had beneficial effects on cardiopulmonary function and quality of life in postmenopausal breast cancer survivors. Exercise also has an impact on risk of breast cancer and death. A lack of exercise can be responsible for up to 50 percent more breast cancer deaths.[7]

A presentation from the 2006 American Society of Clinical Oncology (ASCO) meeting discussed the results of a meta-analysis of studies concerning breast cancer.[8] Among their conclusions were the following:

- Obesity is associated with a significantly higher risk of distant recurrence (almost 200 percent) and a 160 percent higher risk of death.
- A preliminary report suggests that a prudent low-fat diet will help reduce risk of breast cancer recurrence and thereby increase survival.

A prudent diet, weight control, and exercise programs should be a part of every breast cancer protection program (see Part III).

Female Reproductive Organ Cancer

Cervical Cancer

Three years after women begin vaginal intercourse, or at age twenty-one, cervical cancer screening is recommended every three years with a cytological Pap smear and pelvic examination. Using the liquid-based Pap smear, annual screenings are initially recommended after age twenty-one, but after age thirty, with three negative screening examinations, screening can be done every two to three years. Women over thirty may also be tested every three years with a pelvic examination and a Pap test, plus the human papilloma virus (HPV) DNA test. After age seventy, women with three normal Pap tests in a row and no abnormal Pap test in the last ten years may choose to stop having cervical cancer testing. If a patient has had a total hysterectomy with removal of the cervix, screening is not recommended.

It is believed that the early cervical lesion occurs in the surface layer of the cervical lining (intraepithelial neoplasia), which is caused by HPV-16 and HPV-18. HPV is the most common sexually transmitted disease, infecting 20 million Americans each year. Each year 9,700 women are diagnosed with cervical cancer, and 3,700 die. The HPV vaccines now available may also help prevent anal warts, anal and penile cancer, and vaginal and vulvar cancer.

A recent placebo-controlled study of the HPV-16 vaccine (three doses) in 2,400 women aged sixteen to twenty-three followed for 17.4 months showed persistent HPV-16 in 3.8 percent of women in the placebo group and no persistent HPV-16 infection per 100 women-years in the vaccine group, showing 100 percent efficacy.[9]

Two vaccines are available, but vaccination works only before recipients are exposed to the virus.

- Gardasil (Merck) is quadrivalent for HPV-6, HPV-11, HPV-16, and HPV-18. For those with HPV-6 and HPV-11, Gardasil protects against genital warts. For those with HPV-16 and HPV-18, it provides approximately 70 percent protection against cervical cancer. For patients age sixteen to twenty-five, it decreases the rate of cervical cancer approximately 70 percent.
- Ceravix (GlaxoSmithKline) is for cervical cancer prevention in women over age twenty-five. It is bivalent for HPV-16 and HPV-18.

These vaccines are also effective in preventing vaginal and vulvar cancer.

Endometrial Cancer

Since 2001, the American Cancer Society (ACS) has not recommended screening for those with average risk except for those with a history of endometrial cancer, those on replacement estrogen therapy or tamoxifen therapy, or those having late menopause, infertility, no children, obesity, diabetes, or hypertension. Women should be informed of possible risks and advised about spotting and unexpected vaginal bleeding as signs to report to their physicians for an evaluation. After age thirty-five, endometrial biopsy is recommended for women with hereditary non-polyposis colon cancer.

Ovarian Cancer

Ovarian cancer screening has not yet been proven effective and is not recommended. A rectal/pelvic examination is suggested, with routine medical checkups. If there is a history of hereditary ovarian cancer syndrome, an annual or semiannual pelvic examination, a cancer antigen–125 (CA-125) blood test, and a transvaginal ultrasound are recommended. If diagnosed early, ovarian cancer has a high cure rate, but right now only about 20 percent of cases are diagnosed before they have spread outside the ovaries. Early signs can include persistent abdominal bloating, pelvic or abdominal pain, difficulty eating or a feeling of fullness, and frequent urination or change in bowel habits. These signs are also seen in women who don't have cancer, but if they persist, a woman should see her doctor.

A retrospective study was performed at Cedars-Sinai Medical Center in Los Angeles to see whether there was a link between obesity and decreased survival in epithelial ovarian cancer. The study concluded that obese patients were more likely to have cancer limited to the ovaries, and advanced cancer and obesity were independently associated with a short time to recurrence and a shorter overall survival. Patients received optimal surgery by a gynecologic oncologist, chemotherapy as indicated with a gemcitabine combination, with carboplatin for relapsed ovarian cancer, and the use of intraperitoneal (in abdominal cavity) chemotherapy to help promote a prolonged survival. Some patients entered clinical trials with epidermal growth factor drugs and antiangiogenesis drugs such as bevacizumab (Avastin).[10]

It is known that women who are obese have a worse prognosis than those who have an ideal body weight. This may be because of increased comorbidities, such as diabetes or high blood pressure, but also may be related to hormonal factors.

Another factor affecting treatment outcome could be underdosing of chemotherapy because of obesity-related calculations. Also, in obese women it is more difficult to feel the ovaries, making earlier diagnosis more difficult.

Colorectal Cancer and Adenomatous Polyps

A million new cases of colorectal cancer are diagnosed worldwide yearly, with a half million deaths. In the United States, it is the second leading cause of cancer deaths, with about 140,000 new cases and about 60,000 deaths yearly. The cause of colorectal cancer is genetic alterations in several gene sequences in colon-lining cells, which form mutations (transformations) from normal colon-lining mucosa cells to adenomatous polyps to carcinoma.

A study of 35,755 colorectal cancer survivors of age sixty-seven and older found a substantial reduction in life expectancy after diagnosis of early stage colorectal with age and with increasing comorbidity.[11] Survival decreased from 19.5 years to 12.4 years for male survivors with one or two chronic illnesses and to 7.6 years in the presence of three or more comorbidities. For women, survival decreased from 23 to 16 years with one or two illnesses and to 7 years if three or more comorbidities were present. Therefore, screening should be promoted for older people.

The suggested guidelines have been modified over the years and currently include the following recommendations:

- Patients should undergo an annual fecal occult blood test or fecal immunological test (by a doctor or nurse in the office or a take-home test) and a sigmoidoscopy every five years.
- Flexible colonoscopy should be performed every ten years.
- A double-contrast barium enema can also be used every five years and colonoscopy every ten years.
- A rectal examination with a yearly physical examination is also recommended to detect rectal or anal carcinoma.
- Any positive tests should be followed by a colonoscopy.

Screening should be started after age fifty. Those with a family history of nonpolyposis colorectal cancer or familial adenomatous polyposis merit earlier surveillance. Patients with a history of adenomatous polyps or a personal or family history of colorectal cancer (especially in first-degree relatives) are at high risk for colorectal cancer. They should be screened earlier than age fifty (suggested starting age is forty to forty-five).

Lung Cancer

Lung cancer is now killing more women, and earlier diagnosis is the key to survival. ACS statistics predict that about 70,880 women will die of lung cancer in 2007. This is the number one cause of cancer deaths. The number of new cases diagnosed in 2007 was about 98,620. The rise in lung cancer correlates with increased cigarette smoking since World War II, when many women joined the work force. In the 1960s, smoking became a sign of independence, equality, and liberation and was tied to that movement.

About 10 to 20 percent of lung cancer cases involve people who never smoked. In some cases, women stopped smoking twenty or thirty years before lung cancer was diagnosed. Of note is that more than half the women and men diagnosed with lung cancer already have advanced metastatic disease to bone or organs. The five-year survival rate is approximately 15 percent. With earlier diagnosis, the five-year survival rate increases to about 50 percent, with about 38 percent surviving ten years. The cure rate is approximately 25 percent.

Although their success must be proven in clinical trials, new drugs are becoming available. In addition to improved treatments, there is a need for better diagnostic tools for earlier detection. Currently, there are no firm recommendations for screening detection, although studies have been done on sputum and bronchial washing Pap smears and spiral computed axial tomography (spiral CAT) scan in current smokers, which have often led to the early diagnosis of lung cancer. These studies are under evaluation, especially spiral CAT scan assessment. CAT scans appear to be the optimal diagnostic technology currently available. An improved screening strategy is also urgently needed.

Prostate Cancer

A PSA test is recommended after age fifty for people with a ten-year or longer life expectancy. A digital rectal examination is part of the yearly physical examination. Earlier screening beginning at age forty-five is recommended for men of African American descent and those with a first-degree relative diagnosed with prostate cancer. For those with relatives diagnosed before age sixty-five, testing at age forty is recommended.

It appears that PSA levels of less than 4.0 ng/dl are of less concern, although prostate cancer has been detected at lower PSA levels. Continued rising PSA levels above 4.0 ng/dl are related to the PSA velocity, and those with rapidly increasing PSA levels merit a urological evaluation and prostate biopsies. These risks should be discussed with patients.

Osteoporosis

Osteoporosis is responsible for more than 1.5 million fractures annually, mostly of the hip, spine, and wrist. Ten million Americans already have osteoporosis, and 34 million more have low bone mass, placing them at higher risk for this disease. Sixty-eight percent of those affected by osteoporosis are women. One out of every two women and one in four men over fifty will have an osteoporosis-related fracture in their lifetime.[12] Based on hospital and nursing home figures, the yearly cost of direct expenditures for osteoporosis fractures is about $14 billion.

A recent study of 44,000 women showed that 27 percent of those aged sixty-six to seventy were screened in a three-year period, but less than 10 percent of the oldest women, aged eighty to ninety, were screened. Bone density testing (DEXA) was recommended for all women over age sixty-five, with a test every two years; such testing is covered by Medicare. It was also reported that "40 percent of white women aged 50 and older will suffer an osteoporosis-related fracture of the hip, wrist, or spine at some point in their lifetime. More than half of those with hip fractures never fully recover, and 20 percent of women will end up in the nursing home."[13]

Osteoporosis may occur as early as six months after androgen hormone ablation treatment for prostate cancer, with a decrease in testosterone through androgen deprivation treatment. This treatment also increases the risk of diabetes and cardiovascular disease.[14]

4 Toxicities of Selected Chemotherapy and Immunotherapy Drugs

Robert Ignoffo, Pharm.D., and Ernest H. Rosenbaum, M.D., F.A.C.P.

Often as new drugs are developed and used, and the longer they are used, new and unpredicted side effects occur, such as those seen with some of the new biological targeted therapies.

The following table provides an overview of commonly used drugs and their known short- and long-term side effects. Selected drug- and treatment-related toxicities are discussed in greater detail in Part V.

Drug	**Definition and Action**
Albumin-bound paclitaxel (Abraxane)	A different form of Taxol, albumin-bound. Damages DNA by promoting early microtubule assembly. *Early Toxicity Effects* • Flulike symptoms such as fever, chills, malaise, myalgias (muscle and bone pains), arthralgias (joint pains). • Vascular leak syndrome. • Weight gain. • Arrhythmias, tachycardia, hypotension (heart and blood pressure irregularities). • Edema (swelling). • Renal insufficiency. • Pleural effusion and pulmonary congestion. • Myelosuppression (a decrease in blood cell production). • Neuropathy (nerve pain or discomfort).
Amifostine (Ethyol)	An organic thiophosphate used to reduce incidence of kidney toxicity for patients receiving cisplatin-based chemotherapy and radiotherapy of brain, head and neck, and parotid gland. *Early Toxicity Effects* • Nausea and vomiting. • Low blood pressure during intravenous (IV) infusion. • Flushing, chills, fever, and sleepiness during IV infusion.

Drug	**Definition and Action**
Anastrozole (Arimidex)	A nonsteroidal aromatase inhibitor. *Early Toxicity Effects* • Asthenia (weakness) in up to 20 percent of patients. • Hot flashes in 10 percent. Also mild nausea, vomiting, and constipation. • Dry, scaling skin or rash. • Arthralgias (joint pain) in 10–15 percent of patients (in hands, knees, hips, back, and shoulders) and early morning stiffness. • Peripheral leg edema (swelling) in 7 percent of patients. • Occasionally a flulike syndrome, with fever, malaise, and myalgias (muscle and bone pains). *Additional Toxicities* • Can prolong QT interval on electrocardiogram (EKG) in 40–50 percent of patients. An EKG is recommended before use. • A syndrome of fever, shortness of breath, skin rash, fluid retention, weight gain, and pleural and pericardial effusions in up to 3 percent of patients. • Leukocytosis (elevated white blood cell count) is common initially and later. • Musculoskeletal pain, hyperglycemia (high blood sugar), and peripheral neuropathy (nerve pain) are occasionally seen. • Osteoporosis and some increase in fractures have been noted.
Bevacizumab (Avastin)	A humanized monoclonal antibody that binds and blocks vascular endothelial growth factor receptor. Drug is too new to evaluate possible late toxicity effects. *Early Toxicity Effects* • Has been noted to cause moderate high blood pressure, usually controlled well with standard blood pressure medication in 19 percent of patients. • Proteinuria (excess protein in the urine) occurs in 24 percent of patients. • Minor bleeding episodes such as nosebleeds seen in 25 percent of patients. • Venous thrombosis (deep blood clots). • Strokes and arterial thromboses have been reported. • Tumor hemorrhage (low risk). • Some blindness has been reported. • Delayed wound healing after surgery has been noted, and often elective surgery is delayed for six or eight weeks after drug administration. Use of this drug is also delayed for at least four weeks after surgery because of wound healing problems.

Drug	**Definition and Action**
Bleomycin (Blenoxane)	An antibiotic chemotherapy that damages DNA. Potential lung toxicity; pulmonary function tests and chest x-ray should be done before treatment. Lymphoma patients are more susceptible to an anaphylactic reaction. *Early Toxicity Effects* • Skin reaction is most common, with erythema (redness) and hyperpigmentation, thickening of skin and nail beds, and hyperkeratosis (thickening and hardening of the skin). • Pulmonary toxicity usually is dose related, occurring in about 10 percent of patients. This is age related and rarely progresses to pulmonary fibrosis (scarring that is fatal in 1 percent of patients). • Hypersensitivity reaction with fever and chills in about 25 percent of patients. • Vascular events, including myocardial infarction (heart attack), stroke, and Raynaud's phenomenon (vascular spasms, hands turn red, white, then blue), are rarely seen.
Bortezomib (Velcade)	A proteasome inhibitor commonly used in multiple myeloma and non-Hodgkin's lymphoma. *Early Toxicity Effects* • Fatigue, malaise, general weakness, and gastrointestinal toxicity, with nausea, vomiting, and diarrhea. • Myelosuppression with thrombocytopenia (low platelet count) and neutropenia (low white blood cell count). • Peripheral sensory neuropathy (nerve pain), which usually improves after discontinuation of bortezomib. • Fever occurs in about 40 percent of patients, as well as orthostatic hypotension (sudden drop in blood pressure) in about 12 percent of patients.
Capecitabine (Xeloda)	An oral antimetabolite form of 5-fluorouracil (5-FU). Inhibits both DNA and RNA. *Early Toxicity Effects* • Diarrhea in up to 55 percent of patients. • Mucositis (inflammation and reduction of the gastrointestinal lining). • Loss of appetite and dehydration. • Hand–foot syndrome, with hand and foot redness, tingling, numbness, pain, and a dry rash with itching in about 15–20 percent of patients. • Occasional increase in liver enzymes, including bilirubin, and myelosuppression (a decrease in blood cell production). • Neurologic toxicity, with confusion, cerebellar ataxia (poor coordination), and rare brain encephalopathy. • Cardiac symptoms with EKG changes and serum enzyme elevations. • Tear duct stenosis (closure), both acute and chronic conjunctivitis.

Drug	Definition and Action
Carboplatin (Paraplatin)	A heavy metal alkylating agent. Damages DNA. *Early Toxicity Effects* • Myelosuppression (a decrease in blood cell production), which is dose limiting; thrombocytopenia (reduced platelet count) is most common. • Nausea and vomiting that can be delayed, necessitating antinausea medication. • Renal toxicity with high-dose therapy, less common than with cisplatin; careful observation for electrolyte imbalances, including low calcium, potassium, magnesium, and sodium. • Peripheral neuropathy (nerve pain) in less than 10 percent of patients, usually over age sixty-five. • Occasional ototoxicity (inner ear damage). • Alopecia (hair loss) is uncommon.
Cetuximab (Erbitux)	A recombinant, humanized monoclonal antibody directed against the epidermal growth factor receptor (EGFR). *Early Toxicity Effects* • Caution with use in patients with known hypersensitivity to murine (mouse) protein. • Toxicity infusion-related symptoms of fever, chills, urticaria (hives), flushing, fatigue, headache, bronchospasm, dyspnea (shortness of breath), angioedema (swelling and welts), and hypotension (low blood pressure). • Itching, dry skin, and pustular acneiform skin rash, mainly on face and upper trunk. • Pulmonary toxicity: interstitial lung disease with cough, dyspnea, and pulmonary infiltrates.
Cisplatin (Platinol)	Heavy metal alkylating agent. Damages DNA and mitotic spindles. *Early Toxicity Effects* • Nephrotoxicity (impaired kidney function), usually dose limiting, in 35–40 percent of patients. Renal function tests before and after therapy needed. • Nausea and vomiting, both early and delayed. • Neurotoxicity with paresthesias and numbness, often in a stocking–glove pattern. • Ototoxicity with high-frequency hearing loss and tinnitus (ringing in ears). • Hypersensitivity reaction with facial edema, wheezing, bronchospasm, and hypotension (low blood pressure). • Ocular toxicity: optic neuritis, papilledema, cerebral blindness, and altered color perception rarely observed.

Drug	Definition and Action
	• Transient elevation of liver function tests, mainly serum glutamic-oxaloacetic transaminase (SGOT) and serum bilirubin. • Metallic taste of food and loss of appetite. • Vascular events have occurred, including myocardial infarction (heart attack), arteritis (artery inflammation), strokes, and thrombotic microangiopathy (small blood vessel clots), and Raynaud's phenomenon (vascular spasms, hands turn red, white, then blue). • Alopecia (hair loss).
Cyclophosphamide (Cytoxan)	An alkylating agent. Damages DNA. *Early Toxicity Effects* • Myelosuppression (a decrease in blood cell production) dose limiting, mainly neutropenia (reduced white blood cell counts), days 7–14. • Bladder problems such as toxicity with hemorrhagic cystitis, dysuria, and elevated urinary frequency in about 5–10 percent of patients. • Nausea and vomiting, usually on first day. • Alopecia (hair loss), usually two to three weeks after initiation of therapy. • Hyperpigmentation of skin and nails. • Amenorrhea with ovarian failure. • Cardiotoxicity with high-dose therapy. • Elevated risk of infections. *Late Toxicity Effects* • Elevated risk of second malignancy, including acute myelogenous leukemia and bladder cancer (especially in patients with chronic hemorrhagic cystitis).
Darbepoetin alfa (Aranesp)	An erythropoietic growth factor that promotes red blood cell production. Used for anemia caused by cancer or chemotherapy. *Early Toxicity Effects* • Contraindicated in patients with hypertension or cardiovascular disease. • Contraindicated in pregnant and breastfeeding mothers; excreted in breast milk. • Occasional toxicities include diarrhea, nausea, vomiting, local pain at injection site, headache, fever, fatigue, weakness, arthralgias (joint pains), and myalgias (muscle and bone pain). • Rare rash and itching skin.

Drug	Definition and Action
Daunorubicin (Cerubidine)	An anthracycline antibiotic. Damages DNA. *Early Toxicity Effects* • Myelosuppression (a decrease in blood cell production), most commonly thrombocytopenia (reduced platelet count), days 10–14. • Nausea and vomiting in about 50 percent of patients soon after therapy. • Mucositis (inflammation and reduction of the gastrointestinal lining) and diarrhea during the first week, but is not dose limiting. • Cardiotoxicity in the acute form in the first two to three days with arrhythmias and EKG changes, pericarditis, and myocarditis. Usually transient. • Is a strong vesicant (blistering agent), and extravasation (drug leaking into skin at injection site) can lead to tissue necrosis and chemical phlebitis. • Alopecia (hair loss) is universal, and nail hyperpigmentation and occasional skin rash and urticaria occur. *Late Toxicity Effects* • In the chronic form, cardiotoxicity is dose dependent, with a dilated cardiomyopathy and congestive heart failure, usually at dosages greater than 550 mg/m^2. A cardiotoxic effect of daunorubicin may be inhibited by the iron-chelating agent dexrazoxane (Zinecard).
Dexrazoxane (Zinecard)	An iron-chelating agent. Protects anthracycline DNA damage. Dexrazoxane should not be used at the beginning of a doxorubicin therapy because it may decrease tumor response. *Early Toxicity Effects* • A mild, reversible myelosuppression (low blood cell production). • Pain at injection site. • Mild nausea and vomiting.
Docetaxel (Taxotere)	A mitotic microtubule spindle poison and radiosensitizer. *Early Toxicity Effects* • Myelosuppression (a decrease in blood cell production), including neutropenia (low white blood cell count), thrombocytopenia (low platelet count), and anemia (low red blood cell count). • Hypersensitivity reactions with skin rash, erythema (skin redness), hypotension (low blood pressure), dyspnea (shortness of breath), and bronchospasm, which occur early in drug administration. Can be prevented with use of corticosteroids, diphenhydramine, and cimetidine or famotidine. • Fluid retention syndrome with weight gain, peripheral edema, pleural effusion, and ascites.

Drug	**Definition and Action**
	• Alopecia (hair loss) in up to 80 percent of patients. • A macular, papular skin rash with dry, itchy skin and brown fingernail discoloration, often with loss of fingernails. • Mucositis (reduction of the gastrointestinal lining) and diarrhea seen in about 40 percent of patients, with mild nausea and vomiting of brief duration. • Peripheral neuropathy (nerve pain) is uncommon but seen with docetaxel and paclitaxel. • Fatigue, arthralgias (joint pains), and myalgias (muscle pains) seen in about 60 percent of patients.
Doxorubicin (Adriamycin)	An anthracycline antibiotic. Damages DNA. *Early Toxicity Effects* • Similar to daunorubicin, with myelosuppression (low blood cell production), with dose-limiting leukopenia (low total white blood cell count) and with thrombocytopenia (low platelet count) and anemia. • Myelosuppression, most commonly thrombocytopenia, days 10–14. • Both acute and delayed nausea and vomiting. • Mucositis (inflammation and reduction of the gastrointestinal lining) and diarrhea in the first week. • Cardiotoxicity in the acute form, usually within the first two to three days, with arrhythmias and conduction abnormalities with EKG changes, pericarditis, and myocarditis. Usually transient. • It is also a strong vesicant (blistering agent) if injection leaks into skin (burns and scars skin). It can cause hyperpigmentation of nails, skin rash, itchy skin, and urticaria. • Alopecia (hair loss) is universal but reversible about three months after therapy ends. *Late Toxicity Effects* • Chronic form, late dependent dilated cardiomyopathy associated with congestive heart failure (the risk increases with dosages greater than 450 mg/m^2). Dexrazoxane may be used to prevent cardiotoxicity after a cumulative doxorubicin dosage of 300 mg/m^2.
Doxorubicin liposome (Doxil)	A liposomal encapsulated form of doxorubicin. An anthracycline antibiotic. *Early Toxicity Effects* • Myelosuppression (low blood cell production), which can be dose limiting, with lowest blood counts days 10–14 and recovery by day 21. • Nausea and vomiting, usually mild, in 20 percent. • Mucositis (reduction of the gastrointestinal lining) and diarrhea, not dose limiting.

Drug	Definition and Action
	• Cardiotoxicity similar to that of Adriamycin, with arrhythmias the first two to three days. EKG changes and pericarditis and myocarditis. • Similar toxicity for skin, hyperpigmentation, hair loss. • Infusion reactions include dyspnea (shortness of breath), facial swelling, headache, chest tightness, hypotension (low blood pressure), and back pain. This usually occurs in about 5–10 percent of patients in the first treatment. • Palmar–plantar erythrodesia (hand–foot syndrome), with skin erythema (redness), pain, skin dryness, cracking, skin sloughing, painful palms and soles. *Late Toxicity Effects* • In the chronic form, a dose-dependent cardiomyopathy associated with congestive heart failure (rare).
Epirubicin (Ellence)	An anthracycline antibiotic derivative of doxorubicin. Damages DNA. *Early Toxicity Effects* • Similar toxicities to that of doxorubicin; should *not* be used with cimetidine and is incompatible with heparin. • Myelosuppression (low blood cell production), especially in older adults who had prior chemotherapy and radiotherapy. • Mild nausea and vomiting. • Mucositis (reduction of the gastrointestinal lining) and diarrhea. • Cardiotoxicity is similar but less severe than with doxorubicin. Rhythm and conduction disturbances, with chest pain, mild pericarditis syndrome, usually occur in the first two days and are transient. Weekly schedules and continuous intravenous infusion can decrease cardiotoxicity. Dexrazoxane may also be helpful in reducing cardiotoxicity. • Alopecia (hair loss) is less common than with doxorubicin and is observed in about 25–50 percent of patients, starting about ten days after therapy begins. • A potent vesicant (burns and scars skin), its extravasation to tissue causes major problems with inflammation and chemical phlebitis. • Skin toxicity with skin flushing and hyperpigmentation of skin and nails. • Photosensitivity (sensitivity to light). *Late Toxicity Effects* • In the chronic form, there can be cardiomyopathy with congestive heart failure, especially with cumulative dosage greater than 900 mg/m^2.

Drug	Definition and Action
Erlotinib (Tarceva)	A small-molecule inhibitor of the EGFR tyrosine kinase. *Early Toxicity Effects* • Drug interactions with phenytoin, phenobarbital, and St. John's wort. Patients receiving warfarin need careful monitoring. • Skin: pruritus, dry skin, and pustular acneiform skin rash. • Diarrhea and mild nausea and vomiting. • Pulmonary toxicity of interstitial lung disease with cough, dyspnea (shortness of breath), fever, and pulmonary infiltrates.
Etoposide (Etopophos)	Plant alkaloid. Inhibits DNA synthesis. *Early Toxicity Effects* • Myelosuppression (low blood cell production). • Moderate nausea and vomiting in 30–40 percent of patients. • Anorexia (loss of appetite). • Alopecia (hair loss). • Mucositis (inflammation and reduction of the gastrointestinal lining) and diarrhea. • Hypersensitivity reaction with chills, fever, bronchospasm, dyspnea (shortness of breath), tachycardia (rapid heartbeat), facial and tongue edema (swelling), and hypotension (low blood pressure).
Exemestane (Aromasin)	A nonsteroidal aromatase inhibitor. *Early Toxicity Effects* • Transient bone pain in up to 25 percent of patients, usually mild or moderate. • Elevated white cell count. • Transient elevation of liver function tests.
Fluorouracil (Efudex)	An antimetabolite. Inhibits DNA and RNA formation. *Early Toxicity Effects* • Myelosuppression (low blood cell production). • Mucositis (reduction of the gastrointestinal lining) or diarrhea, occasionally severe. • Hand–foot syndrome with tingling, numbness, pain, skin erythema (redness), dryness, swelling, pigmentation and nail changes, and pruritus, usually with infusion therapy. • Neurologic toxicity, with confusion, seizures, cerebellar ataxia (poor coordination), and somnolence. • Cardiac symptoms with EKG changes and serum enzyme elevations are uncommon; occasional ischemic heart disease.

Drug	**Definition and Action**
	• Tear duct stenosis, with blepharitis (eyelid inflammation) and acute or chronic conjunctivitis. • Dry skin and photosensitivity in pigmentation are common.
Gefitinib (Iressa)	A small-molecule binder of EGFR. *Early Toxicity Effects* • Mild hypertension. • Pruritus, dry skin, and pustular acneiform skin rash. • Mild elevation in serum transaminase. • Asthenia (feeling of weakness). • Anorexia. • Mild nausea and vomiting. • Conjunctivitis, blepharitis, corneal erosion, and abnormal eyelash growth. • Rare episodes of hemoptysis (coughing blood) and gastrointestinal hemorrhage.
Gemcitabine (Gemzar)	An antimetabolite. Inhibits DNA synthesis. *Early Toxicity Effects* • Myelosuppression (low blood cell production). • Nausea and vomiting. • Diarrhea and mucositis (reduction of the gastrointestinal lining). • Flulike syndrome. • Transient hepatic (liver) dysfunction, with elevated serum transaminase and bilirubin. • Pulmonary toxicity, with mild dyspnea (shortness of breath) and drug-induced pneumonitis. • Infusion reactions include flushing, facial swelling, headache, dyspnea (shortness of breath), and hypotension (low blood pressure). • Mild proteinuria (excess protein in the urine) and hematuria (blood in the urine) are occasionally seen. • Alopecia (hair loss) is rarely observed. • Macular, papular rash involving trunk and extremities with pruritus.
Ifosfamide (Ifex)	An alkylating agent; alkylation directly damages DNA. *Early Toxicity Effects* • Myelosuppression (low blood cell production), mainly neutropenia (low white blood cell count). • Bladder toxicity, with hemorrhagic cystitis, dysuria, and urinary frequency. • Uroprotection with mesna and hydration must be used to prevent bladder toxicity.

Drug	Definition and Action
	• Nausea and vomiting. • Neurotoxicity, with lethargy, confusion, seizures, cerebellar ataxia, weakness, hallucinations, and cranial nerve dysfunction. • Alopecia (hair loss) in more than 80 percent of cases. • Skin rash, hyperpigmentation, nail changes, and syndrome of inappropriate secretion of antidiuretic hormone. • Amenorrhea, oligospermia, and infertility are seen. *Late Toxicity Effects* • Bladder fibrosis (scarring) may lead to a secondary increase in bladder cancer.
Imatinib (Gleevec)	A small molecule tyrosine kinase inhibitor. *Early Toxicity Effects* • Flulike syndrome. • Nausea and vomiting. • Transient ankle and periorbital (eye) edema (swelling). • Myalgias (muscle pains). • Fluid retention, with pleural effusion, ascites, pulmonary edema, and weight gain. • Diarrhea. • Myelosuppression (low blood cell production), with neutropenia (low white blood cell count) and thrombocytopenia (low platelet count). • Cardiomyopathy, with ventricular dysfunction and congestive heart failure. • A lowering of bone phosphorus, causing osteoporosis.
Irinotecan (Camptosar, CPT11)	A topoisomerase I inhibitor. Damages DNA. *Early Toxicity Effects* • Myelosuppression (low blood cell production). • Early diarrhea within twenty-four hours of drug administration. Prevent with atropine. • Delayed diarrhea after twenty-four hours that may last three to ten days after treatment and can be severe and prolonged. This can lead to dehydration and electrolyte imbalance. • Mild alopecia (hair loss). • Transient elevation of serum transaminases, alkaline phosphatase, and bilirubin.
Lapatinib (Tykerb), investigational	A monoclonal antibody against both HER1 (EGFR) and HER2 (HER2/neu). *Early Toxicity Effects* • Diarrhea has been seen with use of this drug.

Drug	Definition and Action
Letrozole (Femara)	A nonsteroidal aromatase inhibitor. *Early Toxicity Effects* • Mild musculoskeletal pains and arthralgias (joint pains). • Headache and fatigue. • Mild nausea, less frequent vomiting, and anorexia. • Hot flashes in about 6 percent of patients.
Leuprolide (Lupron)	An antihormone, a leuteinizing hormone-releasing hormone analog (LHRH) that suppresses pituitary leuteinizing hormone and follicle-stimulating hormone, thus reducing testosterone production. *Early Toxicity Effects* • Hot flashes. • Impotence. • Gynecomastia (male breast enlargement). • Decreased libido. • Tumor flare-up in up to 20 percent of patients in first two weeks, with increased bone pain, urinary retention, back pain, and occasional spinal cord compression. • Pretreatment with flutamide or bicalutamide is vital. • Elevated serum cholesterol. • Nausea and vomiting are rarely seen.
Methotrexate (Mexate)	An antimetabolite, folic acid antagonist. Blocks DNA replication. *Early Toxicity Effects* • Myelosuppression (low blood cell production). • Mucositis (inflammation and reduction of the gastrointestinal lining). • Acute renal failure after high-dose therapy with urinary retention, increased uric acid, and renal toxicity from intratubular precipitation of methotrexate and its metabolites. • Poorly defined pneumonitis with fever, cough, and interstitial pulmonary infiltrates. • Acute cerebral dysfunction, paresis, aphasia, and seizures with high-dose methotrexate. • Erythematous skin rash, pruritus, urticaria (hives), and photosensitivity (light sensitivity). • Menstrual irregularities.
Mitomycin-C (Mutamycin)	An antitumor antibiotic, like alkylating agent. Blocks DNA synthesis. *Early Toxicity Effects* • Myelosuppression (low blood cell production), leukopenia, and thrombocytopenia (low platelet count).

Drug	Definition and Action
	• Nausea and vomiting. • Mucositis (reduction of the gastrointestinal lining). • Potent vesicant, causing blistering. • Anorexia and fatigue are common. • Uncommon hemolytic uremic syndrome, with microangiopathic hemolytic anemia, thrombocytopenia (low platelet count), and renal failure. • Pulmonary edema. • Neurologic abnormalities and hypertension are additional toxicities. • Interstitial pneumonitis (pneumonia) with dyspnea (shortness of breath), unproductive cough, and interstitial infiltrates on chest x-ray.
Mitoxantrone (Novantrone)	An antitumor antibiotic. Inhibits DNA and RNA synthesis. *Early Toxicity Effects* • Myelosuppression (low blood cell production), leukopenia, and thrombocytopenia (low platelet count). • Nausea and vomiting in 70 percent of patients, mild. • Mucositis (reduction of the gastrointestinal lining) and diarrhea, not severe. • Acute toxicity with atrial arrhythmias, chest pain, and myopericarditis syndrome. • Chronic toxicity, a form of cardiomyopathy with congestive heart failure. *Late Toxicity Effects* • Cardiotoxicity similar but less severe than with doxorubicin.
Oxaliplatin (Eloxatin)	Third-generation platinum compound, alkylating agent. *Early Toxicity Effects* • Neurotoxicity in acute and chronic forms seen in 80–85 percent of patients, with peripheral sensory neuropathy and distal paresthesias, visual and voice changes often exacerbated by cold. • Dysesthesias (pain and numbness) in upper extremities and laryngopharyngeal region. Difficulty breathing and swallowing, often within hours or the first couple of days after therapy. • Exposure to cold causes symptoms that are spontaneously reversible. • Chronic toxicity is dose dependent, with up to a 50 percent risk of impairment in proprioception and neurosensory function at a cumulative dosage of 850–1,200 mg/m^2. • Oxaliplatin-induced neuropathy is reversible, usually within three to four months after oxaliplatin is stopped. • Moderate nausea, vomiting, and diarrhea. • Myelosuppression (low blood cell production).

Drug	Definition and Action
Paclitaxel (Taxol)	A mitotic microtubule spindle poison and a radiosensitizer. Drug interaction: More myelosuppression (low blood cell production) may be observed when platinum is administered before paclitaxel as a result of inhibition of plasma clearance. *Early Toxicity Effects* • Myelosuppression with recovery days 15–21. • Hypersensitivity reaction in 20–40 percent of patients, with skin rash, flushing, erythema (skin redness), hypotension (low blood pressure), dyspnea (shortness of breath), and bronchospasm. Usually occurs within the first two to three minutes of an infusion. • Neurotoxicity: sensory neuropathy with numbness and paresthesias (tingling), dose dependent. • Additional neurotoxicity with cisplatin, diabetes, and chronic alcoholism. • Asymptomatic bradycardia (cardiotoxicity) in about 30 percent of patients. • Occasional heart block and ventricular arrhythmias. • Alopecia totalis (total loss of hair on the scalp). • Mucositis (reduction of the gastrointestinal lining) and diarrhea in 30–40 percent of patients, more common with a twenty-four-hour schedule. • Onycholysis (fingernail damage or loss) seen usually after a weekly schedule of six courses.
Pemetrexed (Alimta)	An antimetabolite, anti–folic acid. Blocks DNA replication. May enhance the antitumor activity of 5-fluorouracil. Caution with abnormal renal function. Check creatinine clearance. Somewhat like methotrexate. Hydration important to ensure urine output. *Early Toxicity Effects* • Myelosuppression (low blood cell production), leukopenia (low total white blood count), and thrombocytopenia (low platelet count). Immunosuppression: Both B- and T-lymphocytes are suppressed. Elevated risk of infections. • Nausea and vomiting, not severe. • Mild elevation of serum bilirubin and transaminases (liver). • Occasional headache, lethargy, fatigue, and allergic hypersensitivity, with fever, chills, myalgias (muscle pains), and arthralgias (joint pains). • Vision and ear problems such as conjunctivitis, photophobia (light sensitivity), diplopia, ototoxicity with ear pain, labyrinthitis, and tinnitus (ringing in ears), uncommon.

Drug — **Definition and Action**

Rituximab (Rituxan)

A monoclonal antibody against CD20 antibody.

Early Toxicity Effects

- Infusion reactions: flulike symptoms with fever, chills, urticaria, flushing, fatigue, headache, bronchospasm, dyspnea (shortness of breath), angioneurotic edema (swelling), and possible hypotension (low blood pressure), usually within thirty minutes to two hours after start of first infusion.
- Tumor lysis syndrome may occur, with hyperkalemia, hyperuricemia, hyperphosphatemia, hypocalcemia, and renal insufficiency. Onset is twelve to twenty-four hours after first treatment.
- Skin reactions including pemphigus, Stevens–Johnson syndrome, and toxic epidermal neurolysis.
- Occasional arrhythmias and chest pain during infusion in those with preexisting cardiac disease.
- Myelosuppression (low blood cell production) is rare, but lymphopenia (low lymphocytes in the blood) is common in up to 50 percent of patients.
- Mild nausea, vomiting, cough, and dyspnea (shortness of breath).

Steroids (cortisone, prednisone, dexamethasone)

May activate resting cancer cells so they can be damaged by chemotherapy. Can block toxic immune effects.

Early Toxicity Effects

- Pneumonitis (lung inflammation) and increased susceptibility to infections have been seen when high-dose steroids have been used.

Tamoxifen (Nolvadex)

A synthetic anti-estrogen drug.

Early Toxicity Effects

- Menopausal symptoms: hot flashes, nausea, vomiting, vaginal bleeding, menstrual irregularities, and occasional vaginal discharge or vaginal dryness.
- Fluid retention with peripheral edema (swelling) in about 30 percent of cases.
- Tumor flare may occur in the first two weeks of initiation of therapy.
- Headache, lethargy, and dizziness, uncommon.
- Visual disturbances, including cataracts, retinopathy, and decreased visual acuity have been described.
- Skin rash with pruritus (itching).
- Hair thinning or partial hair loss.
- Deep vein thrombosis, pulmonary embolism, and superficial phlebitis are rare cardiovascular complications.
- Elevation of serum triglycerides.

Late Toxicity Effects

- Increased incidence of endometrial hyperplasia, polyps, and endometrial cancer.

Drug	**Definition and Action**
Thalidomide (Thalomid)	Inhibits tumor necrosis factor-alpha. Thalidomide is an immunomodulatory agent and antiangiogenic agent. Severe fetal malformations if used during pregnancy. *Early Toxicity Effects* • Severe teratogenic effects (fetal malformations), including loss of limbs. • Neurological consequences, with fatigue, orthostatic hypotension (sudden drop in blood pressure), and dizziness. • Peripheral neuropathy, with numbness, tingling, and pain in feet or hands; not dose related, greater risk with prior neurotoxic agents. • Constipation, a major gastrointestinal toxicity. • Not myelosuppressive, although it does affect tumor necrosis factor-alfa and other cytokines. • Occasional macular, papular skin rash, urticaria, dry skin, and, rarely, Stevens–Johnson syndrome (severe skin inflammation). • Daytime sedation or fatigue, usually with larger initial dosages. • Elevated risk of thromboembolic complications, including deep vein thrombosis and pulmonary embolism.
Topotecan (Hycamtin)	A topoisomerase I inhibitor. Damages DNA. *Early Toxicity Effects* • Myelosuppression (low blood cell production) with neutropenia (low white blood cell count). • Mild nausea and vomiting. • Headache, fever, malaise, arthralgias (joint pains), and myalgias (muscle pains). • Alopecia (hair loss). • Microscopic hematuria (blood in the urine) in 10 percent of patients. • Transient liver function test elevation.
Trastuzumab (Herceptin)	An adjunct immunological therapy often used with chemotherapy. A monoclonal antibody against the HER2/neu receptor, which can block cell reproduction. *Early Toxicity Effects* • Infusion-related symptoms of fever, chills, urticaria (hives), flushing, fatigue, headache, bronchospasm, dyspnea (shortness of breath), angioedema, and hypotension (low blood pressure). • Mild nausea, vomiting, and diarrhea. *Late Toxicity Effects* • Cardiac toxicity, with dyspnea (shortness of breath), peripheral edema (swelling), low left heart ventricular ejection fraction in 5–7 percent of

Drug	Definition and Action
	patients with trastuzumab alone, 25–30 percent with trastuzumab and an anthracycline, and 12 percent with trastuzumab and paclitaxel. Caution with preexisting cardiac dysfunction; careful baseline assessment of cardiac function needed before treatment. • Elevated toxicity risk with Adriamycin/Cytoxan programs. • Myelosuppression (low blood cell production) when administered with chemotherapy. • Side effect of pain, weakness, and headache. • Pulmonary toxicity (rare), with cough, dyspnea (shortness of breath), sinusitis, pulmonary infiltrates, or pleural effusion.
Vinblastine (Velban)	A plant alkaloid. Binds microtubular proteins arresting mitosis in metaphase. *Early Toxicity Effects* • Myelosuppression (low blood cell production). • Mucositis (reduction of the gastrointestinal lining) and stomatitis (mouth canker sores). • Mild nausea and vomiting. • Anorexia and diarrhea may also occur. • Alopecia (hair loss) is common. • Hypertension is the most common cardiovascular effect. • Neurotoxicity with peripheral neuropathy, including loss of deep tendon reflexes, constipation, and paresthesias (numbness and tingling). • Orthostatic hypotension (sudden drop in blood pressure), paralytic ileus, and urinary retention are seen. • It is a vesicant (blistering agent), and extravasation causes major local skin damage. • Headaches and depression have been observed. • Vascular events, including strokes, myocardial infarction (heart attack), and Raynaud's syndrome (vascular spasms, hands turn red, white, then blue), and, rarely, respiratory distress with pulmonary edema, bronchospasm, and interstitial pulmonary infiltrates.
Vincristine (Oncovin)	A plant alkaloid. Binds microtubular proteins arresting mitosis in metaphase. *Early Toxicity Effects* • Neurotoxicity, which can be dose limiting, with peripheral neuropathy, paresthesias (numbness or tingling), paralysis, and loss of deep tendon reflexes. • Autonomic nervous system dysfunction, with sphincter problems, constipation, abdominal pain, paralytic ileus (bowel obstruction). • Uncommon cranial nerve palsies, ataxia (poor muscle coordination), cortical blindness, seizures, and coma. • Bone, limb, jaw, and parotid gland pain occasionally occur.

Drug	**Definition and Action**
	• Orthostasis (sudden drop in blood pressure). • Alopecia (hair loss) with skin rash and fever. • It is a vesicant (blistering agent) and causes local tissue injury if extravasated.
Vinorelbine (Navelbine)	A synthetic derivative of vinblastine, binds microtubular proteins arresting mitosis in metaphase. Abnormal LFTs are associated with increased toxicity, and dose reduction may be needed. *Early Toxicity Effects* • Myelosuppression (low blood cell production), which is dose limiting, mainly neutropenia (low white blood cell count). • Nausea and vomiting, moderate on first day. • Gastrointestinal toxicities: constipation 35 percent, diarrhea 17 percent, stomatitis (canker sores) 20 percent, and anorexia 20 percent. • It is a vesicant (blistering agent), and caution is needed to avoid extravasation. • Neurotoxicity, usually mild and less severe than with other vinca alkaloids. • Alopecia (hair loss) in 10–15 percent of patients. • Fatigue in about 35 percent of patients. • Hypersensitivity or allergic reaction, including dyspnea (shortness of breath) and bronchospasm (wheezing), especially when used in conjunction with mitomycin-C.

5 Cognitive Changes and Psychological Support for Cancer Survivors

Ernest H. Rosenbaum, M.D., F.A.C.P., David Spiegel, M.D., and Patricia Fobair, L.C.S.W., M.P.H.

Cognitive changes resulting from cancer, its treatment, or complications from treatment are not uncommon. Additional factors are the effects of aging, psychological problems, and drug use. Cognitive changes can occur at any time from diagnosis to treatment to posttreatment and can be progressive or can resolve anywhere up to the end of life. Clinicians agree that there is little doubt that even subtle cognitive impairment is a real complication of chemotherapy and brain radiotherapy. Mood change is also associated with cognitive impairment.

Cognitive changes often are seen in children after brain irradiation and intrathecal (spinal canal) chemotherapy and are a result of neurotoxicity. Hormone manipulations, chemotherapy, radiation, and biologic response modifiers are also common causes of cognitive problem in adults and children.

There are few interventions and limited options for treatment. Evaluation may help improve factors such as fatigue, insomnia, and depression, which contribute to cognitive problems and are confounding factors needing attention and correction if possible. Unfortunately, there otherwise is little to offer, for now, except support programs and reassurance.

A recent study[1] concluded that cognitive impairment from chemotherapy usually is a temporary complication. In another study, imaging has shown changes in metabolism.[2] Daniel Silverman of the University of California at Los Angeles has shown that adjuvant chemotherapy for breast cancer can affect the brain, causing long-lasting changes that are shown with positron emission tomography (PET) scans when compared with normal controls. With continued improvement in therapy, more women are surviving longer, and many complain of cognitive impairment after chemotherapy. This is especially noted with multitasking, as shown in neuropsychological testing. Many of the changes were in the brain's inferior frontal gyrus, and this was shown in short-term memory testing. Silverman continues his studies with a five-year plan for longitudinal brain imaging to further test the effect of chemotherapy in women with breast cancer.

Researchers have proposed that oncologists warn patients about this risk, with reassurances that cognitive effects usually are a temporary problem, and include it among the standard informed consents for patients enrolled in clinical trials. Studies of cognitive dysfunction in breast cancer survivors disagree on the prevalence of the condition depending on when the evaluation is performed: before therapy, after therapy, or during the recovery period months later.

Psychological Support

Patients facing a diagnosis and treatment for cancer often have anxiety, depression, psychological distress, loss of control, and fear. These emotions are better controlled with psychological support such as counseling, group therapy, or good supportive care.

Effective medications for depression and anxiety can also help some people reduce their distress. In particular, antidepressants can improve energy and mood, breaking the cycle of despair, hopelessness, and poor self-esteem that can spiral into worsening depression.

Short- and Long-Term Psychological Effects

David Spiegel, M.D., Patricia Fobair, L.C.S.W., M.P.H., and Ernest H. Rosenbaum, M.D.

All patients and survivors not only have medical problems from cancer and its therapy but also challenges to their emotional and social well-being. Problems with anxiety, depression, and difficulty coping can complicate medical symptoms and side effects of treatment. For example, Fobair et al. (1986) found that scores for depression among survivors of treatment for Hodgkin's disease were connected with patient reports of loss of energy or fatigue.[3] Survivors with self-reported energy loss were more likely to be depressed. This result was confirmed in subsequent work by Bloom et al. (1993).[4] A recent study of the impact of cancer-related fatigue on the lives of patients found that 76 percent of 6,125 patients interviewed reported fatigue at least a few times a month and 30 percent on a daily basis. Among those affected, the fatigue prevented a normal life and interfered with their daily routine.[5]

The stress of coping with a cancer diagnosis ranges from mild to severe, often depending on the severity of the diagnosis and treatment and the prior mood of survivors. A third or more of patients report psychological distress during the early months of treatment.[6] Ongoing distress levels may be similar. The prevalence of psychological distress in one study of 4,496 cancer patients at Johns Hopkins Cancer Center was 35 percent.[7] Mood usually improves over time for many survivors.[8] Although some patients have adjusted their lives and actually feel better, others continue to have anxiety, depression, and feelings of isolation, as well as problems interacting with friends and family. Subgroups of survivors remain vulnerable to distress or depression for a long period of time. Clinical depression affects around 18–21 percent of survivors at various points in time.[9] Cancer survivors who were depressed before their diagnosis are at greatest risk for shortened survival time.[10]

Depression and Health[11]

Psychosocial research in the past thirty years has documented the problems of cancer survivors after cancer treatment. Problems such as fatigue (affecting 35–80 percent of survivors), distress (affecting 35–40 percent), depression (20–40 percent), body image (31–70 percent) and sexual problems (30–64 percent), and cognitive and memory losses (20–45 percent) all suggest the need for interventions that help cancer survivors achieve a better quality of life.

A recent analysis[12] of self-report surveys completed by 2,100 cancer patients found a statistically significant relationship between depression and physical and mental health. Researchers identified the domains related to mental health and physical health, including:

- Physical functioning
- Physical limitation
- Pain
- General health
- Mental health
- Limitation caused by emotional problems, altered social functioning, and lack of vitality

Hypertension was found to be a leading comorbidity among cancer patients with depression. Additional comorbidities included arthritis of hips, knees, or hand and wrist. Fifty-four percent of participating patients reported no difficulty with activities of daily living.

In the self-reported survey covering the past two years,

- 21 percent reported periods of depression lasting two weeks.
- Approximately 12 percent reported depression "much of the time."
- Approximately 12 percent reported depression "most of the time."

Twice as many of the unmarried participants reported having depression as married participants, selecting primarily in the "most of the time" depression category. A lower level of education also was associated with more depression for respondents in all three depression categories. Those who reported having depression also had a clinically significant lower quality of life than those who reported no depression at all.

The researchers determined that early screening for depression is very important to help clinicians develop a treatment plan and to help patients cope with their problem, which will reduce their suffering from depression and may increase their quality of life.

Depression Symptoms and Survival Prognosis

Depression has been associated with decreased survival in medical illnesses, specifically for patients with cardiovascular disease or organ transplants. Depression predicts poorer outcome with cancer in a similar manner. Prior research on the association between depression and survival in cancer patients has been limited, but a recent review reported that nineteen of twenty-four major recent studies indicate that depression predicts shorter survival time with cancer.[13] The most comprehensive research has been done in patients with breast cancer and patients undergoing blood stem cell transplants:

- A study of approximately 600 women with newly diagnosed, early stage breast cancer at the Massachusetts General Hospital found that women with depressive symptoms had a 300 percent higher risk of death.[7]
- A study of patients admitted to the hospital for blood stem cell transplant demonstrated that depressive symptoms within the first three to four weeks of admission were associated with an increase in one- and three-year mortality rates.

Studies measuring depression in lung cancer populations have addressed primarily patients with advanced-stage non–small cell lung cancer. Demonstration of a definitive relationship between depression and survival in this patient population could have a large impact on treatment decision making and prognostication. Such a relationship would provide a clear rationale for evaluating the role of treatments for depression on patient survival, which could be a key issue for cancer patients. Patients with advanced non–small cell lung cancer have a median survival of less than a year and high rates of depressed mood, ranging from 16–29 percent. The results of a prospective study evaluating a potential association between depressive symptoms and survival in patients with newly diagnosed advanced non–small cell lung cancer seen at Massachusetts General Hospital were presented at ASCO 2006.[11] The study found that approximately 10–25 percent of all cancer patients experience major depression, and the rates of depression increase with disease severity and symptoms, such as pain and fatigue.

The study also analyzed depression, anxiety, and survival at six months and overall survival in patients who had either advanced Stage IIIB with pleural or pericardial effusion or Stage IV and a poor performance status of 0–1. The majority of patients received chemotherapy as their initial therapy; 11 percent received oral epidermal growth factor tyrosine kinase inhibitor (either erlotinib or gefitinib), 25 percent of patients needed radiation, and 33 percent had brain metastases at the time of diagnosis. A small percentage of those in the study felt quite certain they were going to experience adverse side effects and thus may have entered the study with subthreshold levels of depression or actual depression already in place.

These researchers emphasized the need to distinguish depression from other biological processes and other symptoms, including the following:

- Sickness behaviors that can be linked to cytokines (chemicals that alter body reactions, affecting metabolism or mood, for example), which can show up either as a result of illness or as a result of depression[14]
- Fatigue that can be linked to changes in activity level and a decrease in pleasant activities, which could result from a fatigue symptom that can be mediated by abnormal diurnal variation in cortisol levels[15] and cytokine activity[16]
- Disruptions in sleep and appetite that can be direct consequences of cancer and cancer treatment[17]

The researchers also stressed the importance of identifying the role of depression in compromised quality of life, negative expectations, potentially decreased life span, and increased morbidity and mortality in cancer patients. They recommended the following:

- Assess major depressive disorder using careful diagnostic interviews in addition to self-report measures, including assessment of a lifetime history of depression in order to determine the effects of a premorbid history. Observed effects of increased sensitivity to stress based on prior history of depression suggest a subgroup of cancer patients who are in greatest need of intervention and at greatest risk.
- Develop a self-report survey based on consistent measures of depressive symptoms.
- Assess genetic vulnerabilities to begin to identify a subset of depressed cancer patients who are at greatest risk of depression.[18]

Simple Cancer Patient Screening for Depression

The Depression Screening Form on page 50 is designed to help determine whether a person is depressed and to what degree. Scores averaging 4–5 should be a warning sign that distress and depression may be significant, meriting a psychological assessment.[19] Cancer survivors are vulnerable to both acute and posttraumatic stress, a result of the life threat and loss of control experienced after diagnosis and treatment.

Posttraumatic Stress Disorder Symptoms

These responses are similar to those of the acute and posttraumatic stress syndromes, seen in soldiers on the battle front or returning from war or among those who have experienced extreme psychological or physical problems. In a study of traumatic stress symptoms among women with recently diagnosed primary breast cancer, Koopman et al. (2002) found that the intensity of postsurgical treatment and lower emotional self-efficacy among

Depression Screening Form

Sex (male/female)										
Age										
	1	2	3	4	5	6	7	8	9	10
Fatigue										
Nausea										
Pain										
Depression: genetic predisposition										
Depression: family history										
Depression: prior history										
Unhappiness or sadness										
Thoughts of suicide										
Hair loss										
Sleep problems										
Weight loss or malnutrition										
Activities of daily living (exercise)										
Scale goes from low (1) to high (10) severity										

breast cancer survivors were important factors predicting their traumatic stress symptoms.[20] A later study showed that the degree of traumatic stress, emotional self-efficacy, and social support could lead to poor interactions with medical staff.[21] Problems interacting with physicians and nurses were associated with greater levels of cancer-related traumatic stress, less emotional self-efficacy, and less satisfaction with support from family, friends, and spouse.

Recent work places importance on mood disorders among the medically ill and finds a bidirectional link with many medical illnesses. Although further studies are needed, there is evidence that posttraumatic stress–related disorders affect the course of medical illnesses.[22] Symptoms are of three types: intrusion, avoidance, and hyperarousal. They include constant preoccupation with the disease, nightmares, and difficulty concentrating on anything else. Others suffer from numbing and avoidance, an inability to enjoy previously pleasurable activities, and efforts to escape thinking about or dealing with their illness. Finally, some may become irritable, have difficulty sleeping, or respond excessively to everyday annoyances.

Group and Psychological Support

Patricia Fobair, L.C.S.W., M.P.H., and David Spiegel, M.D.

Many cancer survivors desire psychosocial attention to their problems during and after treatment. Three interventions have demonstrated effectiveness in reducing depression or improving the quality of life:

- Group therapy
- Journal writing
- Physical exercise

Counseling and educational programs offered immediately after diagnosis and after treatment can reduce stress and lead to a better adjustment to the consequences of having cancer and its therapy. For example, Classen et al. (2001) found that women with metastatic breast cancer who participated in the supportive–expressive group therapy program showed significantly fewer traumatic stress symptoms than the control group.[23] A secondary analysis showed greater decline in total mood disturbance and traumatic stress symptoms among patients in the treatment condition. This result is similar to that of earlier work by Spiegel et al. (1981).[24]

The Cancer Center and the Center for Integrative Medicine at Stanford University Hospital & Clinics has been a leader in offering group support, individual counseling, massage, medical qigong, restorative yoga, healing and guided imagery, expressive art and imagery, creative writing, healing touch, and exercise programs. Educational programs are provided, such as "Managing and Understanding Your Chemotherapy" and "Look Good and Feel Better," as are nutritional consultations. Support groups are provided for patients with breast cancer, brain cancer, ovarian cancer, colorectal cancer, leukemia, and lymphoma; patients with multiple diagnoses; and husbands of women with cancer. Such emotional support can be helpful both psychologically and physically.

Group Support

Participation in support groups and other activities is a normalizing experience, exposing cancer patients to others in the same boat. Group members take pride in their newfound abilities to help one another and cope more masterfully with their cancer. They quickly form strong bonds of mutual support and come to see such groups as places where they can discuss anything no matter how difficult or frightening. They also learn that their emotions are not enemies to be suppressed but rather signals regarding aspects of life that need attention. Fear, anger, and sadness are normal companions during the course of cancer, but they need not take over one's life. Rather, patients can address specific problems. Even fears of dying and death are best handled openly, focusing on the aspects that one can do something about, such as the manner of one's dying, important priorities in life, and intensifying relationships that matter.[25] Improving means of communicating with family, friends, and healthcare professionals is another important task that can be promoted by various kinds of support programs. Finally, there are a variety of means of improving physical comfort, from gentle exercise to yoga, massage, meditation, and training in self-hypnosis. Such techniques can help those with cancer to control their symptoms and enhance physical and emotional well-being.[26]

Group support has been helpful to survivors in lowering emotional suppression, allowing greater adoption of a fighting spirit, and lowering mood disturbance. In one group studied, patients showed significant decreases in reexperiencing and avoidance symptoms, which are components of posttraumatic stress disorder.[27] Psychological and social educational care have been found to decrease anxiety, depression, nausea, vomiting, and pain in adults with cancer and to improve patients' mood and knowledge.[28]

Journal Writing

Journal writing focused on expressing emotions significantly decreases the survivor's physical symptoms and medical visits for cancer-related morbidities. Written emotional disclosure has been shown to buffer the effects of social constraints on distress among cancer patients.[29]

Psychological Effects of Physical Exercise

Physical exercise helps survivors find more positive attitudes toward their physical condition and sexual attractiveness, less confusion, fatigue, depression, and total mood disturbance, and greater vigor when compared with sedentary women. Sexual functioning among men with prostate cancer improved as a result of increased physical activity. Improved survival among women who walked three to five hours per week indicated that physical activity after a breast cancer diagnosis might reduce the risk of recurrence or death from this disease.[30]

Psychosocial, Spiritual, and Religious Support

Cardiovascular research has shown that patients who gain comfort and strength from religion or spirituality and who participate in social and community groups had a lower mortality rate during the six months after cardiac surgery than those who were deficient in these categories, although a recent study found that knowledge of receiving intercessory prayer was actually associated with a *higher* rate of complications.[31]

In a recent article in the *Journal of the National Cancer Institute,* Edward Creagan, M.D., of the Mayo Clinic wrote that "cancer survivors may be spared for reasons that are not clearly understood" and that "among the coping methods of long-term cancer survivors, the predominant strategy is spiritual."[32] It is still recognized that the biology of a cancer is the most important determinant in the life history of a cancer course, but religion or spirituality may be an important component of successful coping with the course of the cancer.

The Role of Spirituality, Religious Faith, and Medical Practice[32]

There is much interest in spirituality and religious faith as resources for those with cancer. In ancient times, shamans in Egypt, Greece, and Mesopotamia had priestly duties and often acted as physicians. Later, Hippocrates, in some respects, led the way toward more modern, scientifically based medicine by relying more on physical and empirical observations of patients, rather than spiritual causes. During the Renaissance, medicine further became separated from religion as the science developed with knowledge. However, as Dale A. Matthews, M.D., associate professor of medicine at Georgetown University School of Medicine, noted, "An historic reconciliation between medicine and spirituality has occurred. Spiritual and religious practices can help those with serious illness feel connected and valued, and can help them with the struggle for meaning that affects many cancer patients." It is important to ask patients about their sense of spirituality and what gives their life meaning. Christina Larson, M.D., of George Washington University School of Medicine Department of Health Care Sciences, wrote, "When you ask that kind of question, you are engaging on a more intimate level with a person. In some cases, the effect is to inspire closed-mouthed patients to volunteer information that could be important to their care, for instance, a patient who believes that his or her faith is up to God may not willingly accept chemotherapy."

Although claims have been made that religious patients live longer, there is no robust evidence that this is the case, above and beyond the effects of the health-related practices of certain religious groups. Dr. Matthews draws a few conclusions, such as, "Some religious communities have healthier behaviors because their creed tells them to. Seventh-Day Adventists have lower rates of cancer, because they don't smoke, drink little, and pursue a vegetarian diet." Noting that regular religious practices can lower blood pressure and perception of pain, Dr. Matthews reviewed a small study by University of Vermont researchers in which thirty-six patients with advanced cancer who were religious were found to report lower levels of pain. According to Matthews, "Social support, in turn, has been shown to enhance recovery and reduce depression in cancer patients."

Religion and spirituality play a role in most people's lives, their decision-making practices, and their hopes for the future. There is a spiritual struggle, trying to rationalize how the world acts for both good and evil, suffering and pain, and faith and justice. Sometimes, the emotional trauma of a cancer diagnosis is so severe that it creates doubts about religion and spirituality, and it is a struggle to keep the faith against what can be grave doubts of reality. However, having faith and devotion is often what carries people through a cancer diagnosis or other adversity in life. Religious and spiritual practices may offer opportunities for social support, self-soothing, and a sense of being protected and cared about that can be helpful to many cancer patients.

PART II

A Survivor's Road Map to Health and Longevity

6 Strategies and Solutions for Cancer Survivors

Ernest H. Rosenbaum, M.D., F.A.C.P., and Isadora R. Rosenbaum, M.A.

"There is a doctor inside each patient. [Let us] give the doctor who resides inside a chance to go to work."

—*Albert Schweitzer, physician and Nobel Prize winner*

Survivors are a large group of diverse people with different prognoses depending on many factors. The main goal is to maintain the best possible quality of life while living with cancer. You, the survivor, are not alone: Although each person has his or her own struggle coping with the many challenges of trying to attain healthy longevity and survival, you have a lot of company.

Quality of life is difficult to define and is different for each person. Generally, we think of it in terms of companionship with family and friends, rewarding work, health, and financial security. Through awareness of these and other factors that you define for yourself, we hope to help you maintain or regain your quality of life. The feeling of loss of control can be overwhelming. To complicate things even more, the quality of life can diminish very quickly when one is fearful or fatigued, is enduring therapeutic side effects, or is contemplating the possibility of treatment failure or death. However, by addressing these very real issues and creating a support system with lifestyle choices tailored to meet your needs, you can empower yourself and your body. We in the medical community have consistently seen that survivors have more resilience than they at first believe; they surprise themselves by drawing on previously untapped reserves of courage and determination to prevail over their illness.

> Serious illness is a reminder that life is not infinite. Those who respond creatively to a life-threatening illness hear it as a wake-up call, a reminder of how time is short and life is precious. They do what matters most while they can, experience the joys of living and loving, and let the people around them know how much they are loved and appreciated. To feel embedded in a network of caring at a time of serious illness is deeply reassuring. The will to live is not the denial of death. Rather, it is the intensification of life

experience which comes when you realize how finite life is.

—*David Spiegel, M.D.*

Health professionals believe that a combination of medical therapy and supportive care offers the best chance to maintain a patient's quality of life. Such comprehensive care addresses a wide range of needs, from relieving the physical symptoms of cancer and cancer therapy to satisfying the craving for intellectual, creative, and spiritual sustenance. Satisfaction of these diverse needs demonstrates the powerful connection between mind and body. Obtaining relief from pain, nausea, or fatigue, for example, restores a sense of calm. Sufficient sleep, appropriate exercise, and good nutrition are energizing. Discussing one's negative feelings candidly with others can diminish their effect. Learning to control blood pressure and heart rate through such means as biofeedback and self-hypnosis can foster a sense of personal power. Exploring one's creative potential can lead to joy and transcendence.

Cancer is an assault on your life: It can affect every aspect of your life, from your faith and the quality of your relationships to your physical being and your career. Yet, as we have seen with so many of our patients, it need not destroy the quality of your life.

Remember, You're Not Alone!
Mastery of courage is the challenge.
Quality of Life is the goal!

—*Ernest H. Rosenbaum, M.D.*

Living with Cancer

Beyond the medical surveillance and treatment partnership, an essential concept for survivors is supportive care. Supportive care includes such elements as nutrition; exercise; mind and body control such as biofeedback, tai chi, and self-hypnosis; individual or group counseling for the survivor, family, and friends; spiritual guidance; and creative pursuits such as art and music.

Learning to recognize what you need is the most important key to survivorship. Supportive care activities and services can help you increase your ability to cope and to identify the lifestyle choices that will enable long-term survival with this chronic disease. We believe that supportive care services are essential to the quality of life while one is living with cancer and that they contribute to the quality of life even during the events that lead to death. Set short-term goals to attain emotional satisfaction and peace of mind. Often the confrontation with death allows one to appreciate the true meaning of life. Seek ways to cope with or to overcome physical, emotional, or financial obstacles presented by the disease and the side effects of treatment. There are always people you can turn to for help.

Knowledge Is Power

Knowledge about your type and grade of cancer, the treatment alternatives, and the proper supportive care is essential. It will allow you to make informed decisions, to anticipate potential problems, and to feel a sense of control over your life.

Support Begins with Knowledge

Make an effort to learn about your illness (through the Internet, library books, survivors, support groups, and doctors) and how it may affect your life. Your physician is one of your primary sources of information. However, it can be difficult to fully absorb all the details you might discuss in the course of a consultation with your doctor. It may be helpful to request permission to tape-record these discussions or to ask a friend or relative to accompany you and take notes. This will enable you to review the information at a later time.

A Shared-Care Plan Approach

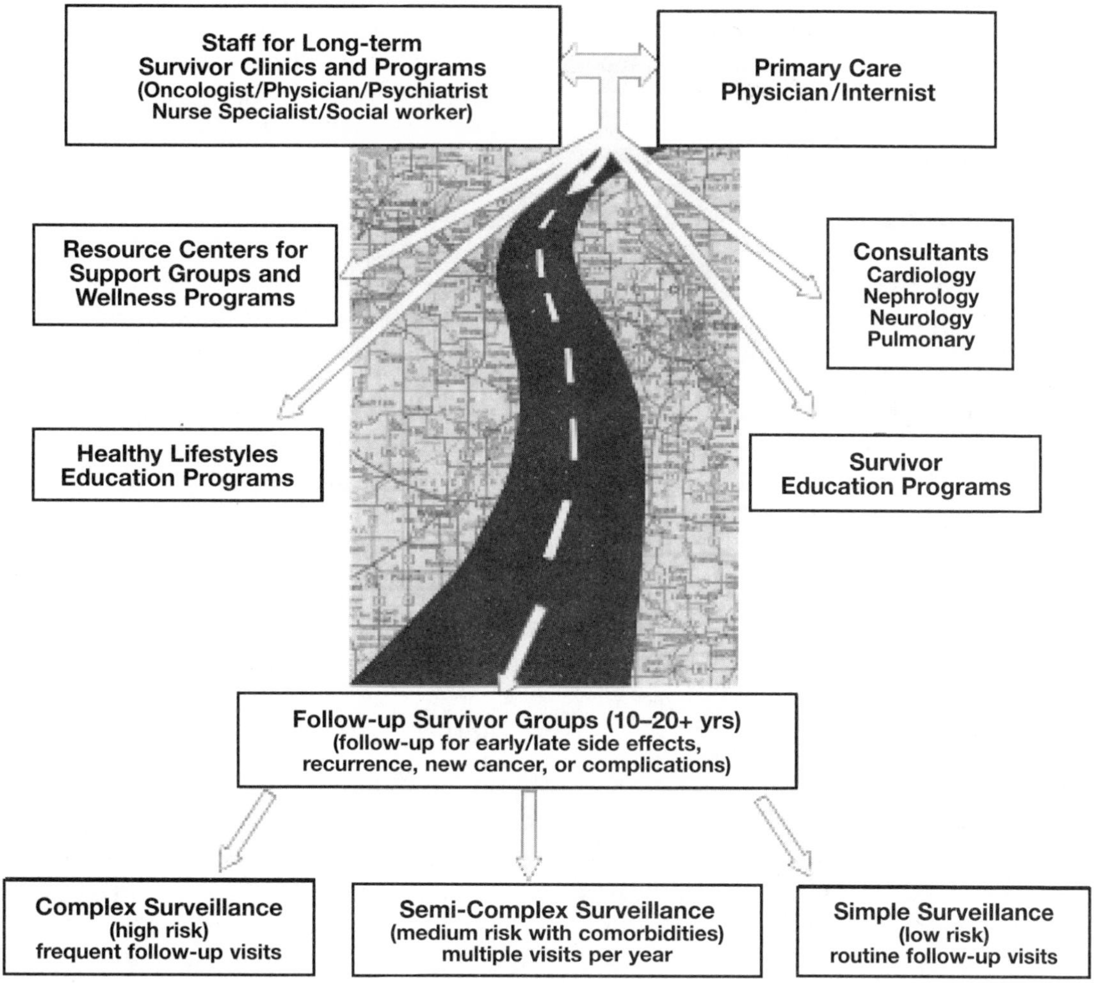

Staff for Long-term
Survivor Clinics and Programs
(Oncologist/Physician/Psychiatrist
Nurse Specialist/Social worker)

Primary Care
Physician/Internist

Resource Centers for
Support Groups and
Wellness Programs

Consultants
Cardiology
Nephrology
Neurology
Pulmonary

Healthy Lifestyles
Education Programs

Survivor
Education Programs

Follow-up Survivor Groups (10–20+ yrs)
(follow-up for early/late side effects,
recurrence, new cancer, or complications)

Complex Surveillance
(high risk)
frequent follow-up visits

Semi-Complex Surveillance
(medium risk with comorbidities)
multiple visits per year

Simple Surveillance
(low risk)
routine follow-up visits

Other sources of information include the medical libraries or cancer resource centers that most major hospitals or institutions maintain for their patients. They typically have the latest books and periodicals. Most of these centers also issue newsletters with up-to-date articles on medical therapy and coping techniques. They also have lectures on supportive care, offer individual and group support sessions, and conduct classes on pertinent subjects. We also suggest that you check out the Internet (see Appendix C).

Realistic, Achievable Goals

Whatever your health status, setting reasonable goals and achieving them is an important part of maintaining your quality of life. Survivors often find that they need to reevaluate at least their short-term goals because of their disease and its treatment. By setting reasonable short-term goals—even limited ones such as getting out of bed, walking to the bathroom, or leaving the hospital and going home—you will reduce your sense of frustration and powerlessness. If you are able to achieve these goals, begin to set longer-term goals, such as going back to work or taking a vacation.

It is not uncommon for people with cancer or some other serious disease to experience a reordering of priorities. In reevaluating your long-term goals, you may decide on some new ones. Discovering something that you want to achieve or do, something that has special meaning to you, can be very empowering. As difficult as it may seem, setting your affairs in order can also help to relieve stress. Put together financial and other records, write your legal and ethical wills, complete an advance directive, and discuss your end-of-life care with your family, medical team, and attorney.

No matter what stage your cancer is in, setting short-term, long-term, and lifetime goals will help you define and achieve your life's purposes. By doing what gives you pleasure and fulfillment, you will gain a greater sense of control over your life and add meaning to your life.

The Importance of Developing Strategies

In keeping with Plato's discovery more than 2,000 years ago that the physical and psychological elements of human life are inextricably linked, health professionals today believe that a combination of medical therapy and supportive care offers the best chance to maintain a survivor's quality of life. Such comprehensive care addresses a wide range of needs.

Pain, insomnia, nausea, forgetfulness, sexual problems, and muscle atrophy can reduce a person's quality of life. For cancer survivors, who may experience several or all of these difficulties at once, the pleasure can seem to drain out of life. Knowing whether the disease itself or its treatment causes these problems is an essential part of achieving a better quality of life. The good news is that many of these problems can be addressed through medication, open communication, and adjustments to your daily routine (including lifestyle choices). If you are experiencing one of these problems, talk with your healthcare team, a family member, a friend, or a member of the clergy. Solutions for many of these problems are reviewed in this book.

> Anything is possible. You can be told you have a 90 percent, or a 1 percent chance. But as long as you take that chance and believe in yourself and are a brave person, and then want to be better than before. . . . I'm living proof that you get a second chance, and the second time around is better than the first.
>
> —*Lance Armstrong, cancer survivor, winner of the Tour de France*

Coping

Fifty years ago, there was little discussion on how to cope. Survivors just dealt with their problems, feeling isolated and distressed. Now the concept of developing coping skills has received much attention from healthcare professionals.

Coping refers to the attitudes you develop and the actions you take to maintain your equilibrium and adjust to the stresses caused by cancer. Different people cope in different ways. It is normal to feel frustrated at times, but how you cope can make a difference. By externalizing your frustrations, you can improve your quality of life. Of course, the nature of your psychological and emotional needs will change as you proceed from your initial diagnosis through cancer therapy into survivorship.

You can benefit from talking about your concerns and seeking help. Fortunately, a number of people can serve as your sounding board. These can include a social worker, psychiatrist, or psychologist, a clergyperson, a sex therapist, a friend, another cancer patient, or a support group. In essence, your relationships need not change. You can have the same give-and-take dynamic with family and friends that sustained you in the past. The exchange of love and support will improve your ability to fight for your life. You don't have to try to cope alone. You might even derive an inner strength from your understanding and support that can enable you to help others find solutions to *their* problems. Feeling good about yourself will help you cope better.

Some ways of coping that you may find helpful include the following:

- Relying on others for support and assistance
- Sharing your feelings with others
- Seeking professional counseling
- Keeping a journal
- Setting realistic goals and readjusting them when necessary
- Controlling fear and anxiety with stress reduction techniques
- Adopting a "mantra," or a reassuring phrase for meditation
- Giving yourself time to adjust to and recover from bad news
- Accepting your limitations (both physical and emotional)
- Recognizing that you still have control over many aspects of your life
- Avoiding procrastination
- Moving on from mistakes rather than letting them debilitate or destroy you
- Alleviating day-to-day stress
- Helping a friend
- Being compassionate and understanding toward yourself

Attitudes That Can Help

Once you are diagnosed with cancer, your life has been changed forever, and although you have hopefully gone through successful treatments and achieved a remission or cure, you still may live with fear of a recurrence, a new cancer, latent side effects or the possibility of functional disability, emotional changes, and even death. *Your attitude, your philosophy of life, and how you manage your health care needs can make a big difference in how you cope and recover following the diagnosis and treatment of cancer.* Remember Saint George and the Dragon. Everyone faces crises and problems in life that may seem insurmountable, and yet with courage, faith, and hope it is possible to confront the "dragon," not be overwhelmed, and to go forth in life with better health and survival. Your attitude can make a difference in how you cope. Courage, compassion, forgiveness, and positive thinking are four attitudes that can help you cope with the difficulties of living with cancer.

"Attitude"

The longer I live, the more I realize the impact of attitude on life. Attitude, to me, is more important than facts. It is more important than the past, than education, than money, than circumstances, than failures, than successes, than what other people think or say or do.

It is more important than appearance, giftedness or skill. It will make or break a company, a church . . . a home. The remarkable thing is we have a choice every day regarding the attitude we will embrace for that day. We cannot change our past . . . we cannot change the fact that people will act in a certain way. We cannot change the inevitable. The only thing we can do is play on the one thing we have, and that is our attitude!

I am convinced that life is 10% what happens to me and 90% how I react to it. And so it is with you. . . . We are in charge of our Attitudes.

—*Charles Swindoll*

Courage

Courage is the ability to face seemingly insurmountable crises with determination and fortitude. By courage we do not mean stoicism. Plato defined courage as *knowing when to be afraid.* Courage is about recognizing the difficulties we face and deciding to move forward in a way that reflects our personal philosophy and our moral standards. In doing so, one takes certain gambles or risks.

> Courage is resistance to fear, mastery of fear—not absence of fear.
>
> —*Mark Twain*

Compassion

Compassion is the desire to diminish or eliminate the suffering of another. It involves our inner spirit, how we feel toward other human beings, and how we support them during times of trial and difficulty. Acting with compassion entails giving of yourself, your warmth, your inner strength, to help sustain another. People who are ill often find that their own suffering enhances their sense of compassion and that feeling and expressing compassion for others becomes a sustaining force for them. Compassion for oneself, especially in a time of great difficulty, can also be a powerful healing force.

Forgiveness

It is not uncommon for people to hold onto past hurts, prior grievances, and old grudges. When you can forgive past disappointments and struggles, you increase your chances for healing and present-day happiness. Forgiveness does not mean that you have to condone actions that were painful, reconcile with people who have seriously wronged you, or give up your right to judgment and your quest for justice. Forgiveness means making peace with things you cannot change and turning your thoughts to the matters in your current life that need your attention. Let the past stay where it belongs.

Research shows that when people practice forgiveness they experience less physical and emotional stress, depression, and anger. When forgiveness is implemented, people also show greater physical vitality, optimism, spiritual connectedness, and confidence about managing their emotions. The benefits of forgiveness are lasting. Start by forgiving something small and practice until the little things no longer bother you. Then work on bigger issues that distress you.

Positive Thinking

A positive and optimistic outlook will not only improve your quality of life but also increase your chances of long-term survivorship. Studies suggest that a negative or pessimistic outlook may actually decrease your chances of recovery. When you have cancer, it can be difficult to maintain a positive attitude. Every day you are confronted with many obstacles, including the side effects of the illness and treatment and feelings of fear, anger, depression, and loneliness. All of this can affect even the most buoyant personality. One way you can help yourself maintain a positive attitude is by setting reasonable, achievable goals. Another helpful hint is to put your energy into activities that bring satisfaction to your life. Doing your best to maintain a positive attitude will help you cope with your illness.

Hope

Hope is a precious commodity that is often hard to define but is very important to keep alive. It often gives a person a glimpse of the future and is supported by fortitude, courage, and ingenuity, often in the face of adversity.

For patients with cancer, the future is often unknown, and hope is what keeps them alive to endure treatments and social and personal adversities. It is supported by the positive attitudes of the medical team but can be very fragile. Anything that demoralizes a person can negate the feeling of hope, which can make a difference in a person accepting or denying the next set of treatments if failure has occurred. The feeling of hope and the will to live vary daily depending on one's physical status, psychological outlook, and treatment success or failure. The hope is to be kept alive, to live, and to recover through a resilient attitude rather than a feeling of hopelessness. It is often a shared feeling with one's personal team—family and friends—because the future is often nebulous, and it is hope that keeps one alive to fight for another day, a month, a year, and a return to better health.

Support Groups

Support groups provide patients with an opportunity to see the problems they are confronting through the eyes of others. This can give patients a new perspective on their situation, reduce any inappropriate guilt, and help patients recognize that their problems are the result of the cancer rather than some personal failing. Questions such as "Why me?" take on a new meaning in a group of people wondering the same thing.

Although support groups may not be right for everybody, they help most survivors develop more active coping strategies and dispel feelings of isolation. Group discussions can lead to the discovery of new domains of potential control. Taking charge of treatment decisions and lifestyle choices, working to improve family relationships, and setting priorities can be powerful antidotes to the helplessness engendered by illness. Group members can also develop and consolidate their own sense of personal competence in dealing with cancer by helping other group members. Helping others enhances one's own sense of self-esteem and purpose in life. Such programs are available in oncology centers, private practices, and supportive care programs such as those of the American Cancer Society and the Lymphoma and Leukemia Society.

Friends and Family

The support of family and friends is an essential part of maintaining your quality of life. Family and friends provide you with emotional support, physical comfort, spiritual guidance, a welcome diversion, and assistance with logistics. Even friends and family who do not live in your area can be a part of your support team through telephone calls, e-mails, letters, care packages, or occasional visits. Find out who can help you with various tasks—such as driving you to the doctor, shopping, cooking, or helping with childcare—and enlist your team.

Spending time with your friends and family will enrich your life. Share a meal, play a game, or look through an old photograph album together. Some of our patients have participated in the Life Tapes Project. Patients find that the process of telling their stories is a way to express love and talk about family legacies, and the videotape or DVD becomes a permanent record of these legacies. Some patients also record their family genealogies. Writing an ethical will, or your philosophy of life, is another way to share important beliefs with your family. For more information on End of Life Care and Life Tape Project, visit www.cancersupportivecare.com.

Spirituality, Faith, and Religion

> Faith is often an invisible force which carries great healing power. . . . It is a supremely potent belief.
>
> —*From* The Relaxation Response, *Dr. Herbert Benson, Harvard University*

At times of extreme vulnerability, we all tend to pay more attention to our innate spirituality and seek to restore a feeling of being connected with the universe or a spiritual idea beyond ourselves. We may seek this liaison through prayer and a renewed devotion to God and our religion or through ritual exercise such as yoga, tai chi, or qigong.

One aspect of your quality of life is your sense of peace or acceptance. Patients who do not participate in a formal religion but who nonetheless consider themselves spiritually involved often feel that their spirituality has been deepened through their experience with cancer. Some reflect on the suffering of humankind through the ages and feel that by having cancer they are participating in one aspect of what it means to be human. Some patients find peace in a surrender to mystery and a trust in some larger reality—a divinity or intelligence, or a purpose—that gives meaning to their suffering.

Spirituality also plays a role in end-of-life care, helping patients use their remaining time to achieve a sense of peace and purpose, even in their final weeks, days, or hours. Spiritual practices can strengthen feelings of hope or give meaning to life before death.

Diversions

You will probably find that now, more than ever, diversions are an important part of your quality of life. Seek out the activities that you would normally do to lift your spirits, stimulate your mind, and tap into your creative potential, or explore new activities. Attend concerts, go to sporting events, play board games, enroll in a class that you have always wanted to take, do crafts, play an instrument, exercise, or take a vacation. There may be classes or activities available to you at your medical center or in your community, or you may be able to work with an occupational therapist or art therapist. See Part VI, "Improved Survival with Creative Expression."

7 What Survivors Need to Know After Anticancer Therapy

Despite the uncertainties, as a survivor after therapy, each person needs to participate in a self-protection plan in order to map out a feasible future, knowing the risks and knowing their options to reduce those risks.

For cancer treatment survivors, emotions such as denial, anger, and fear can subside as life normalizes. When one is facing the next chapter of life, a reevaluation of one's priorities and direction in life is common. There are many questions to be addressed, such as:

- How will I survive?
- Will the cancer come back?
- How do I improve my relationships?
- Is my career satisfying?
- How secure will I be in the future?

At this turning point in life, lifestyle changes are more feasible in part because the potential of a new cancer or cancer recurrence motivates survivors to make choices to decrease those risks and in part because of the potential to reduce the toxic side effects of therapy. A review of the most commonly used drugs, showing early and late side effects from treatment, can be found in Chapter 4. Survivors also need guidance, resources, and an understanding that life can be as good as they make it. After cancer therapy, a patient should receive a cancer survivorship care plan summary that has all the vital information from the time of diagnosis to the time therapy is completed and follow-up, which can also be available as a summary of cancer care for other doctors the patient may visit. Guidelines for the cancer survivor care plan are being developed by a group representing the major cancer organizations in cooperation with the American Society of Clinical Oncology, the American Cancer Society, the National Cancer Institute, the Oncology Nursing Society (ONS), and the National Coalition for Cancer Survivorship. This knowledge will help patients with their follow-up care over the next ten to twenty years. For more information on cancer survivorship plans, see Chapter 2.

The following sections provide knowledge, strategies, and solutions that will help.

Lifestyle Changes to Improve Health and Longevity

There is a definite relationship between our lifestyles and our survival after cancer therapy. It has been well established that through exercise and a prudent diet, one can decrease the risk of recurrence, increase survival and longevity, and reduce the risk of treatment-related side effects. These topics are reviewed in several sections in this book, including the prudent diet, the rationale for exercise, smoking cessation, limiting alcohol consumption, and supportive care plans for osteoporosis, pain, lymphedema, sunshine exposure, sexual dysfunction, fatigue, and other problems.

Postcancer Survivorship Measures

Survivors of cancer graduate to a new life but may face many consequences related to their therapy, both psychological and physical. The challenges they face can best be overcome with a team approach, including their medical team, family, friends, community resources, and, most importantly, themselves.

The knowledge and participation needs include the following:

- Conscious participation in your medical care through the recommendations and schedules in your cancer survival care plan
- Knowledge about potential short- and long-term side effects and possible cancer recurrence or a new cancer, and self-observation for warning signs
- Knowledge and implementation of lifestyle changes to reduce the risk and severity of side effects and comorbidities
- A list of community resources for psychosocial and group therapy support and aid in obtaining benefits, insurance, employment protection, and life support needs
- Ongoing communication of new advances in medicine and current research that could be of aid in reducing the aftereffects (sequelae) of cancer and cancer therapy

Armed with this knowledge, survivors can be proactive, initiating necessary lifestyle changes to promote better health and longevity. With greater awareness of possible late side effects, survivors can anticipate potential problems and take earlier action to prevent adverse outcomes.

A Surveillance and Screening Program

Although many survivors want to forget their cancer experience at the end of their therapy, many others need the reassurance of having a plan and knowing how to recognize what may be side effects of their disease or its treatment or a new or secondary cancer. After you complete anticancer treatment, the oncologist will recommend a follow-up program for doctor visits and screening tests. This cancer survivorship care plan provides a summary of your medical treatment record and follow-up recommendations. Knowledge of this plan makes it possible for survivors to truly understand the lifelong scope of their condition and become "partners" in their medical care.

The essential elements of a posttherapy surveillance and screening program include the following:

- Periodic doctor visits for routine checkups
- Identification of specific blood tests and x-rays, computed axial tomography scans, magnetic resonance imaging as needed
- Disease-specific follow-up screening guidelines
- A review of the short- and long-term potential side effects and the signs and symptoms of a possible cancer recurrence or a new cancer

There is no one specific follow-up guideline schedule because each patient is different and will need a specific cancer survivorship care plan, in part depending on the type of cancer, its risks, and its aggressiveness.

Cancer Risk Factors: Percentage of Total Diagnoses

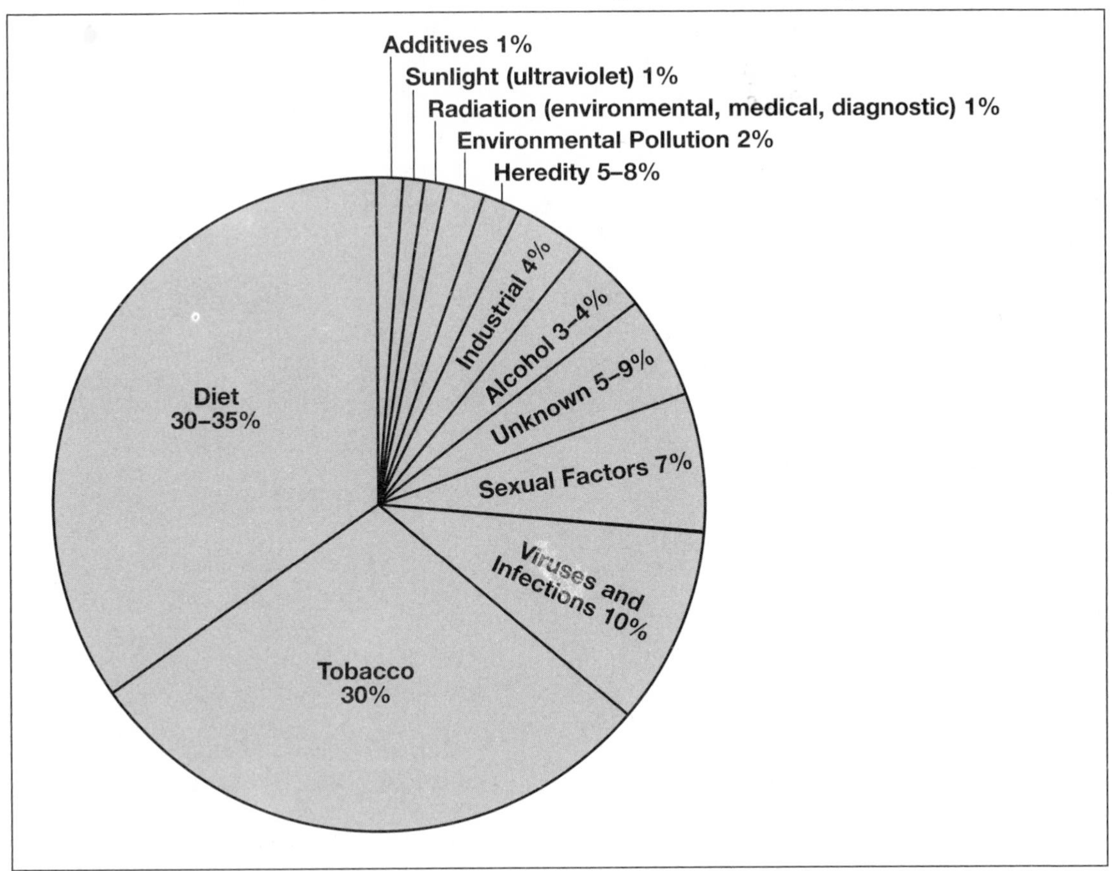

Warning Signs and Symptoms of a Potential New or Secondary Cancer[1]

Learning that there is a risk of developing a new or a second cancer can cause anxiety and provoke fear in survivors. After completing treatment, this is the last thing patients want to hear. Unfortunately, the risk of cancer increases for everyone as they age. A survivor's risk of developing a new or a secondary cancer is comparable to that of people of their same age in the general population except for some specific factors that can increase their risk:

- The type of cancer
- The person's age at diagnosis
- The specific treatment (surgery, chemotherapy, or radiation therapy)
- The person's genetic and family history
- The drugs used for treatment (second cancer risk is related to certain chemotherapy drugs and the field and dosage of radiotherapy)

Healthy Living After Treatment for Cancer

A family history of cancer in some patients who have inherited gene changes (mutations) increases the chances of getting a new primary cancer or a secondary cancer. But overall, these inherited changes are uncommon and account for less than 10 percent of patients with cancer.

Rarely, for example, people can develop acute myeloid leukemia after treatment. Secondary leukemia usually occurs, if at all, within the first ten years after treatment of the original cancer. The risk of developing a secondary leukemia is higher for people who were treated with high dosages of alkylating agents (e.g., cyclophosphamide or nitrogen mustard), epipodophyllotoxins (e.g., etoposide or teniposide), and anthracycline chemotherapy drugs (e.g., doxorubicin, daunorubicin, or epirubicin).

Your family medical history will indicate whether genetic counseling or testing is needed. Your doctor will advise you if you need genetic counseling, but it is a good policy to ask whether genetic counseling or testing is needed. A review of your cancer treatment (drugs and radiation therapy) and family history with your healthcare provider or a cancer specialist and more frequent screening may be recommended to increase the likelihood that second cancers or a new cancer are detected early, when they are most effectively treated. Be sure to get all the screening tests that are recommended for you.

By practicing better health maintenance behaviors, you become aware of changes in your body and increase the likelihood that problems will be detected at earlier stages. By developing a relationship with a primary care provider who knows your cancer treatment history, risks of late complications, and recommended screening evaluation, you will improve your chances of catching problems at an earlier, more treatable stage.

These and any new or persistent symptoms should be reported to your healthcare provider promptly:

- Pulmonary
  - Persistent cough or hoarseness
  - Shortness of breath
  - Coughing up bloody sputum
- Oral, head, neck
  - Discolored areas or sores in the mouth that do not heal
- Breast
  - Lump or breast mass
- Neurological
  - Persistent headaches
  - Vision changes
  - Persistent early morning vomiting
- Hematological
  - Easy bruising or bleeding
  - Paleness of the skin
  - Excessive fatigue
- Bone
  - New or persistent bone pain
- Skin
  - Changes in moles or sores that do not heal
  - New lumps or skin changes
- Gastrointestinal
  - Difficulty swallowing or changes in stomach or gastrointestinal symptoms such as nausea, vomiting, constipation, or diarrhea
  - Changes in bowel habits
  - Persistent abdominal pain
  - Blood in the stools
- Genital and urinary
  - Blood in the urine
  - Painful urination or defecation (constipation)
  - Mass (lump) in testes

Suggested Dietary Modifications

- Follow a low-fat, high-fiber diet, with five or more portions of fruits and vegetables daily. About 6–8 oz. of whole grains and cereals per day is recommended.
- Diets rich in fruits and vegetables provide vitamins C and A (which have been shown to reduce cancer risk in animal studies).
  - People whose diets are rich in vitamin C appear less likely to get cancer, especially cancer of the stomach and

esophagus. The best way to get these nutrients is to eat lots of colorful, fresh fruits and vegetables. Citrus fruits, melons, cruciferous vegetables, and greens are high in vitamin C.

- Good sources of vitamin A are dark green and deep yellow or red vegetables and certain fruits. If your diet is low in vitamins, a multivitamin supplement may help, but avoid extra high dosages (especially of beta-carotene and vitamin E) because these can cause serious side effects and beta-carotene has been shown to increase the risk of lung cancer. High dosages of supplements (antioxidants such as vitamins C and E) will block and reduce the effectiveness of many chemotherapy drugs and radiation therapy and should not be used during cancer therapy.

- Avoid preservatives such as nitrites, commonly found in cured meats such as lunchmeats, hot dogs, bacon, and sausages, which can increase the risk of cancer in the stomach and esophagus. Some of these foods, especially lunchmeats, are also high in fat. Foods of this kind should be eaten rarely and in small portions.

To lower the risk of getting a second cancer, avoid cancer-promoting habits:

- Survivors should not smoke or chew tobacco and should avoid exposure to secondhand smoke when at all possible.
- Because skin cancers are one of the most common second cancers, especially for those treated with radiation therapy, survivors should take extra care to protect their skin from sun exposure. This includes regularly using sunscreen with a sun protection factor of 15 or more, wearing protective clothing, avoiding outdoor activities from 10 a.m. to 2 p.m., when the sun's rays are most intense, and not tanning.
- Drink alcohol only in moderation. Heavy drinkers, especially those who use tobacco, have a high risk of cancer of the mouth, throat, and esophagus. Women weigh less, have a higher body fat ratio, and metabolize alcohol more slowly than men and therefore experience stronger effects. The risk of breast cancer appears to be slightly higher in women who drink alcohol. Limiting the use of alcohol can reduce these cancer risks and decrease the chances of other alcohol-related problems, such as liver disease. The use of a multivitamin with folic acid may help offset the adverse effects of alcohol in those who do drink, even in moderation.
- Eat right. A high intake of dietary fat has been linked to the risk of several common adult cancers and cardiovascular disease. People who eat high-fat red meat diets have a greater risk of getting breast and colon cancer; this may also be true for breast and prostate cancers.
  - High-fat diets are also associated with obesity, heart disease, and other health problems. To reduce all of these risks, daily fat intake should be limited to 30 percent or less of your total calorie intake.
  - Dietary fiber is found in whole grains, several types of vegetables, and certain fruits. Fiber reduces the time it takes for wastes to pass through the intestinal tract, thus lowering the risk of colorectal cancer. High-fiber foods also tend to be lower in fat and richer in nutrients.
  - Eating cruciferous vegetables also helps reduce cancer risk. Cruciferous vegetables include cabbage, brussels sprouts, broccoli, and cauliflower. Eating these vegetables is thought to protect against cancer by blocking the effects of cancer-causing chemicals in other foods. Cruciferous vegetables are also high in fiber and low in fat. These foods should be abundant in the diet.
  - Some chemicals used to preserve foods are cancer promoting (carcinogenic) in

large quantities. Diets high in salt-cured and pickled foods and lunchmeats that contain preservatives such as nitrites can increase the risk of cancer in the stomach and esophagus.

Start today by taking time to review your health habits and practice healthy behaviors that will help keep your risk of second cancers or a new cancer to a minimum and promote your survival.

Late and Long-Term Effects of Cancer and Its Therapy

Ernest H. Rosenbaum, M.D., F.A.C.P., and Patricia Fobair, L.C.S.W., M.P.H.

A 2003 Surveillance Epidemiology and End Results (SEER) study found disparities in the long-term or late side effects of cancer and its treatments among those receiving follow-up care. According to the study findings, "Survivors of childhood acute lymphoblastic leukemia are at a higher risk for cardiotoxic problems; Latina breast cancer survivors may suffer more physical symptoms from their illness than Caucasian, Asian, or African-American women; rural cancer survivors worry more about the financial impact and isolation associated with their illness than their urban counterparts, and poverty is associated with high risk for psychosocial morbidity regardless of gender, age, culture, or geography."[2] Thus, in addition to the many side effect differences posed by the various types of cancer and their corresponding therapies, side effects differ according to age, ethnicity, geography, poverty, and other factors. Despite these differences, gathering all possible knowledge about the possible latent side effects of cancer therapy can arm survivors with knowledge and a plan. By providing and promoting lifestyle interventions, it is possible to reduce the rate of current and late comorbidities and adverse therapy-related toxic side effects.

Late effects of therapy involve unrecognized toxicities that occur from a few months to many years after treatment.

With the current five-year survival rate of more than 64 percent, the majority of cancer survivors will live years or decades longer. At the same time, they face various challenges after potential curative or remission therapy, affecting personality, emotions, and social relations. Surgery, radiation therapy, chemotherapy, and immunotherapy can cause physical changes that result in limitations and challenges to quality of life. Horning et al. (1994) looked for toxic effects of treatment in a prospective study of three-year survivors' of Hodgkin's disease and found that patients treated with mediastinal radiotherapy had a more pronounced reduction in pulmonary function and less complete recovery than those treated with chemotherapy alone.[3]

Prostate cancer is the most common form of male cancer. The most common androgen deprivation therapies to treat metastatic prostate cancer or to prevent recurrence are surgical orchiectomy (removal of the testicles) and medical orchiectomy with gonadotrophin-releasing hormone. The objective is to lower testosterone levels, either surgically by removal of the testicles or medically with hormone injections to block the pituitary gland stimulation of testosterone production. The anticancer benefit of androgen deprivation therapy brings with it many endocrine-related side effects that affect quality of life. They include osteoporosis, sexual dysfunction (loss of libido, impotence), hot flashes, gynecomastia (enlarged breasts), metabolic syndrome (insulin resistance with type 2 diabetes is also related to lower testosterone concentrations), and body composition changes (decreased lean body mass, increased fat mass).[4] For more information on these topics, see Chapters 11, 16, and 23. Men with prostate cancer have a higher rate of noncancer mortality than men in the general population, and some of this is believed to be related to treatment.[5] Adverse effects and late complications affect not only overall health and quality of life but also survival. Therefore, evaluation of risk factors is an important part of treatment decisions.

Often, there may be changes five or ten years after treatment from delayed side effects, such as heart problems after doxorubicin, epirubicin, or trastuzumab therapy. Research is ongoing to evaluate better and safer treatments and ways of coping and reducing these side effects. In addition, lifestyle changes for improved health have been recommended because most cancer patients die of other comorbidities, usually related to age, such as heart, lung, kidney, gastrointestinal, or liver problems. Those who have had amputations, disfiguring surgery, or colostomies, for example, have limitations on daily living activities, self-esteem, and coping and may suffer from depression.

Often, long-term complications from toxic side effects of therapy not only bring back fears and physical problems but also may necessitate specialized treatments to help alleviate these symptoms. For example, patients who undergo brain radiation therapy and receive some chemotherapy drugs can have both short- and long-term memory problems, often called "chemobrain." Knowing that this could happen can help reduce the resulting anxiety. After appropriate evaluation, the patient needs to know that this is not a recurrence of the cancer but a delayed side effect of the treatment. Another example is thyroid failure after neck radiation that included the thyroid gland.

Long-term effects are side effects or complications of therapy that persist when therapy is completed, requiring patients to develop compensatory treatment programs to relieve or control them. In contrast, *late effects* occur months or years after treatment.

Surgery, radiation therapy, chemotherapy, and immunotherapy can cause damage to vital organs, such as the heart, lungs, kidneys, and gastrointestinal tract. Hancock and Hoppe (1996) found that long-term complications of treatment after Hodgkin's disease included early cardiovascular disease, pulmonary dysfunction, thyroid dysfunction, infertility, gastrointestinal problems, soft tissue changes, alterations in immunity and risk of infection, and secondary cancers.[6] These results have been confirmed and were summarized in an international collaborative report for the Rockefeller Foundation in 2003.[7]

Older adults may have preexisting heart, lung, kidney, gastrointestinal, neurological, or liver problems, which can be aggravated by anticancer therapy because these organs may be more susceptible to side effects from treatment. For example, peripheral neuropathy, with pain, numbness, tingling, loss of sensation (mainly in hands or feet), or heat and cold sensitivity, is a common side effect for patients receiving paclitaxel, docetaxel, platinum compounds, vincristine, vinblastine, vinorelbine, and oxaliplatin chemotherapy.

Cardiac dysfunction can occur early or late in treatment with anthracycline drugs, such as doxorubicin, daunorubicin, epirubicin, and mitoxantrone. Though they may cause long-term problems, anthracyclines are used to treat a variety of cancers. For example, younger, premenopausal women frequently receive anthracycline combination therapy (with or without Herceptin), despite the known possible risk of future cardiac disease as it still remains the standard of therapy. An evaluation of cardiac risk factors, including prior heart disease, hypertension, age, smoking, diabetes, obesity, increased cholesterol and cardiac lipids, left chest wall radiation, and an assessment of familial cardiac disease is essential. Postmenopausal women who could be at risk for future cardiac problems now have the option of omitting risky anthracycline drugs and substituting a combination of Taxol (or taxatere) with carboplatin with similar results for reducing the risk of recurrence and improving survival.

Long-term follow-up is recommended for possible congestive heart failure twenty or more years after treatment.

For those who already have cardiac problems, radiation to the heart and treatment with these drugs can also cause progressive cardiac problems. Protective drugs are being developed to delay or prevent damage (e.g., dexrazoxane). In addition, changes to a healthier diet and scheduled routine exercise are important for promoting better health and preventing disease.

Platinum compounds can cause decreases in kidney function, and this effect can be exacerbated by abdominal radiation involving the kidneys. Platinum compounds may also cause high-frequency hearing loss. For those undergoing head radiation therapy, cataracts, dry eyes, and dry mouth are common side effects. Abdominal radiation can cause chronic diarrhea, malabsorption, lactose intolerance, bowel dysfunction, and weight loss.

8 Genetics and Cancer Survivorship

Ernest H. Rosenbaum, M.D., F.A.C.P.

Familial Cancer

Cancer is caused by a genetic change in the cell's DNA from specific DNA mutations. Gene damage and its relationship to cancer cell growth and maturation can be caused by an inherited or acquired DNA defect. Genetic relationships have been established for breast, endometrial, and colon cancers. It generally takes at least two "hits" (a cell's DNA genetic mutation) for a cell to initiate the change to a cancer cell. People born with a familial genetic mutation already have the first "hit," so environmental gene damage (e.g., from tobacco, alcohol, asbestos, diet, or sunlight) can be the second hit, causing the cell to become a cancer cell. Once a cell's DNA has made the initial mutation to a cancer cell, the cancer cell undergoes multiple, complex genetic and metabolic changes as the cells multiply, grow, and possibly metastasize. Thus, a combination of environmental effects and genetic changes can proceed to develop cancer.

Who Is at a Genetic Risk for Cancer?

- Those with a history of being diagnosed with cancer before age fifty
- Those who have two or more close relatives or a child, uncle, aunt, or grandparent with one or more cancers diagnosed before age sixty
- Those who have three or more relatives with the same or different forms of cancer
- Those who have one or more relatives with multiple cancers, such as breast and ovarian cancer

Seek genetic counseling and testing to evaluate your hereditary history and obtain appropriate recommendations. Genetic testing is not for everybody; it is designed primarily for those in certain risk categories. Even negative test results do not rule out the chance that a different gene mutation exists but has not been detected. Thus far, no assurance from a negative test is possible.

Patients with a potential cancer risk can do several things:

- Increase surveillance, such as doing mammograms and colonoscopies at an earlier age, and adopt healthy lifestyle

modifications, drug therapy (e.g., tamoxifen for breast cancer prevention), and possibly prophylactic breast surgery (mastectomy) to reduce the cancer risk.
- Become informed about which surveillance programs are the best options for you.

Genetics and Breast Cancer

More than 90 percent of familial breast cancer cases are caused by DNA mutations in the BRCA1 or BRCA2 genes, which normally become cancerous through interactions with other genes. If a person inherits a BRCA gene mutation, it predisposes her to breast or ovarian cancer. In BRCA carriers, radiation exposure has been found to have a large effect on breast cancer risk, at least an order of magnitude greater than in previously studied medical radiation exposure cohorts.[1] These results must be confirmed, but with their greater radiosensitivity, women with BRCA 1 or BRCA 2 genes must be especially cautious about mammograms and radiation exposure, chiefly women aged forty years and younger and women born after 1949, particularly those exposed only before the age of twenty years.[2]

Some families have a history of endometrial or colon cancer or multiple polyps at an early age. Melanoma and pancreatic and gastric cancers may also have a hereditary link.

Biomarkers for Cancer

The future of early diagnosis, cancer detection, and treatment may well rely on biomarkers. Early diagnosis can lead to more efficient and effective treatment. For example, in a standard blood test, if the hemoglobin is below 11 g/dl, or in the anemic range, this is a biomarker indicating that something is wrong.

The human genome has been mapped, and this allows us to investigate various areas of DNA for possible biomarkers that can be very significant in diagnosis and treatment. Genes and protein abnormalities that indicate disease, and other biomarkers, have limited clinical value thus far because we are still learning more about them and how to use them. As biomarkers become quantified, their value will be more exact and relevant to the stage of disease and the speed of progression of the disease. Cost-effective tests are being developed, and new biomarkers hold great promise for cancer and many other diseases.

These biomarkers have been used for many generations, but only recently have they been found to have a qualitative and quantitative value that help characterize the disease process. For example, in colon cancer, when a carcinoembryonic antigen (CEA) test is positive (increased), it can reflect the presence of occult disease that can lead to an appropriate workup and possible surgical resection, radiation therapy, or chemo-immunotherapy and cure, or other treatments as indicated. The same can be said of the cancer antigen–125 (CA-125) test for ovarian cancer or of the prostate-specific antigen (PSA) test for prostate cancer. Unfortunately, there have been many disappointments because the biomarkers may not always reflect the true status of disease, so refinement in the detection and quantification of these biomarkers is part of current research.

What will be of great advantage is the use of new diagnostic techniques, such as microarray tests, in which hundreds or thousands of genes are analyzed. These genes can become biomarkers, helping to distinguish those who should and should not be treated and indicate how they should be treated. Thus, biology, chemistry, and immunology are being coordinated. They are powerful tools that will be of great use in the future.

The use of targeted therapies is emerging, and biomarkers will be very important in testing the sensitivity of targeted therapy, its use, its value, and its prognostic implications. New treatments will be enhanced by the use of biomarkers to help refine the usefulness of therapy and predict how it will affect cancer growth and thus survival. In addition, as technology is perfected, the tests could take

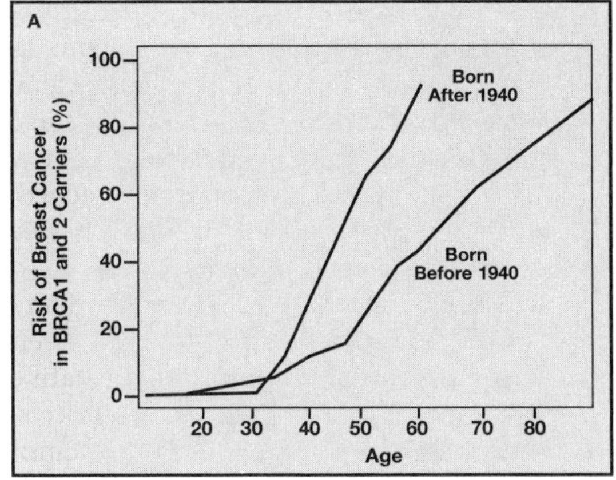

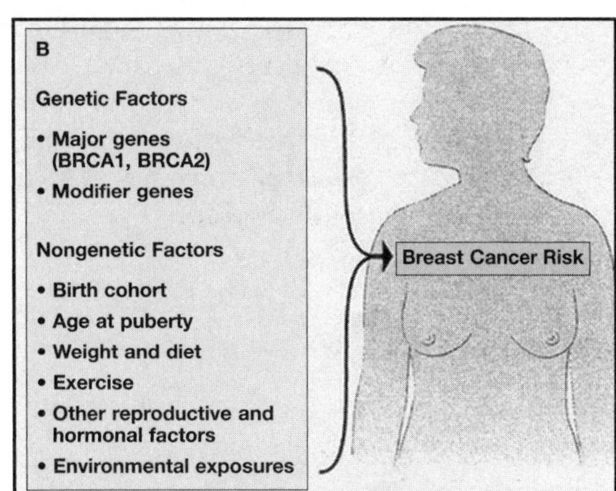

Reprinted with permission from King MC, Marks JH, Mandell JB, New York Breast Cancer Study Group. Breast and Ovarian Cancer Risks Due to Inherited Mutations in BRCA1 and BRCA2. *Science* 2003; 302(5645):643–6. Copyright 2007 AAAS.

just minutes or hours rather than weeks, days, or years to yield appropriate results. Also, new tests (e.g., the commercially available immunohistochemistry tests developed by Genentech and Dako to detect HER2 protein overexpression) not only reflect the aggressiveness of disease but also can be important as biomarkers for disease progress or failure. The fluorescence in vitro hybridization (FISH) test is more exact than the Hercept test, and as research progresses, we will certainly have more information on the use of these tests and their value in prognosis. The U.S. Food and Drug Administration has developed a committee for biomarker development.

This is the beginning of a new era, and new biomarkers will be found and studied and will help greatly in the treatment of cancer patients. There are many biomarkers for cancer. A few examples are as follows:

- C-reactive protein (CRP) is a marker for inflammation, which may also reflect cancer growth or other disease activity. Those with an elevated blood CRP have a higher risk of colon cancer and possibly breast cancer. Additionally, the bacterium *Helicobacter pylori* causes chronic stomach inflammation and ulcers that can also increase the risk of stomach cancer.
- Insulin and insulinlike growth factor–1 (IGF-1) appear to stimulate cancer cell growth through cell cycle progression and by preventing premature death of cancer cells.[3] Research indicates a synergistic effect between IGF-1 and estrogen[4] and between IGF-1 and insulin resistance[5] in breast cancer. A prospective cohort study observed a 310 percent higher risk of breast cancer in premenopausal women who had the highest quartile of IGF-1, compared with women in the lowest quartile.[6] A weaker association was found with fasting insulin levels, such that premenopausal women in the two highest quartiles had a 70 percent greater risk of breast cancer. Other studies support a stronger link between IGF-1 and breast cancer in premenopausal women.[7] Recent studies indicate that high insulin levels increase the concentration of IGF-1. These higher levels of IGF-1 and greater abdominal fat are associated with higher risk of breast cancer.[8] IGF-1 has also been implicated in several other cancers, such as prostate, colorectal, non-Hodgkin's lymphoma, and lung cancer. Among other factors, a diet low in fiber may favor the development of insulin resistance and hyperinsulinemia.[9]

Hyperinsulinemia may contribute to the development of breast cancer in overweight or obese women.[10] Additionally, obesity and fasting hyperinsulinemia have been associated with a poorer prognosis in women with established breast cancer.[11]

- One-quarter of patients with colorectal cancer have a family history of the disease; 3–4 percent of these patients have a genetic autosomal dominant inheritance pattern called Lynch's syndrome. The formal name for Lynch's syndrome is hereditary nonpolyposis colorectal cancer (HNPCC).

In the last fifteen years, genetic research has revealed that mismatched DNA repair genes (MLH1, MSH2, MSH6, and PMS2) conferred a high susceptibility to colon and endometrial cancer and an elevated risk for ovarian, stomach, small bowel, hepatobiliary system, urethral, brain, and other cancers.[12]

Colon cancer is a common malignancy with a prognosis based on stage: Stage I has a greater than 90 percent five-year survival, and Stage IV metastatic has less than 5 percent five-year survival. Therefore, early diagnosis is critical for survival. Having three affected family members involving two generations and at least one person diagnosed before age fifty helps identify high-risk HNPCC patients (Amsterdam criteria). Screening for polyps over age fifty is essential. Both diet and lifestyle factors and genetic factors influence the risk of colorectal cancer.

Healthful lifestyles and behavior modification with diet, physical activity, and weight control are believed to have a favorable impact on the development of colon cancer.[13] A diet low in animal fats and high in fruits, vegetables, and fiber is associated with a lower risk of colon cancer. Thus far, there are no significant data on diet and exercise for Lynch's syndrome, and recently, an oral calcium supplement program failed to demonstrate effective preventive benefits. Tobacco use has been implicated as a risk factor for colorectal cancer, but alcohol use did not influence colon cancer risk.[14]

More studies are needed to assess the effect of diet, exercise, and smoking cessation on patients with the Lynch syndrome, but a diet high in fruits, vegetables, and fiber, with physical activity, weight control, and avoidance of tobacco is certainly a reasonable approach and should be recommended for patients with Lynch's syndrome.

Genomic Methods to Identify Appropriate Treatment Choices

Genomic therapy allows personalized "signature" therapy with molecular profiling using gene microarrays and genomic proteomics. This profiling is used to help identify which people are at higher risk of recurrence independently and more accurately than the standard clinical criteria, such as tumor size, receptors, and pathology. Distinguishing those who are at low risk, medium risk, or high risk helps physicians determine who should receive adjuvant chemotherapy. Gene expression profiling microarray analyses can be used to predict survival in patients with breast cancer. The assay also helps predict which patients will benefit from hormonal therapy or chemotherapy. European studies use a seventy-gene predictor of prognosis.[15]

In the United States, the Onco*type* DX method analyzes twenty-one genes, of which sixteen have predictive value. The 21-Gene Recurrence Score allows a gene expression profiling assay, including sixteen cancer genes and five reference genes, to provide a risk score. The score for low risk is less than 18, intermediate risk is 18–30, and high risk is greater than 31. A major advantage of the 21-Gene Recurrence Score is that it was found to predict the risk of failure and the value of chemotherapy for patients with node-negative, estrogen receptor–positive disease who could be treated with tamoxifen rather than chemotherapy. Thus, the Onco*type* DX can help physicians and patients make more informed treatment decisions and reduce chemotherapy overtreatment and inadequate levels of treatment for patients who could benefit from chemotherapy. It helps in making better decisions where there is uncertainty. This is an example of a pharmacogenomic predictor of response to therapy.

The DNA genomes and certain mutations within the cancer suppressor P53 gene have been implicated in the production of cancer. Groundwork at the Johns Hopkins Kimmel Cancer Center in Baltimore by Tobias Sjoblom led to the identification of these genetic changes. It takes multiple genetic changes to cause mutations in a cell to form cancer. For example, in typical colorectal cancer, an average of fourteen to twenty mutant genes have been identified. In the future, studies of gene sequencing will help identify the events that lead to the cellular changes that evolve into cancer.[16]

A gene expression signature helps identify patients with Stage I, non–small cell lung cancer who do or do not need chemotherapy depending on their risk of relapse. Thus, it is a way of personalizing lung cancer care using a molecular signature. Molecular signatures help identify high-risk lung cancer patients, which appears to be a better way of assessing overall survival than the current clinical criteria depending on tumor size, stage, and pathology.[17] The study, CALGB-9741, helped predict which patients would relapse with a 79 percent accuracy rate (68 percent sensitivity, 88 percent specificity). Additional studies are in progress to help validate the model.

Genomic Methods to Determine Breast Cancer Treatment

The use of molecular genetic analysis (microarrays) of tumors from patients in adjuvant and metastatic trials probably will provide additional guidelines for patient management in the future.

For patients receiving adriamycin (anthracyclines) and/or trastuzumab (Herceptin), careful cardiac monitoring with the application of appropriate stopping rules in order to obtain maximal benefits with minimal risk for the greatest number of patients is needed.

Use of anti-angiogenic targeted therapy strategies for breast cancer has recently been shown to be effective. Anti–vascular endothelial growth factor (VEGF) antibodies, such as bevacizumab (Avastin), are now available for adjuvant and metastatic cancer treatment. These selected targeted agents, such as bevacizumab, combined with chemotherapy are also used for recurrent or metastatic disease. This has resulted in improvement in progression-free survival, although overall survival improvements have not been validated.

Side effects of bevacizumab include hypertension (which is usually controlled with standard treatment), proteinuria, occasional tumor bleeding, nephropathy (kidney damage), fatigue, and neutropenia (low white blood cell count).

Patients with VEGF-positive receptors appear to have a poorer prognosis. New research has shown that sunitinib, sorafenib, and pazopanib are potent inhibitors of VEGF receptors, and trials are ongoing—and have shown some preliminary promise—with inmunotherapy to improve survival.[16,17] Thus, antibodies that target VEGF and oral tyrosine kinase inhibitors of VEGF receptors have been shown to be effective in treating metastatic breast cancer. Research is ongoing to test for the most optimal treatment schedules.

Recent research has been done on lapatinib (Tykerb), which is a novel oral dual tyrosine kinase inhibitor for the arbB-1 and arbB-2 receptors. Lapatinib can be used as final therapy or with chemotherapy for metastatic breast cancer and also for patients progressing on trastuzumab therapy. Lapatinib is also used for brain metastases in HER2-positive patients (approximately 20–25 percent of breast cancer cases are HER-2 positive). The time to progression is longer, but the overall survival thus far has not been affected. Trials with lapatinib and capecitabine have shown improved responses (29 percent) over capecitabine alone (16 percent). Lapatinib toxicity includes nausea, vomiting, stomatitis, fatigue, and dyspepsia.

9 Work and Insurance Issues

Patricia Fobair,
L.C.S.W., M.P.H.

Workplace and Disability Issues

Unfortunately, many people do not understand that cancer is not contagious, and their fears may cause problems in the work area. Misconceptions and prejudices can influence how employers and coworkers treat survivors. Fears that cancer survivors will be less productive have not been borne out. In a study by MetLife Insurance and Bell Telephone, cancer survivors showed no difference in job performance compared with those who had not had cancer. In fact, survivors often worked harder to prove their worth.[1]

Supervisors may make changes in a cancer survivor's duties, often for fear that he or she will not be able to meet current responsibilities. Coworkers and supervisors may treat the person differently or not promote him or her as merited. It is important to take notes on such problems because if you're discriminated against and legal action is necessary, you will need documentation. The Americans with Disabilities Act (ADA) of 1990 makes it illegal to discriminate against any qualified applicant who is disabled, has a history of disability, or is perceived to have a disability. Therefore, survivors have recourse if they have legitimate complaints (contact the Equal Employment Opportunity Connection, 1801 L Street, NW, Washington, DC 20507). A good resource is the National Coalition for Cancer Survivorship, Silver Springs, Maryland (www.canceradvocacy.org). More information is also available in the following publications:

- The Institute of Medicine and National Research Council report "From Cancer Patient to Cancer Survivor, Lost in Transition," published in November 2005
- *A Cancer Survivor's Almanac,* by Barbara Hoffman of the National Coalition for Cancer Survivorship, published in 2004

These two references also have extensive information about health insurance and employment issues for survivors.

Protecting Your Employment

Work is an important part of our lives. Before the 1970s cancer survivors often faced employment discrimination.[2] The good news is:

- There are fewer barriers to employment today and greater legal protections for problems when they come up.

- Cancer survivors have become greater advocates for themselves in the workplace.
- Healthcare providers have also responded to survivors' demands for greater flexibility in scheduling medical care to accommodate their work schedules.[2]
- More than two-thirds of survivors return to work. For example, when Short et al. (2005) interviewed 1,433 working survivors between 1997 and 1999, 73 percent had returned to work within one year.[3]
- Most cancer survivors are able to continue working or return to work without limitations resulting from their diagnosis or treatment. Wheatley et al. (1974) found that the work performance of employees who were treated for cancer differed little from that of others hired at the same age for similar assignments.[4] Their turnover, absence, and work performance rates were so satisfactory that Wheatley et al. concluded that hiring people with a cancer history was sound industrial practice.

Some survivors do have difficulty with employment after treatment for cancer:

- Cancer survivors have poorer outcomes in employment than matched control subjects.[2,5]
- One estimate found that 16.8 percent of working-age survivors (compared with 5 percent of matched controls) were unable to work because of a physical, mental, or emotional problem; of those who could work, 7.4 percent (compared with 3.2 percent of matched controls) were limited in the kind or amount of work they could do.[6]
- In 2001, Short et al. found that 16 percent of men and 21 percent of women who were working at diagnosis reported limitations in their ability to work that they attributed to cancer.[3]
- Cancer has an impact on survivors' physical capabilities. Bradley and Bednarek (2002) found that 18 percent reported problems completing some physical tasks.[7]
- Fatigue limits some survivors' ability to perform mental tasks, such as concentrating for longer periods of time (12 percent), learning new things (14 percent), and analyzing data (11 percent).[2,7,8]
- Five characteristics predicted those most likely to be working a forty-hour week among 403 survivors of Hodgkin's disease: male gender, less depression, age over thirty years, less fatigue, and lack of evidence of advanced disease.[9]

Job discrimination has been a problem, but the situation may be getting better:

- In 1982 Feldman found that 54 percent of white-collar and 84 percent of blue-collar survivors reported discrimination at work.[10]
- In the 1980s Fobair et al. found that 43 percent of 403 survivors of Hodgkin's disease reported difficulties at work that they attributed to their cancer history.[9]
- In the 1990s Yankelovich Clancy Shulman found that 20 percent of 503 survivors reported discrimination, including changed job responsibilities, forced early retirement, denial of expected promotion, and termination.[11]

Types of problems encountered by cancer survivors include the following:

- In 1986, Fobair et al. found that employment discrimination problems included denial of insurance, 11 percent; denial of other benefits, 6 percent; not being offered a job, 12 percent; termination of employment after medical treatment, 6 percent; conflicts with supervisors or coworkers, 12 percent; and rejection by the military, 8 percent.[9]
- In 1988, Bloom found that eighty-five male patients with Hodgkin's disease had more work-related problems than patients treated for testicular cancer.[12] The Hodgkin's group was more likely to report that employee benefits such as sick leave, disability insurance, and health insurance were inadequate. They cited more problems

concerning relationships with coworkers and supervisors or, if self-employed, loss of clients. These problems were considered to be treatment related rather than work related.

- Work problems can be divided into two groups: those with negative evaluations by others and those with a negative self-evaluation. Fobair found that 67 percent of Hodgkin's survivors experienced a negative evaluation by others, and 33 percent experienced a negative self-evaluation. Adverse job selection was a problem for 32 percent. Loss of benefits was a problem for 32 percent. Nine had a negative performance appraisal (4 percent). The 33 percent with a negative self-evaluation said "no" to future options and career advancement.[13]

What can be done about employment problems and job discrimination?

- According to federal law and many state laws, an employer cannot treat a survivor differently from other workers in job-related activities because of his or her cancer history as long as the survivor is qualified for the job.
- Four federal laws provide some job protection to cancer survivors: The ADA, the Federal Rehabilitation Act, the Family and Medical Leave Act (FMLA), and the Employee Retirement and Income Security Act (ERISA).[2]
  - The ADA prohibits some types of job discrimination by employers, employment agencies, and labor unions against people who have or have had cancer. The ADA covers private employers with fifteen or more employees, state and local governments, the legislative branch of the federal government, employment agencies, and labor unions.[14] The ADA prohibits not hiring an applicant for a job or training program, firing a worker, or providing unequal pay, working conditions, and benefits on the basis of disability; punishing an employee for filing a discrimination complaint; or screening out disabled employees.[2]
  - The Federal Rehabilitation Act bans public employers and private employers that receive public funds from discriminating on the basis of disability. Employees covered by this law include those of the executive branch of the federal government, employees of employers that receive federal contracts and have fewer than fifteen workers, and employees of employers that receive federal financial assistance and have fewer than fifteen workers.[15]
  - The FMLA was enacted in 1993 to provide job security to workers who must attend to the serious medical needs of themselves or their dependents. The FMLA requires employers with fifty or more employees to provide up to twelve weeks of unpaid, job-protected leave for family members who need time off to address their own serious illness or to care for a seriously ill child, parent, or spouse or a healthy newborn or newly adopted child. An employee must have worked at least twenty-five hours per week for one year to be covered. The law allows employers to exempt their highest-paid workers.[16]
  - The ERISA may provide a remedy to an employee who has been denied full participation in an employee benefit plan because of a cancer history. ERISA prohibits an employer from discriminating against an employee for the purpose of preventing him or her from collecting benefits under an employee benefit plan. All employers who offer benefit packages to their employees are subject to ERISA.[17]
- State employment discrimination laws have been written in many states to parallel the requirements of the ADA. California expressly prohibits discrimination against

cancer survivors. Qualified workers are entitled to relief. California prohibits discrimination in the "terms and conditions of employment," such as salary, benefits, duties, and promotional opportunities. Employers are required to provide reasonable accommodation of an employee's disability. Employers are prohibited from asking about an applicant's medical history before offering employment.[2]

- State medical leave laws relate to paid or unpaid medical leave for employees with cancer. Employees who do not receive medical leave as a job benefit may have a right to medical leave under state law.[2]

Avoiding Employment Discrimination

Professor Barbara Hoffman is a member of the Legal Research and Writing Faculty, Rutgers University School of Law, Newark, New Jersey. As a lawyer and cancer survivor, Hoffman advises, "Lawsuits are neither the only, nor usually the best, way to fight employment discrimination. The state and federal laws help cancer survivors by discouraging discrimination and offering remedies when discrimination does occur. But, these laws should be used as a last resort because enforcing them can be costly and time consuming and does not necessarily result in a fair solution."[2] Hoffman advises cancer survivors to take the following measures to lessen the chance of encountering employment discrimination:

- Do not volunteer information about a cancer history unless it directly affects qualifications for the job.
- Do not lie on a job or insurance application.
- Be aware of your legal rights.
- Suggest specific reasonable accommodations where appropriate.
- Keep the focus on current ability to do the job in question.
- Apply only for jobs for which you are qualified.
- Provide an employer with a physician's letter that explains your current health status, prognosis, and ability to perform the essential duties of the job in question.
- Seek help from a job counselor with résumé preparation and job interviewing skills.
- Do not ask about health insurance until after you receive a job offer.
- Look for jobs with state or local governments or large employers (fifty or more employees) because they are less likely than small employers to discriminate.
- Seek information and assistance from organizations that advocate for cancer survivors, such as the National Coalition for Cancer Survivorship, Cancer Care, Inc., and the American Cancer Society. Contact information for these organizations can be found in Appendix C.
- Consider consulting local disability lawyers, listed in the yellow pages of your phone book under *Attorneys*.
- *A Cancer Survivor's Almanac* by Barbara Hoffman is an excellent resource.

Work and career continue to be important aspects of the lives of cancer survivors. Although continuity in work roles may be limited by cancer treatment, and some work problems continue to exist, there are now more federal and state laws to support survivors in their return to employment. Studies tell us that survivors returning to work are more likely to have more energy, better body image, and better mood, positive coworker support, and a desire to return to the job. If problems arise, survivors may want to consider advice from the organizations listed in this chapter and consider ways to renegotiate and protect their employment.

When Going to Work Is Not Possible!

Employee Benefits

Employee benefits often include time off for illnesses, medical insurance, and partial payment contributions for disability, if needed. Some employers encourage first using your sick leave days, followed by vacation time, before asking for time off without pay. Large employers (more than fifty employees) are able to accommodate your leave better than smaller companies.

Short-Term Disability Programs

States sometimes make disability insurance available to employees in the private sector, providing short-term monetary benefits to workers who experience a decrease in income after a disability. This disability must be a non–work-related illness or injury. Benefits may be paid to replace part of the disabled person's wages. A few exceptions to eligibility are railroad employees, nonprofit organizations, government employees, and those who claim religious exemptions. Research specific disability programs in your state.

Long-Term Disability Programs

The Social Security and Supplemental Security Income disability programs are the largest of several federal programs that provide assistance to people with disabilities. Social Security Disability Insurance (see www.socialsecurity.gov) is a federally financed program designed to provide funds to those with long-term disabilities. Eligibility is determined by the extent and permanence of the disability and a base number of years of employment covered. (Working five out of the last ten years has been required in the past.) Social Security Disability Insurance pays benefits to you and certain members of your family if you are covered, meaning that you worked long enough and paid Social Security taxes. Supplemental Security Income pays benefits based on financial need. Applicants need to obtain medical validation that they are totally and permanently disabled. This program is not designed for applicants who plan to return to employment within a year. In recent years, the refusal rate of Social Security disability claims has increased, and applicants have had to reapply several times before their claims were accepted. If needed, consider consulting local disability lawyers, listed in the yellow pages of your phone book under *Attorneys*.

Health Insurance

Although many working-age cancer patients have health insurance coverage through their employment, and many survivors over age sixty-five are covered by Medicare, 15 percent of all Americans lack health insurance: 18 percent of adults thirty-five to forty-four and 13 percent of adults aged forty-five to sixty-five.[18] A study of insurance records reveals a disparity in treatment. Breast-conserving surgery with axillary dissection and radiotherapy has been the standard of practice as an alternative to mastectomy and provides similar results. A study of treatment and outcomes for disabled women diagnosed with Stage I breast cancer between 1989 and 1999 showed that women with Social Security Disability Insurance and Medicare coverage had fewer breast-conserving surgeries (43 percent vs. 49 percent) and axillary lymph node resections. They were less likely to receive standard therapy, and their survival rates were lower. Although many did not receive radiotherapy (generally a part of standard therapy) and therefore would experience a higher rate of recurrence, differences in treatment did not explain the mortality difference. The difference may result from poor physician communications or inadequate access to care because of disability.[19]

Additional problems exist for the homeless and the impoverished members of our population who cannot afford adequate care, nursing, home care visits, or nursing home care as indicated. Geriatricians are now working with oncologists to resolve some of these problems.[20]

Handling Problems for Those Who Have Health Insurance

Survivors can have problems with health insurance and medical coverage. For example, eligibility and coverage for cancer care may be denied employees for various technical reasons. Resolving insurance denials for employed people entails locating the appropriate person in the workplace or insurance company who has the responsibility for employee medical benefits and the authority to change the negative decision. The longer the worker has been employed with the company, the more likely it is that the dispute will be resolved in the employee's favor. Hospital social workers often are successful in negotiating the patient's situation with line supervisors, employer benefit staff, or management staff and with insurance companies. There are several negotiating points that the employed patient's representative can use in lobbying for a favorable outcome, including the importance of the job to the patient, the worker's loyalty to the employer and eagerness to return to work, or the seriousness of the patient's medical situation.

The Patient Advocate Foundation is a national nonprofit organization that serves as a liaison between patients and their insurers, employers, and creditors to resolve insurance, job retention, and debt crisis matters related to their diagnosis through case managers, doctors, and attorneys. Mediation is provided to ensure access to care, maintenance of employment, and preservation of financial stability. The foundation also provides financial assistance to patients who meet certain qualifications to help them pay for prescriptions and treatments. You can search for advocates by state and type of service needed at www.patientadvocate.org.

People over age sixty-five on Medicare may have gaps in their Medicare coverage. If supplemental insurance has not been obtained before the diagnosis, a Kaiser health maintenance organization (HMO) plan may be purchased to cover the gap. For those with inadequate funds, an application for Supplemental Income and Medicaid could lead to the assistance needed.

Helping Survivors Without Medical Insurance

In most states, all patients without funds or insurance may use the county hospital medical services, available in each county. Eligibility workers at the hospital will help the patient locate the state and federal benefits available to them. For patients and survivors over sixty-five without Medicare, the county hospital can be a lifesaver. Veterans in good standing may be eligible for medical care in Veterans Administration hospitals. For those with funds but no insurance, some states have a sponsored plan to cover people unable to get medical coverage through regular insurance companies or HMOs.

Additional Programs Providing Financial Assistance to Help Pay for Care

Some hospitals may have funds from a federal program called the Hill-Burton Care Program. If available, Hill-Burton funds provide free or reduced-cost medical services through obligated facilities. In exchange for federal funds for construction and modernization, hospitals agree to provide a reasonable volume of services to people unable to pay. Applicants for assistance must meet income eligibility requirements, and assistance may be denied once a facility has given out its required amount of free care.[18]

The American Cancer Society offers services that can offset some patient costs. Transportation from home to hospital is one service. The costs of staying away from home may be covered in some locations. See Appendix C for contact information.

CancerCare, a nonprofit voluntary agency provides financial assistance for treatment-related expenses such as transportation, child care, home care, and pain medication. See Appendix C for contact information.

The Leukemia and Lymphoma Society offers financial aid to patients who have leukemia, non-Hodgkin's lymphoma, Hodgkin's disease, or multiple myeloma.

The AVONCares Program, in partnership with CancerCare, provides limited financial assistance for women with breast cancer for transportation, child care, and home care services.

Sharing Hope, a program started by advocacy organization Fertile Hope, offers cancer patients significant price reductions for sperm banking and egg or embryo freezing through participating reproductive service providers. The Lance Armstrong Foundation provides administrative funding for the Sharing Hope program.

Many pharmaceutical companies have patient assistance programs to help people afford expensive prescription drugs. There are eligibility requirements and limitations on what can be provided, but such programs are vital to survivors because their drugs can be so costly. The American Cancer Society call center links people to pharmaceutical companies that provide financial assistance and helps them with the paperwork. Most counties in the United States have an American Cancer Society office.

In summary, problems with medical coverage and health insurance must be faced immediately after diagnosis. In many instances problems can be resolved with the help of the social services within the hospital or county or a nearby veterans hospital.

PART III

Ways to Improve Lifestyle and Quality of Life

10 Diet and Cancer Survivorship

Natalie Ledesma,
M.S., R.D., and
Ernest H. Rosenbaum,
M.D., F.A.C.P.

A cure does not mark the end of the healing process. Sometimes it's a difficult transition from the state of illness to one of well-being. The goal is to resume as normal a life as possible, but major changes follow the crisis of a cancer diagnosis and treatment. Physical, psychological, and social problems may come to light or persist after the completion of cancer treatment.

Functional status may deteriorate during cancer therapy but usually recovers with time after therapy. Older cancer patients who have one comorbidity have twice the risk of experiencing functional debility; with two comorbidities the risk increases up to fivefold. Some of the problems survivors face after surgery, chemotherapy, and radiation therapy include a decrease in immune functioning, cardiopulmonary toxicity, kidney, liver, and neurological side effects, and, in many cases, weight gain.

To promote better health and reduce the risk of premature morbidity and mortality, survivors need to improve their physical and emotional quality of life and lifestyle. Unfortunately, with aging new risk factors are constantly emerging, necessitating new solutions, constant vigilance, and care. The diagnosis of cancer not only poses a challenge for survivors but also necessitates many changes in lifestyle for both the patient and family, including preventive activities such as psychosocial support, healthful diet, exercise, sun protection, osteoporosis prevention, smoking cessation, and alcohol limitation or abstinence.

Factors Influencing Lifestyles

Physicians and nurse specialists are best situated to recommend the screening and preventive medicine programs that will promote a better quality of life for posttherapy cancer patients. Most cancer data are for the risk of developing cancer. That speaks directly about the potential effects of diet after diagnosis and the risk of recurrence and death. Survivors often adopt behavioral changes, although it has been shown that men with less education, people over age sixty-five, and urban occupants make fewer behavioral changes.

Improving lifestyle may reduce comorbid health risks and can help reduce therapy side effects. By controlling their weight with a diet low in saturated fats and high in fruits, vegetables, and whole grains and implementing exercise, survivors can increase their longevity. Exercise also promotes psychological and emotional well-being and improves quality of life. Smoking cessation and limited alcohol intake also help.

American Cancer Society Guidelines

The American Cancer Society (ACS) recently released new guidelines for cancer prevention, emphasizing a healthy weight, weight control, healthful diet, and community support and encouraging more physician activity in implementing community-based interventions promoting healthful lifestyles.[1]

Lifestyle factors can influence the risk of cancer and its recurrence. Body weight management and a prudent healthy diet are extremely important. It is estimated that one-third of more than 500,000 cancer deaths that occur annually in the United States result from poor diet and physical inactivity. The major ACS guidelines include the following:

- Consuming a healthful diet, emphasizing plant-based foods including fruits, vegetables, beans, legumes, and whole grains. Reduce dietary fats, saturated fats, trans fats, and the ratio of omega-6 fatty acids to decrease the risk of breast cancer and other cancers, heart disease, and stroke. The value of soy is still being studied because, as a weak phytoestrogen, it has the potential to increase the risk of breast cancer for estrogen receptor–positive patients.
- Maintaining a healthy weight throughout life by balancing caloric intake with physical activity. For women, this is especially important after menopause.
- Adopting a physically active lifestyle. Exercise at least 30 minutes a day (e.g., brisk walking).
- Limiting consumption of alcoholic beverages to no more than one drink per day for women and two drinks for men.
- Recognizing the factors that call for individual control or community interventions: longer working days, more households with two full-time workers, less time for food preparation, and greater family reliance on convenience foods that may have less nutrition value.

In addition to these fundamental guidelines, it is also important not to smoke or chew tobacco. Pesticides are another common concern among health advocates. Research hasn't proven the risk of pesticides, and thus far, no link with PCBs or DDT is proven, but other pesticides are still under investigation.

Diet for Survivors

The foods you consume and the weight you carry are controllable risks that can be overcome with a prudent diet and regular exercise.

Postcancer diet modifications are followed by 30–60 percent of survivors. These changes generally include decreased consumption of meats, saturated fats, trans fats, and sugar and increased consumption of fruits, vegetables, beans, nuts, and whole grains. Additionally, decreased calorie intake and increased exercise are important for weight control, longevity, and survival. Unfortunately, it has been estimated that only 25–42 percent of survivors consume adequate amounts of fruits and vegetables and that 70 percent of breast and prostate cancer survivors are overweight or obese. Men who are older and less educated adopt few of the necessary changes.

In particular, survivors need to acknowledge the dangers of obesity. In addition to diabetes, cardiovascular disease, and stroke, obesity increases the risk for breast (postmenopausal), prostate, colon, leukemia, pancreatic, endometrial, kidney, and esophageal cancers.

Obesity is defined as a body mass index (BMI) higher than 30 and is associated with a higher risk of death. In a study of more than 527,000 people followed over ten years (through 2005), 61,317 participants (42,173

Healthy Lifestyle Diagram

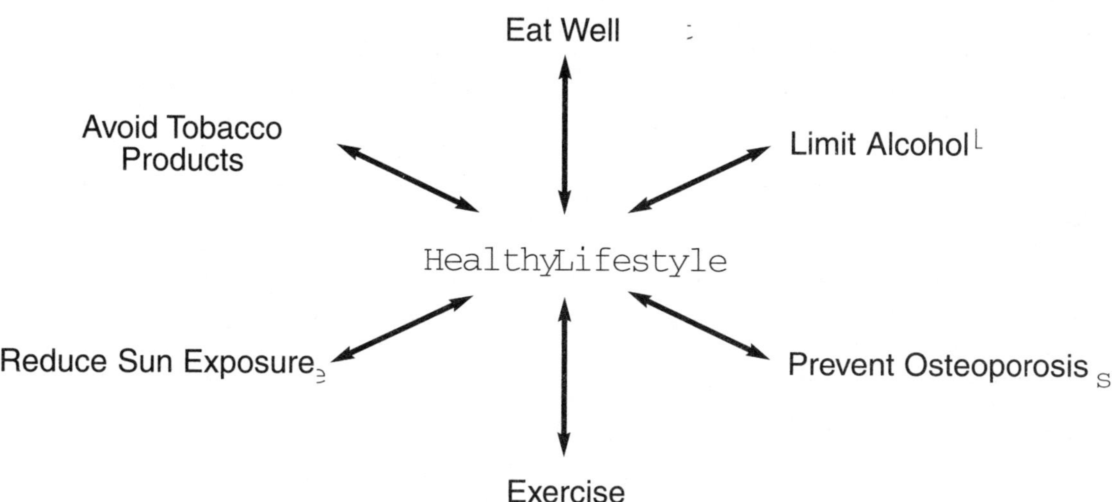

men and 19,144 women) died.[2] Among otherwise healthy people who never smoked, greater mortality was associated with overweight and obesity. The risk of death was three times higher among obese people than among underweight people. Thus, midlife overweight increases the risk of death. The study's findings included the following:

- Even moderate elevations in body mass index (BMI) increased the risk of death. Those who were overweight at age fifty were at 20–40 percent higher risk than participants with a BMI of 23.5–24.9 at that age. Excess body fat is thus recognized as a harbinger of disease and early death. The debate is whether those with moderate elevations in BMI are at higher risk.
- Smoking was associated with a lower BMI but a higher risk of death. Preexisting disease is linked to both lower weight and higher risk of death.
- Weight loss is a behavioral challenge. It takes a lot of determination to achieve a healthier weight.

Survivors must persist in their efforts to avoid obesity. Even small weight losses can bring substantial health benefits, and physician direction and support are vital in helping patients choose a weight loss program.

The standard formulas for calculating BMI in metric and U.S. measurements are as follows:

$$\text{BMI} = \text{weight (kg)}/\text{height (m)}^2$$
$$\text{BMI} = \text{weight (lb)}/\text{height (in.)}^2 \times 703$$

The following table shows the National Institutes of Health classification of BMIs.[3]

Underweight	<18.5
Normal	18.5–24.9
Overweight	25.0–29.9
Obese	30.0–39.9
Extremely obese	>40

There is a continuing controversy in the medical community about the methods used to determine obesity and the mortality risks associated with the condition. Although it is important for older adults to maintain a healthy weight because of their more fragile condition,[4] BMI is a poor predictor of risk for underweight people because age, frailty, and loss of muscle mass affect the calculation.

Because BMI does not differentiate between body fat and lean muscle mass, it is not considered an adequate measure of visceral fat, which appears to be a major contributor to cardiovascular risk. Health providers use a waist-to-hip ratio to verify those with an at-risk physiology.[5]

The waist-to-hip ratio is simply the waist measurement divided by the hip measurement. In one study, those with a waist-to-hip ratio of 1 or higher were shown to be 40 percent more likely to die of cardiovascular disease than those with a ratio of 0.8 or lower.[6]

The Prudent Healthy Diet

- Eat a well-balanced diet.
- Eat eight to ten servings of a variety of fruits and vegetables daily.
  - Opt for vibrantly colored fruits and vegetables.
  - Increase cruciferous vegetables, such as broccoli, cauliflower, cabbage, kale, brussels sprouts, bok choy, collard greens, radish, and watercress.
  - Increase vegetables high in carotenoids, such as orange and dark green vegetables.
- Consume a high-fiber diet (30–35 g/day). Increase beans and whole grains (brown rice, oatmeal, quinoa, millet, barley, spelt, corn tortillas, and whole grain breads and pastas).
- Avoid processed and refined grains, flours, and sugars.
- Eat a low-fat diet (about 20 percent fat calories). Limit saturated fats to 8 percent of calories and avoid trans fats.
- Decrease animal fats and processed meats.
- Increase cold-water fish.
- Include healthful fats in the diet, such as flaxseed, avocado, olive oil, canola oil, fish, soybeans, and nuts.
- Limit salt-cured, smoked, and nitrate-cured foods.
- Limit fried and barbecued foods.
- Limit alcohol consumption.
- Drink 1–4 cups of green tea daily.

A comparison of the prevalence of types of cancers in developed and undeveloped countries shows that people in developed countries tend to have a much higher incidence of colon, breast, stomach, prostate, and lung cancer.[7] Much of current research implicates diet and sedentary lifestyles as major contributing causes.[8]

At a Cancer Research function in the United Kingdom, Timothy Key argued that diet is second to tobacco as the leading cause of cancer in developing countries, and obesity increases the risk of breast, bowel, prostate, kidney, and uterine cancer.[8] When overweight or obesity is combined with alcohol consumption and tobacco use, the risk of mouth, throat, and liver cancer increases.

The New York Breast Cancer study group reported that women with mutated BRCA1 or BRCA2 genes (which confer a high lifetime risk of breast and ovarian cancer) who maintained a healthy body weight and who exercised "clearly delayed" the onset of cancer.[10]

Diets that contain too much sugar and refined foods lead to higher blood sugar and blood insulin levels, which have been associated with a higher cancer incidence.[11] Elevated blood sugar levels have been found in patients with stomach, larynx, colorectal, bladder, pancreas, liver, and kidney cancers.

Patients are more likely to be successful in adopting a prudent diet when they work with trained professionals, commercial programs, or a solo counselor or support group.

Nutrition: Factors for Prevention, Factors for Risk

Just as the foods we eat can increase the risk of developing cancer, nutrition can also play a vital role in helping to prevent cancer and perhaps reduce the risk of cancer recurrence.

Age-Adjusted Rates of the Most Common Cancers[9]

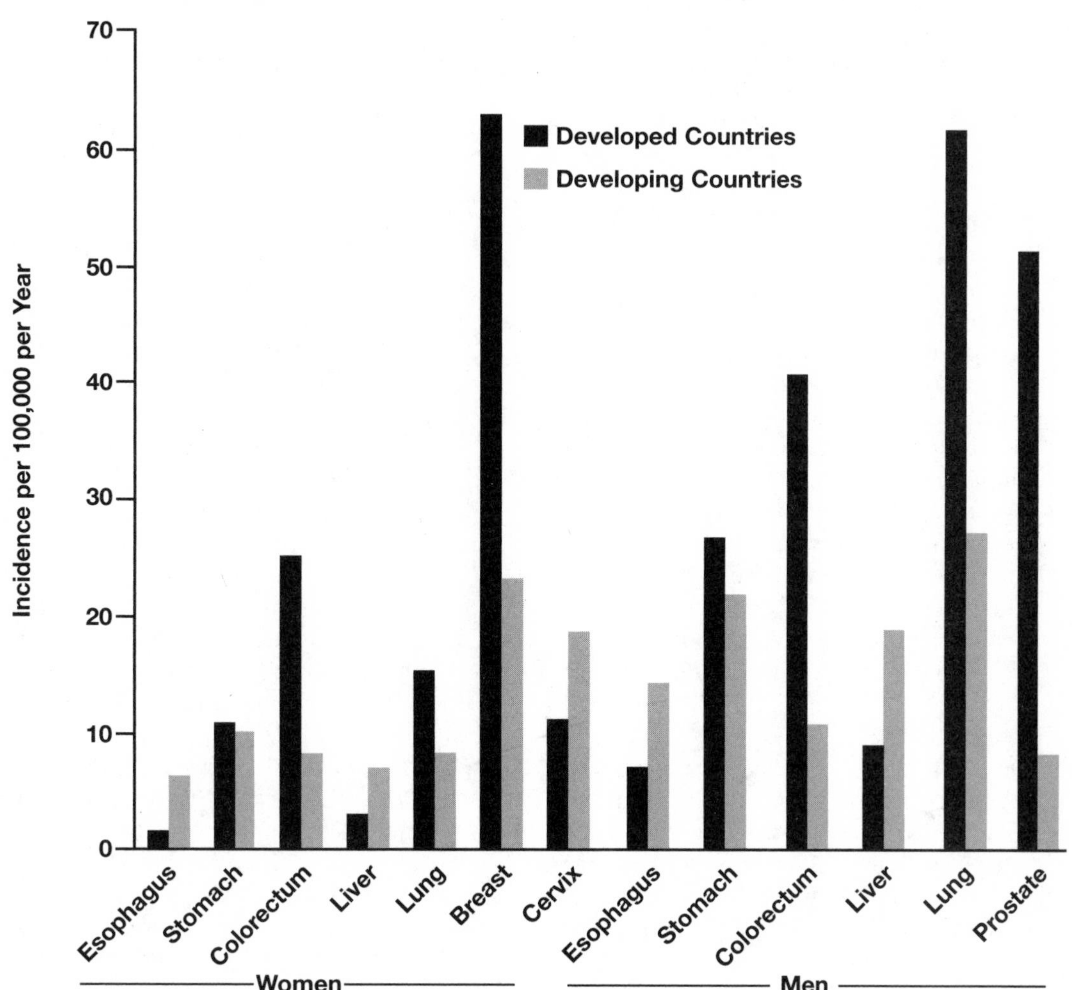

Protective Nutritional Factors

Plant foods appear to protect against breast, prostate, pancreatic, and colon cancer. Scientists estimate that people can lower the risk of these cancers 30–40 percent by eating a diet containing mainly plant-based foods (e.g., vegetables, fruits, whole grains, and beans), exercising regularly, and maintaining a healthy weight.[12] Such a diet may also help to reduce and prevent prostate cancer progression and recurrence and perhaps breast and colon cancer recurrences as well.

- *Carotenoids:* Dietary carotenoids may offer protection against cancer. In various studies, serum beta-carotene levels were lower among breast cancer patients than among women without cancer.[13] This is also seen in prostate and other cancers. Carotenoids are found in colorful fruits and vegetables, including carrots, winter squash, sweet potatoes, cantaloupe, and mangoes. Beta-carotene is one of the antioxidants chemically related to vitamin A and is associated with a lower risk of cancer.

- *Lycopene:* The phytochemical lycopene, a carotenoid and another cancer preventive substance, is found in tomatoes. It is most abundant in cooked tomato products. The strongest data is in prostate cancer, but some prevention evidence has been shown in other cancers.
- *Selenium:* Selenium may also decrease the risk of various cancers, including breast and prostate cancer.[14] A recommended dosage of 200 mcg per day can be achieved by eating two Brazil nuts daily or by including a high-potency multivitamin supplement.
- *Flax:* Flaxseeds contain various protective compounds, including lignans. Lignans appear to bind to estrogen (in women) and testosterone (in men), thus lowering circulating hormone levels.[15] Flax is also a source of omega-3 fatty acids, which may be beneficial. Aim for 2 tbsp ground flaxseed daily.
- *Soy:* There is controversy on the value of soy products. Soy contains various nutrients and phytonutrients that may help inhibit cancer cell growth and tumor development. Studies have suggested a protective effect of soy against prostate cancer.[16] However, recent evidence suggests soy may increase insulin-like growth factor 1 (IGF-1) levels, so there is some concern about taking too much soy. There has also been controversy on the potential of soy to conflict or interact with treatment of estrogen receptor–positive breast cancer. Overall, studies suggest that whole soy foods do not appear to have a negative effect on postmenopausal women with estrogen receptor–positive breast cancer.[17] Additionally, soy consumption may exert cancer preventive effects in premenopausal women, such as increased menstrual cycle length and sex hormone–binding globulin levels and reduced estrogen levels.[18] Dietary sources include soybeans, tofu, tempeh, edamame, miso, soy nuts, and soymilk.
- *Green tea:* Green tea provides phytonutrients, with anticancer and antioxidant properties.[19] A recent study followed 40,000 people consuming green tea over an eleven-year period. The study concluded that green tea protects against overall mortality of all causes, reducing risk of death due to cardiovascular disease. No reduced mortality for cancer was established.[20] More research is needed, but the addition of green tea to the diet is encouraged.
- *Folate:* Folate is a B vitamin found in vegetables, beans, fruits, and whole grains. There is evidence that it can reduce cancer risk. Folate helps to offset the increased risk of breast and colorectal cancer due to alcohol consumption. The pathway data is fairly strong based on genetic-diet studies.
- *Whole grains:* Whole grain foods are low in caloric density and contribute to energy balance. They provide more fiber and certain vitamins and minerals. A high-fiber diet lowers the risk of many chronic illnesses, including cardiovascular disease, diabetes, and diverticulitis. Processed grains and refined flour are of less dietary value.
- *Vegetables and fruits:* There is evidence that eating more vegetables and fruits can lower the risk of cancer. The best advice is to eat five or more 4-ounce servings of a variety of colorful vegetables and fruits each day. Fresh fruits and vegetables are preferred, although frozen produce can still be very nutritious and offer great convenience. Canning often reduces the amounts of heat-sensitive and water soluble nutrients because of the high temperatures used in the canning process. Canned tomatoes are an exception. Cook-

ing also may reduce water soluble vitamins through leaching. Steaming appears to be the best way to preserve the nutritional content of vegetables. Juicing may offer a convenient way to consume vegetables and fruits, especially for those who have difficulty swallowing. It may also increase the body's absorption of nutrients in vegetables and fruits, but juices are less filling because they lack fiber. Juices can also add calories to one's diet, especially if large amounts are consumed.

Cruciferous vegetables contain various helpful compounds, such as indole-3-carbinol. These vegetables appear to improve estrogen metabolism.[21] Cruciferous vegetables include broccoli, cauliflower, cabbage, kale, brussels sprouts, bok choy, collard greens, radish, and watercress.

Vegetarian diets are promoted for better health, and they tend to be lower in saturated fats and high in fiber, vitamins, and phytochemicals. Whether they are helpful in preventing cancer is still being studied. Diets including lean meat in small amounts are also healthful. Strict vegetarians avoid all animal products, including milk and eggs, and they should consider vitamin B_{12}, zinc, and iron supplementation, especially children and premenopausal women.

- *Fats:* Omega-3 fats are found in fish, flaxseed, walnuts, canola oil, soybeans, and leafy green vegetables. Omega-3 fatty acids help suppress cancer formation and hinder cancer progression. Omega-3 fats also reduce the risk of cardiovascular disease. The most favorable fish include salmon, black cod, herring, trout, tuna, sardines, and, to a lesser degree, mahimahi and halibut. Although some types of fish contain high levels of mercury and other toxic chemicals, research has concluded that for healthy adults the health benefits of eating fish are greater than the potential risks of contaminants. Farm-raised fish may carry more toxins than fish caught in the wild. Women who are pregnant or considering pregnancy should not eat farm-raised fish. Fish to be avoided on the basis of mercury exposure include shark, swordfish, golden bass, and king mackerel.[22]

  Monounsaturated fatty acids, such as olive oil, avocados, almonds, and canola oil, may also reduce cancer risk.
- *Fiber:* Plant food carbohydrates that are not digestible by humans, such as oat bran, wheat bran, and cellulose, provide fiber in the diet. Although the association between fiber and decreased cancer risk is weak, fiber is recommended because it contains other nutrients to help reduce cancer risk, and it tends to reduce stool transit time in the colon, thus reducing one's exposure to possible carcinogens in the stool. Furthermore, fiber is satiating and helps with weight control.

General Nutritional Risk Factors

- *Meats:* Red meats, such as beef, pork, and lamb, and processed meats, such as cold cuts, bacon, and hot dogs, can increase the risk of colon, pancreas, rectum, breast, and prostate cancer. Carcinogenesis may well result from the cooking process because heterocyclic amines and polycyclic aromatic hydrocarbons are produced through cooking at high temperatures, and DNA mutations in the meat can be caused by charcoal grilling. Also, free radicals are produced in the colon that can cause DNA damage. The fat content in meat can also contribute to the risk, or the increased risk could also be hormonally influenced (farmers give hormones to cattle to increase their weight).

  In a Harvard University study of more than 90,659 female nurses aged twenty-six to forty-six in the Nurses' Health Study–II, those who ate more red meat in their twenties to forties had a greater risk of breast cancer, probably because of hormonal changes. A study in *The Archives of Internal Medicine* reported that the women who ate the most red meat had approximately twice the risk of breast cancer as those who ate meat infrequently.[23]

- *Fats:* There is evidence that the total amount of fat consumed can increase cancer risk. In addition to watching the amount of fats consumed, one should be aware of the type of fats consumed. Omega-3 fats and monounsaturated fats are better choices. Omega-6 fats, trans fats, and saturated fats should be avoided.

  Omega-6 fats are found in meats, butter, egg yolks, whole milk, and vegetable oils in processed snacks, baked products, and commercial salad dressings. The consumption of omega-6 fatty acids has increased dramatically in the American diet, increasing the risk of cancer, heart disease, and stroke. The increase is the result, in part, of the fast food industry's super-sized portions and very fatty foods.

  The consumption of excess omega-6 fatty acids could promote tumor formation. Recent research at the University of California at San Francisco's Comprehensive Cancer Center by Millie Hugh-Fulford on polyunsaturated fats has shown that when mice were fed omega-6 fatty acids, mice prostate cancer tumor cells grew twice as fast in the laboratory experiments.[24] When mice were fed omega-6 fatty acids, their tumors grew twice as fast. Hugh-Fulford has conducted experiments with omega-3 fatty acids, which appear to block the harmful effects of omega-6 fatty acids. Thus, an optimal balance between the omega-6 and omega-3 fats may play a critical role in the prevention and treatment of cancer.

  In the United States, diets have a ratio of 15:1 omega-6 to omega-3 fatty acids. Current research estimates that a 1:1 ratio of omega-6 to omega-3 is ideal.[25] When these fats are not balanced in the diet, various detrimental effects can occur, such as increased inflammation, proliferation of cancer cells, and a decline in the immune function.[24] When people from Japan and China (who are thinner in general and have a lower incidence of prostate and, for women, breast cancer) adopt the American-style diet after migration to Hawaii and San Francisco, their prostate and breast cancer rates increase to those of the Caucasian population.[26]

  Trans fats are produced during manufacture of hydrogenated oils, such as margarine and shortening, and various processed foods and make them solid at room temperature. Trans fats increase the risk of cardiovascular disease and raise blood cholesterol levels, but there is no proven risk for cancer. To maintain cardiovascular health, the recommendation is to consume minimal amounts of trans fats.

- *Alcohol:* Alcohol increases the risk of many cancers. Alcohol consumption is related to pharynx, larynx, esophagus, liver, and mouth cancers. When mixed with tobacco, it is a potent carcinogen for head, neck, and esophageal cancer. It also has been implicated as a modest risk factor for breast cancer. There is a relationship between overweight or obesity, alcohol, and breast cancer, believed to be caused by increased estrogen production in extra adipose (fat) tissue after menopause and low folic acid levels. Women at high risk, who are overweight and taking postmenopausal hormone therapy, should abstain from or limit alcohol consumption.
- *Soda:* A research report by the Jean Mayer U.S. Department of Agriculture Human Nutrition Center at Tufts University stated that two-thirds of Americans drink sodas, accounting for 14 percent of all calories

consumed daily, and that sweetened drinks account for 11 percent of all calories.[27] Sweets not only add calories and weight but also affect blood sugar levels, placing an added burden on the pancreas to produce insulin.

Supplements, Complementary and Alternative Medicine Concepts, and Generally Held Beliefs

Diets rich in fruits and vegetables and other plant-based foods are preferable to nutritional supplements as cancer preventives because nutritional supplements are not equivalent to the vitamins, minerals, and phytonutrients found in fruits, vegetables, beans, and whole grain foods. There is no evidence that routine supplements increase cancer risk, although megadoses of particular supplements may increase cancer risk.

A National Institutes of Health panel recently reviewed many studies on the use of multivitamins, some of which produced conflicting results. Their summary included the following:

- Supplements of beta-carotene, vitamins C and E, and zinc do help prevent age-related macular degeneration.
- Childbearing women should take folic acid to prevent birth defects.
- Calcium and vitamin D supplements to help reduce bone fractures in postmenopausal women are recommended.
- Beta-carotene was not recommended in general, and there has been a link to increased lung cancer in smokers.
- A healthful diet was recommended rather than high-potency, single-nutrient supplements.

In the absence of scientific evidence, megadose vitamins should be avoided. If you take vitamins, choose one providing the equivalent to the U.S. Department of Agriculture recommended daily dosage.

- *Vitamin A:* The human body can derive vitamin A from animal sources and plant-based foods. It is needed to maintain healthy tissues, but whether beta-carotene or retinol lowers the risk of cancer is still under study. Preliminary evidence indicates that retinoic acid may have anticarcinogenic effects. High-dose supplements may have an adverse effect in former smokers.
- *Vitamin E:* Vitamin E supplements are being tested for potential benefits. The combination of gamma- and alpha-tocopherol may offer greater protection from DNA damage than alpha-tocopherol alone.[28] Studies have shown that vitamin E may reduce the risk of some cancers, most notably prostate cancer.[29]
- *Vitamin D:* Vitamin D is believed to be important in the prevention of various cancers. Cancer prevalence and mortality have been associated with low vitamin D status.[30] Vitamin D probably has beneficial effects for some types of cancer, such as colon, prostate, and breast cancer. Vitamin D can be obtained through sun exposure (twenty minutes daily, depending on skin type), diet (particularly foods fortified with vitamin D, such as milk and cereals), and supplements. Many Americans are deficient in vitamin D, and people need at least 200 IU per day. Research is in progress, and current recommendations range from 200 to 2,000 IU per day depending on one's age. A balanced diet, supplements, and limited sun exposure are recommended.[31]

Additionally, a recent review observed higher cancer risk and mortality among people with low exposure to ultraviolet-B for thirteen cancers, including breast, colon, ovarian, and prostate cancer, non-Hodgkin's lymphoma, and cancer of the bladder, stomach, and uterus.[32] More research is needed, but compelling evidence indicates that vitamin D plays an important role in health and probably in cancer prevention.

- *Calcium:* Studies show that a high-calcium diet may reduce the risk of colorectal cancer and reduce the formation of colorectal adenomas. Daily intake of 1,000 mg for younger people and 1,200 mg for people over age fifty is recommended. However, calcium has been reported to increase the risk of prostate cancer.
- *Antioxidants:* Fruits and vegetables appear to protect the body against damage to tissues that occur during normal oxidative metabolism. Antioxidants, such as vitamins C and E, carotenoids, and other phytochemicals, may be protective. A diet rich in fruits and vegetables can lower the risk of certain types of cancer. Studies on antioxidant supplements are still ongoing and thus far have not demonstrated a reduction in cancer risk.
- *Aspartame:* The artificial sweetener aspartame, which is 200 times sweeter than sugar, has not been shown to have a relationship to the risk of cancer in studies thus far. However, it definitely does not act as an anti-cancer agent.
- *Bioengineered foods:* Thus far, there is no evidence that bioengineered foods (made by adding genes from other plants or organisms to increase a plant's resistance to insects and pests, retard spoilage, and improve transportability) increase cancer risk.
- *Coffee and caffeine:* Coffee does not have a role in causing cancer. Caffeine may heighten symptoms of fibrocystic breast lumps. In addition to coffee, caffeine is found in soft drinks, chocolate, and other foods.
- *Fluorides:* There is no evidence that fluorides cause cancer.
- *Food additives:* There is no convincing evidence that food additives cause human cancers.
- *Garlic:* Garlic and other vegetables in the onion family have widely publicized benefits, but there is insufficient evidence to support this vegetable as a cancer preventive.
- *Soy:* Estrogen receptor–positive breast cancer survivors may want to limit their amount of soy products as part of a healthy plant-based diet.
- *Water and fluids:* It is recommended that one drink 8 cups of a liquid such as water per day, and more may be beneficial. Prioritize water, vegetable juices, and green tea.

Nutritional Risk Factors for Specific Cancers[33]

Colorectal Cancer

This is the second leading cause of cancer death in American men and women. Family history plays a role, as do tobacco use and possibly alcohol intake. Vigorous physical activity may reduce the exposure to possible carcinogens in the stool by helping reduce stool transit time in the colon. A diet high in fruits, vegetables, and fiber also has preventive value, decreasing the risk. Limiting red meat and processed meats also helps decrease risk. Aspirin and nonsteroidal anti-inflammatory drugs, postmenopausal hormone therapy, and possibly increased calcium may reduce the risk of colon cancer.

Endometrial Cancer

Endometrial cancer is the fourth most common cancer in women and the most common female reproductive cancer. Often, it is hormonally related to endometrial hyperplasia (excess of growth of the endometrium), caused by excessive exposure to estrogens unopposed by progesterone. Obesity and endometrial cancer are related, and the increased risk is believed to be related to insulin resistance, elevation of ovarian androgens, and progesterone deficiency associated with overweight. Weight loss and physical activity decrease estrogens in the body and, correspondingly, reduce the risk of endometrial cancer.

Kidney Cancer

The rate of kidney cancer has been rising since 1975. There is evidence of a relationship between excessive weight and renal cell cancer. Although it is less strong, a relationship with tobacco use has also been demonstrated. The best advice is to maintain a healthy weight and avoid tobacco use.

Leukemias and Lymphomas

There are no known nutritional risk factors. Although obesity appears to increase risk of leukemias and lymphomas, dietary intake of fish has been shown to reduce risk.

Lung Cancer

Eighty-five percent of lung cancer cases involve tobacco smoking; 10–14 percent are attributed to radon exposure. Smokers who consume five servings each of fruits and vegetables have a lower risk. Therefore, healthful eating may reduce the risk of lung cancer.

Beta-carotene derived from fruits and vegetables consumed as part of a daily diet is considered protective, but supplemental beta-carotene is not recommended because it increases the risk of lung cancer.

Ovarian Cancer

A typical Western diet (high in meats and low in vegetables) may increase the risk of ovarian cancer. There also appears to be some association between dairy intake and ovarian cancer risk, but more research is needed. Additionally, obesity modestly increases ovarian cancer risk.

Pancreatic Cancer

Pancreatic cancer is the fourth leading cause of cancer death in the United States. Increased risk for pancreatic cancer is associated with tobacco smoking, adult-onset diabetes, and impaired glucose tolerance. Avoiding tobacco, being physically active, and eating a healthful diet are recommended.

Prostate Cancer

Prostate cancer is the most common cancer in American men. There is a strong relationship with male sex hormones, although how diet affects prostate cancer is still uncertain. Diets including tomato products, cruciferous vegetables, soybeans, and fish appear to be associated with a lower prostate cancer risk. There is also evidence that vitamin E, selenium, beta-carotene, and lycopene may reduce prostate cancer risk. Current clinical tests are being conducted to establish the role of vitamin E and selenium. Being overweight appears to be associated with a worse prognosis after a prostate cancer diagnosis and treatment, especially for aggressive prostate cancer. Weight loss and exercise may be beneficial.[34] That said, there is some controversy on the BMI as indicator of risk.[35]

Stomach Cancer

Uncommon in the United States, this is the fourth most common cancer worldwide. A diet with fresh fruits and vegetables can reduce the risk of stomach cancer. Salty, preserved foods are associated with higher risk. There is evidence that a chronic stomach infection, *Helicobacter pylori,* increases the risk of stomach cancer. Following a prudent diet with reduced salt in preserved foods may reduce the risk of stomach cancer.

Upper Digestive and Oral Cancers

Smoking and alcohol are high risk factors for head, neck, and esophageal cancers. Obesity can increase acid reflux and may contribute to initiation of esophageal cancer (metaplasia and dysplasia). A prudent diet high in fruits and vegetables and a decrease in very hot beverages may reduce the risk of oral and esophageal cancers.

11 Lifestyle Recommendations for Controlling Weight

Natalie Ledesma, M.S., R.D., and
Ernest H. Rosenbaum, M.D., F.A.C.P.

Obesity is on the rise, and it's estimated that the increased longevity gained over the last two centuries may now come to an end because of the increased death rate due to obesity. It has been estimated that 112,000 deaths in the year 2000 were due to obesity in the United States, and 2.9 million deaths worldwide were attributed to diabetes.

Recommendations for Losing Weight and Controlling Obesity

- Avoid further weight gain.
- Adopt a prudent diet with low–calorie density foods. To reduce calorie intake:
  - Limit sugar, saturated and trans fats, and alcohol consumption.
  - Reduce the serving size of meals.
  - Limit high-calorie foods and beverages, fats, and refined sugars (cookies, cakes, candy, ice cream, fried foods, and soft drinks).
  - Increase use of fruits, vegetables, and whole grains in place of high-calorie foods.[1]
- Increase physical activity to forty-five to sixty minutes or more of moderately intense physical activity several days per week. Progress from slow walking to a moderate speed if you are very sedentary. If lymphedema is present, get a physical therapy consultation.

American Cancer Society Definition of "Serving" Sizes[1]

Fruits

- 1 medium apple, banana, or orange
- ½ cup of chopped, cooked, or canned fruit
- ½ cup of 100 percent fruit juice

Vegetables

- 1 cup of raw leafy vegetables
- ½ cup of other cooked or raw vegetables, chopped
- ½ cup of 100 percent vegetable juice

Grains

- 1 slice bread
- 1 oz. ready-to-eat cereal
- ½ cup cooked cereal, rice, pasta

Beans and nuts

- ½ cup cooked dry beans
- 2 tablespoons peanut butter
- ⅓ cup nuts

Dairy foods and eggs

- 1 cup milk or yogurt
- 1.5 oz. natural cheese
- 2 oz. processed cheese
- 1 egg

Meats

- 2–3 oz. cooked lean meat, poultry, or fish

Importance of Exercise for Successful Weight Loss

For a weight loss diet, exercise is vital. Although it is not essential for weight loss, aerobic exercise is the most effective because it expends more calories. Aerobic exercise is exercise that rhythmically uses the large muscles of the legs and arms to elevate the heart rate within a certain range. Examples include brisk walking, jogging, swimming, bicycling, gardening, dancing, playing actively with children, and sexual activity.

As a nation, we are exercising less and eating more. One should "burn" about 3,000 calories a day, and the national average is now about 2,000, leaving 1,000 calories to go to fat storage. Not only are we exercising less, but many jobs are no longer physical work but rather sedentary desk jobs. Ten years ago in China, everyone rode bikes; now the number of cars in China has grown from 6 to 20 million in the last six years, and there has also been an increase in the use of motorized bikes. People who use motorized vehicles have a much higher obesity rate than those who still ride bikes.

Exercise is correlated with improved quality of life, improved physical functioning (oxygen capacity, strength, flexibility, and general health), blood pressure, heart rate, reduction of insulin and insulinlike growth factor-1 (IGF-1), and control of circulating hormone levels. Thus, exercise has many benefits for survivors, including increased longevity and survival and potentially reduced risk of a recurrence or new cancer. Furthermore, a prospective observational study reported that physical activity after a breast cancer diagnosis may reduce the risk of a recurrence or death from this disease.[2] The greatest benefit occurred in women who performed the equivalent of walking three to five hours per week at an average pace. The benefit of physical activity was particularly apparent among women with hormone-responsive tumors.

Preexisting comorbidities (arthritis, cardiovascular disease, chronic obstructive pulmonary disease) may limit physical and social functioning. For survivors with these conditions, alternate exercise programs such as tai chi, qigong, and yoga will promote muscle strength, flexibility, coordination, balance, and body function.

Overweight and Obesity Risk Factors for Cancer

Americans in general are gaining weight, and it is estimated that 65 percent of adults in the United States are overweight or obese. The health risks of being overweight range from cardiovascular disease to several cancers, including liver, colorectal, stomach, breast, and esophageal (adenocarcinoma). Obesity has become a pandemic; the risk could become greater than the existing risk for tobacco use.

More than 20 percent of cancers in the United States are associated with obesity and lack of exercise. Obesity is related to 10 percent of breast and colon cancers and approximately 25–40 percent of kidney, esophageal, and endometrial cancers.[3] An article in *Oncology* reported obesity as a risk factor for cancer, with a worse outcome and a higher recurrence rate.[4] Obesity may also mask the cancer, resulting in a delayed diagnosis. Obese patients may receive lower dosages of chemotherapy and therefore have a suboptimal response.[5] Moreover, obese people often are diagnosed with more aggressive cancers.[6]

Obesity and overweight are estimated to account for 90,000 cancer deaths in the United States every year.[7] The healthcare cost for obesity-related medical care has risen from 2 percent in 1987 to 11.6 percent in 2002.[8] The cost of obesity in California alone in the year 2005 was more than $28 billion for healthcare, workers' compensation, and lost workplace productivity.[9] Workplace programs such as stocking low-fat foods in vending machines and providing exercise classes are being instituted, based on the assessment that if one in twenty employees were to slim down, the state would save $6 billion annually.

A recent report from *The Journal of the National Cancer Institute* reviewed the percentages of normal weight, overweight, and obese adults from 1971 to 2002. The majority of the population had gained weight or become overweight or obese. In the study, 33 percent were at a healthy weight, and 65 percent were overweight or obese; 30 percent were obese. Furthermore, a large prospective study found that obesity is strongly associated with the risk of death in both men and women in all racial and ethnic groups and at all ages.[10] Overweight people at the age of fifty years had a 20–40 percent higher mortality risk than those at a healthy weight. Mortality risk was two to three times higher for obese people. In overweight people, many cytokines (chemicals) are released from fat cells, which may promote cancer growth.

Eating out presents a problem for everyone; in the last thirty years restaurant meal portions have become larger, with up to 60 percent more calories. This is one of the causes of the obesity epidemic. The amount of food served in restaurants influences how much people eat, and big portions are hard on people who want to lose or maintain an average weight. It is the diner's responsibility to eat an appropriate amount, but it is also the chef's responsibility not to serve excessively large portions. A reduction in portions by 25 percent is recommended.[11]

The number of children who are overweight or obese has doubled in the last few decades, and an obese adolescent has a 70 percent chance of becoming an obese adult.[12] Currently, about 25 million kids, one-third of U.S. children and teens, are overweight or obese, with an elevated risk of diabetes, high cholesterol, cardiovascular disease, and stroke. The Institute of Medicine reports that food and beverage companies spend $10 billion a year marketing high-sugar, low-nutrition foods directly to children.

It is believed that the carcinogenic process may well begin early in life. Because it takes many years for a cell to become cancerous, cancer prevention programs should include children. Strategies are needed to help fight obesity in youth. It is important to get kids "off the couch" and into exercise activities. Getting our youth to join gym programs and exercise while watching television could help curtail the epidemic of overweight and obesity. There is a need to promote behavioral changes and activities and to offer more healthful food options, including more fruits, vegetables, and grains. Although there is no miracle diet, a healthful lifestyle including a prudent diet should be started early in life.

A Commentary on a Fat World

Lifestyles are changing internationally. As countries such as Japan have adopted some of the habits of Western industrialized nations, the incidence and mortality of breast cancer have risen toward the same level. An article by Tominaga and Kuroishi documents that the low incidence of breast cancer in Japan has risen to the higher level of Western industrialized countries because Japanese are marrying later, having fewer children, consuming more fat, dairy products, and meats, and experiencing an increase in body mass index (BMI) in menopausal women.[13] A review of risk factors indicates that obesity after age fifty is an important risk factor for postmenopausal breast cancer and will be a leading cause of cancer in Japan in the twenty-first century.

In the past forty years, the world population has doubled, but the food production has grown even more. We no longer have general food scarcity. Poverty and infant mortality are receding. The world in general is getting fat. In China, for example, 20 percent of the adults are overweight, and children are much heavier than their counterparts were two decades ago. Heart disease and diabetes also go along with obesity, as shown by rising disease rates in countries such as Thailand, Tunisia, and Kuwait.

Middle- and high-income Americans are becoming obese (approximately 30 percent are), but for lower-income Americans the rate is higher, at 35 percent. Middle- and low-income teenagers are now more overweight. In Brazil, the poor have become fatter than the rich; it is no longer a rich man's disease.

In our industrial era, famine and infections are no longer killers; we are killing ourselves with the effects of being overweight and obese. Now, you can order in from a restaurant, and generally the food is full of fat and carbohydrates; faced with cooking versus delivery, people are choosing delivery. What's left over can be refrigerated or made into a snack later. In general, there has been a decrease in consumption of grown foods and an increase in processed foods, which contain more refined grains, salt, trans fats, and sweeteners. Fast-food restaurants and high-calorie drink manufacturers lead the way. The price of food has become lower in relation to income, increasing the risk of dying what was once a rich man's death: obesity and its comorbid problems.

We need to change our diet, using more fruits, vegetables, and whole grains, and we need to exercise more. This should start with children and toddlers. We need to stop trying to fatten up our children and accept behavior modification rather than obesity.

Obesity and Breast Cancer

There are several relationships among diet, obesity, and breast cancer:

- Women who are obese usually present with a more advanced stage of breast cancer and therefore a poorer prognosis. Excess fat in the breast tissue may mask tumor development until the tumor is larger and more advanced.
- Chemotherapy dosages often are lower in obese patients, producing a less optimal response.
- Being overweight or obese alters hormone levels, mainly estradiol and sex hormone–binding globulin (SHBG). Excess fat, especially abdominal fat, converts adrenal gland hormones into estrogens. There are higher circulating levels of free estrogen in postmenopausal women because of their higher peripheral aromatization of androstenedione from adrenal glands to estriol and estradiol, and lower circulating levels of SHBG.
- Body weight is associated with clinical outcome in women with breast cancer. Those who are overweight or obese or who gain weight after breast cancer are at greater risk of therapy-related complications, recurrence, and death than lighter women.[14] Studies have documented the favorable effect of weight loss on clinical outcome and other comorbid conditions and support the recommendation that breast cancer patients enter a program for weight loss if needed.

Breast Cancer and Diet

Women who are overweight or who gain weight after diagnosis or treatment for breast cancer are at greater risk for several therapy-related complications and for breast cancer recurrence and death than lighter women. Evidence is accumulating that weight can affect clinical outcome and the risk of several comorbid conditions. There is also a relationship between a high-fat diet and higher levels of estrogen and estradiol, which can promote breast cancer. It is believed that low-fat diets lower estrogen levels in postmenopausal and premenopausal women.[15] Therefore, a weight loss program is recommended for overweight patients.[16]

The role of diet in breast cancer development and prevention has been debated for the last thirty years. Recently, Roman Chlebowski of the Los Angeles Biomedical Research Institute completed the first randomized clinical trial showing that diet may have an impact on breast cancer outcome. He showed that the risk of recurring breast cancer was lower for low-fat dieters whose original tumors were not sensitive to estrogen. These estrogen receptor–negative cancers account for one-quarter of all breast cancers. In a presentation at the 2006 meeting of the American Society of Clinical Oncology, Chlebowski presented results showing an adverse prognostic effect of obesity in premenopausal and postmenopausal women for both hormone receptor–positive and hormone receptor–negative breast cancer with or without systemic adjuvant therapy. It was also found that the adverse prognostic effect of obesity was greater in tumors with favorable prognostic factors (small tumor, negative lymph nodes, positive hormone receptors), but adverse effects were also seen in unfavorable prognostic factors. Obesity was also noted in more advanced-stage breast cancer with larger tumors and more axillary node involvement, suggesting that adverse effects of obesity could have large clinical effects. It was also noted that weight gain could be producing a secondary effect of reduced physical activity, and a weight gain of more than 5 kg was associated with a poorer breast cancer outcome. In an update in the January 2007 *NCI Cancer Bulletin,* it was noted that although the study may have been affected by weight loss or other dietary factors in the intervention group, findings still suggest that consuming less fat seems to reduce the risk of breast cancer recurrence.

Women with early-stage breast cancer are highly motivated to seek a more healthful diet. In a study of 531 breast cancer survivors, 52 percent of patients wanted nutritional guidance at diagnosis or soon thereafter, and only a few reported ever receiving dietary recommendations from their physicians.[17] The prudent diet and lifestyle approach can help reduce the risk of comorbidities, improve quality of life, and reduce the risk of breast cancer recurrence in many of the postmenopausal and some premenopausal breast cancer survivors in the United States who are overweight. It can also reduce the risk of second primary breast cancers, cardiovascular disease, diabetes, and osteoporosis.

Dietary studies are in progress, such as the Women's Healthy Eating and Living (WHEL) Study and the Women's Intervention Nutrition Study (WINS).

The WHEL Study, with more than 3,000 premenopausal and postmenopausal women participating, began in 1995, ended randomization in 2000, and is scheduled to be completed in 2007. This study is based on the idea that a high-vegetable, high-fiber diet can slow the progression of breast cancer by markedly raising circulating carotenoid concentrations from food sources and thus reducing hormone levels, helping to regulate breast cancer cell growth. Preliminary results are not available, but early data indicate a statistically significant difference in diet between the intervention and control group.[18] Counseling and food intervention were done. The diet intervention consists of increased vegetable and fruit intake (five vegetable servings, 16 ounces of vegetable juice, three fruit servings), 15–20 percent energy from fat, and 30 grams of dietary fiber daily.

The WINS trial involved 2,500 postmenopausal women randomized to either the control group or the intervention group. Based on the theory that dietary fat is one of the factors involved in the progression of breast cancer and that hormonal factors may respond to the dietary changes, the goal was to change fat intake from the national average of about 34 percent to 22 percent of calories. Preliminary results in the WINS trial have shown a 24 percent decrease in breast cancer recurrence for patients with a good weight loss dietary program and demonstrated a significantly better relapse-free rate in postmenopausal women who lowered their fat intake to approximately 20 percent fat calories.[19] Nineteen of twenty-seven postmenopausal breast cancer survivors in the six-month feasibility study achieved an average weight reduction of 2.3 kg and reduction in serum estradiol of 37 percent.

The Nurses' Health Study demonstrated a lower risk of breast cancer recurrence and death in women who participated in moderate exercise for three to five hours per week.[20] The study also found a higher risk of breast cancer recurrence and death in women who were overweight at the time of diagnosis or who gained weight after diagnosis.

All of these studies led their authors to recommend that physicians caring for patients with early stage breast cancer counsel their patients regarding weight loss, diet, and physical activity.

Hormones and Weight Gain

The higher risk of both breast cancer and prostate cancer associated with weight gain may be related to higher hormone levels. Women taking estrogen, either for birth control or hormone replacement therapy, often gain weight, which appears to increase their risk of breast cancer. The use of estrogen pills has obscured the link between breast cancer and weight. Women who gain the most weight after age twenty are at a higher risk for breast cancer, according to studies at the Harvard University School of Public Health.[21] A recent case control study of 2,000 women found that women who gain weight, particularly after age fifty, significantly increase their risk of breast cancer.[22] Conversely, women (young and middle-aged) who lose weight may decrease the risk of breast cancer. Furthermore, overweight or obesity is associated with poorer prognosis in the majority of the studies that have examined body mass and breast cancer.[23] Many American women take hormones and gain weight during adulthood, increasing their breast cancer risk, and risk begins even before they gain significant weight. Gaining two to three pounds a year after age eighteen leads to a substantial amount of excess weight by menopause. A quarter pound a year adds up to 8 pounds by menopause.

It is believed that in overweight and obese women the extra fat cells raise the risk of breast cancer because they produce hormones that the body converts into estrogens. "Blood estrogen levels are three times higher in overweight women than in lean women."[21] Androgens from the adrenal glands also appear to raise breast cancer risk in overweight women, a relationship particularly predominant in overweight postmenopausal women. The higher risk of breast cancer caused by elevated body weight may also be related to elevated insulin and IGF levels, which can stimulate cancer cell proliferation.[24] Additionally, recent findings indicate that oxidative damage, measured by urinary biomarkers, is significantly greater in women with a higher BMI.[25]

A high-fiber diet is associated with less obesity. Furthermore, a high-fiber diet reduces hormone levels that may be involved in the progression of breast cancer.[26] Interestingly, eating foods high in vitamin C, such as fruits and vegetables, may reduce breast cancer in overweight women (BMI greater than 25).[27]

Studies have shown that Asian women who gained more than ten pounds in the prior decade had a three times greater risk of breast cancer than leaner Asian women, particularly among overweight postmenopausal women.[28] Staying trim reduces the risk of cancer but doesn't eliminate it. Nonetheless, the link is strong between higher weight and postmenopausal breast cancer. Additionally, substantial health benefits can be achieved by even a small reduction in body weight.[29]

Women who have had two pregnancies, had their first child before the age of twenty, breast-fed for more than one year, had late menarche (over fifteen years old), or had early menopause have a lower risk of breast cancer. Therefore, the risk reduction is believed to be related to fewer menstrual cycles. It is believed that estrogens combined with progesterone increase breast cancer risk. Other factors contributing to breast cancer risk in the United States are an abundant food supply (leading to earlier menarche) and the American tendency to begin childbearing later than age thirty.

Special Facts on Breast Cancer

- The older a person, the higher the risk of breast cancer. The average age of diagnosis is about sixty-two.
- The risk is twice as high in women with one first-degree relative (mother, sister, daughter) with breast cancer, and women with two first-degree relatives with breast cancer have five times the risk. Any relative with breast or ovarian cancer raises the risk.
- Five to 10 percent of women with breast cancer have a gene mutation. The most common are BRCA1 and BRCA2 mutations; these women have up to an 82 percent lifetime risk of breast cancer. The lifetime risks of ovarian cancer were 54 percent for BRCA1 and 23 percent for BRCA2 mutation carriers. Physical exercise and lack of obesity in adolescence were associated with significantly delayed breast cancer onset.[30] Removing the fallopian tubes and ovaries reduced the risk of breast cancer risk by 47 percent and the ovarian cancer risk by 89 percent. In women with BRCA2 mutations, removing the fallopian tubes and ovaries lowered the risk by 72 percent, and in women with BRCA1 mutations it lowered the risk by 39 percent.[31]
- Ashkenazi (Jewish) women of European descent are at higher risk because they are more likely to have the BRCA gene mutations.
- Women with early menstrual periods (before age twelve) and late menopause (after age fifty-five) are at higher risk, probably because they have had more hormone (estrogen) exposure by having more menstrual periods. Hormonal exposure also includes a small risk from birth control pills, which contain both estrogen and progesterone.
- Women who have two or fewer children or who have children after age thirty are at higher risk.
- Women who breast-feed for at least a year (all babies combined) have a lower risk because of their lower number of menstrual periods and the accompanying reduction in hormone exposure.
- Women who take estrogens for even a year or two after menopause are at higher risk. This risk normalizes after five years of no estrogens. Recent studies have modified these beliefs and have found that for women with menopausal symptoms (such as severe hot flashes) estrogen therapy for symptom relief for a few years was safe. (Consult your doctor for recommendations.)

- Benign breast hyperplasia lesions increase the risk of breast cancer because more cells appear abnormal.
- Taller women are at higher risk. The reason is unknown.
- Women who consume as little as half an alcoholic drink per day may have a slightly higher risk; drinking more increases risk further. Women are more sensitive to alcohol because they metabolize alcohol more slowly than men. Additionally, alcohol increases endogenous estrogen levels.

The best time to start healthful lifetime habits or changes is in early childhood. A sensible diet, frequent exercise, and an attitude of wellness for a lifetime could help prevent or delay cancer, heart disease, and other health problems.

Prostate Cancer and Diet

The number-one cause of death in the United States and in most countries around the world is cardiovascular disease, and the number-one or number-two cause of death in prostate cancer patients is also cardiovascular disease. The ultimate goal of healthful lifestyle recommendations is to reduce the burden of both of these major causes of death, especially after definitive prostate therapy. Patients should not smoke, and they should reduce their intake of saturated and trans fats, increase their consumption of a variety of fruit and vegetables, consume moderate quantities of dietary soy and flaxseed, increase their consumption of fish or fish oils and other omega-3 fatty acids, and maintain a healthy weight, getting at least thirty minutes a day of physical activity and lifting weights several times a week.[32]

For men with prostate cancer, a variety of beneficial lifestyle changes and over-the-counter agents may have an enormous impact on their health during androgen deprivation therapy (ADT). Vitamin D supplements, aerobic and resistance exercise, cholesterol awareness and reduction, weight loss, and other individual changes can have an enormous impact on the quality and quantity of life. Some of these recommendations help men participate in their overall health rather than just picking up and using a prescription drug for side effects, and this role is just as critical in improving the probability of living longer and better.[33]

Metabolic Syndrome

Metabolic syndrome is an independent risk factor for prostate cancer patients on ADT. Studies have shown that men on ADT experience metabolic syndrome at much greater rates than those not on ADT or in control groups. Hyperglycemia (elevated blood sugar) and abdominal obesity were the main determinants of metabolic syndrome.[34,35]

Metabolic syndrome, which is also a risk factor for cardiovascular disease, consists of having at least three of the following five criteria:

- Fasting blood glucose level greater than 110 mg/dl
- Serum triglyceride level at least 150 mg/dl
- Serum high-density lipoprotein level less than 40 mg/dl
- Waist circumference greater than 102 cm
- Blood pressure at least 130/85

Insulin Resistance and Hyperglycemia

The side effects of hypergonadism (small testicles) include type 2 diabetes and insulin resistance. Studies have shown that insulin resistance and type II diabetes are related to low testosterone concentrations.

Noncancer deaths exceed the cancer death–related mortality among cancer survivors, and cardiovascular disease is the most common cause. Insulin resistance has been known to develop a few months after ADT begins. ADT results in a 63 percent increase in fasting insulin levels without changes in fasting glucose, with some insulin resistance and a significant increase in glycosylated hemoglobin. This suggests hyperinsulinemia with insulin resistance, which can develop a few months after initiation of ADT.[34]

Dyslipidemia (Cardiac Disease)

Hyperlipidemia is a known risk factor for cardiovascular disease. Men with low serum testosterone usually have adverse lipid profiles, with elevated total cholesterol, low-density lipoprotein, and triglycerides. These side effect changes merit a therapeutic program with a low–saturated fat diet and exercise.

Cholesterol-lowering agents are also of help, depending on the lipid panel. The results of current cardiovascular ADT studies are not yet available.

Obesity and Prostate Cancer

A large prospective study observed a significant positive association between BMI and prostate cancer risk.[36] A study by Calle and colleagues[37] reported obese men to have a 20 percent elevated risk of dying from prostate cancer, and men who were severely obese had a 34 percent elevated risk. This research was further supported by recent evidence that obesity is a risk factor for aggressive prostate cancer.[38]

A recent study by Christopher Amling addressed the relationship between obesity and prostate cancer risk.[39] Those with a BMI of 30 had about a 20 percent higher risk of recurrence of cancer. There is a relationship between obesity and a higher-grade cancer and a higher recurrence rate after radical prostatectomy. Black men were found to have a higher recurrence rate and a greater BMI than white men. This supports the hypothesis that obesity is associated with progression of latent to clinically significant prostate cancer and suggests that an elevated BMI may account in part for the racial variability in prostate cancer risk.[40] Obesity is associated with several hormonal alterations, including lower levels of SHBG, and may increase the fraction of biologically available testosterone.[41]

Prostate cancer patients receiving hormone ablation therapy (which prevents production of testosterone) should strive to maintain normal weight. Like women in menopause, men often report greater fat mass, accompanied by a decrease in lean body mass while on ADT.[42] In one study, the average BMI increased by 2.4 percent, and the lean body mass decreased by 2.7 percent.[43] This change is concerning given the association between BMI and prostate cancer risk.

Two studies by Moyad found that what is good for the heart is also good for the prostate. Prostate cancer risk can be reduced by lifestyle changes such as eating less saturated and trans fat, more fruits and vegetables, dietary soy and flaxseed, and more fish, fish oils, and other omega-3 fatty acids; maintaining a healthy weight; and getting thirty minutes of exercise per day. The Moyad studies found that these lifestyle changes can improve overall health after prostate cancer therapy.[44]

Thus, lifestyle factors may play an important role in the development of clinically significant prostate cancer. In Asia, the incidence of prostate cancer and associated mortality rates are lower. When Asians migrate to the United States, their cancer rates approach those of the U.S. population as they adopt Western-style diets.

Comorbidities: Obesity, Diabetes, and Cardiovascular Disease

Obesity is a major comorbidity for breast (postmenopausal), prostate, colon, kidney,[45] esophageal (adenocarcinoma), stomach, and endometrial cancers. The proportion of newly diagnosed obese cancer patients is increasing, as is the number of patients who gain weight during and after therapy. The number of obese children has tripled since 1980. There appears to be a link between abdominal girth and cancer. Thus, heavier children today are at risk for higher rates of cancer in the future. Obesity is also associated with cancer recurrence (breast and prostate), cardiovascular disease, stroke, diabetes, and lower quality of life. Thus, weight control through diet and exercise is crucial for healthy survivorship. However, an American Cancer Society survey found that 83 percent of Americans recognized the link of being overweight to heart disease, 57 percent knew the link to diabetes, but only 8 percent understood the connection between being overweight and cancer risk.

Gradual weight loss in overweight patients is beneficial for control of hypertension, lipid dysfunction, and impaired physical function. The American Cancer Society recommends maintaining a "healthy weight." Diabetes and cardiovascular disease, two diseases associated with obesity, are responsible for a higher number of non–cancer-related deaths among survivors. In survivors, one-half of non–cancer-related deaths are related to cardiovascular disease.

Breast cancer patients receiving chemotherapy and targeted therapies (doxorubicin, epirubicin, or trastuzumab) are at a higher cardiac risk and can benefit from lifestyle changes such as exercise, a low–saturated fat diet, and increased consumption of fruits, vegetables, beans, nuts, and whole grain foods.

Recommendations for Gaining and Maintaining Weight

Some cancer survivors lose weight as a result of their treatments. Maintaining or gaining weight throughout treatments can be challenging. However, it is essential for maintaining a strong immune system. Therapies for some cancers, such as head and neck tumors, may create problems such as anorexia, mucositis (reduction of the gastrointestinal lining), or nausea and vomiting, often necessitating intravenous or tube feeding to maintain adequate nutrition. For patients with these conditions, it is essential to choose nutrient-dense foods, foods that provide the most nutrition in the smallest volume. It also helps to eat small, frequent meals and snacks (four to six times daily).

Nutrient-dense food ideas include the following:

- Fruit smoothies made with protein powder
- Dried fruits
- Energy bars
- Avocados
- Nuts and seeds
- Peanut butter or other nut butters
- Olives
- Hummus
- Coconut milk

12 Exercise and Survival

Francine Manuel, R.P.T.,
Ernest H. Rosenbaum, M.D., F.A.C.P., and
Jack LaLanne

Exercise plays a key role in reducing cancer risk and can be very beneficial in promoting better health, survival, and longevity. It is now well established that exercise promotes longevity and potentially disease control for breast cancer, prostate cancer, and colon cancer; more than half of the survivors in the United States have had one of these three types of cancer. The risk reduction has been confirmed in many studies, which also provide an understanding of the physiological mechanisms by which exercise reduces breast, prostate, and colorectal cancer risk and fatigue and improves quality of life while promoting survival.

Over the past twenty-five years, a growing number of evidence-based scientific studies have compared patients who exercise with sedentary patients. In general, those exercising thirty or more minutes per day with moderate or more vigorous activity will have a higher survival rate, a lower risk for cancer recurrence or a new cancer, better quality of life with less fatigue, lower rates of overweight and obesity, and treatment benefits in undergoing cancer therapy. Exercise improves long-term health by reducing the risk of several comorbid conditions, including disease progression, possible second primary cancers, obesity, osteoporosis, cardiovascular disease, diabetes, and functional decline. Those who exercise also have less fatigue, shortness of breath, depression, and pain during treatment, less disturbed sleep, fewer memory problems, and a better quality of life.

The results of a recent study of exercise and side effects among cancer patients showed that participants who exercised during chemo or radiation therapy and after treatment reported less severe side effects during and especially after treatment. There was less fatigue, shortness of breath, depression, and pain during treatment and less fatigue, shortness of breath, pain, depression, weight loss difficulty, hair loss, disturbed sleep, and memory disturbance in the six months after treatment. Although it is possible that healthier patients with fewer side effects were more likely to exercise, these results suggest that a structured exercise intervention may enhance recovery and quality of life during and after cancer therapy.[1]

Physical activity programs improve cardiorespiratory fitness during and after treatment, lessen fatigue, pain, and nausea, improve vigor and quality of life, decrease depression and

U.S. Cancer Survivors by Cancer Type, 2002

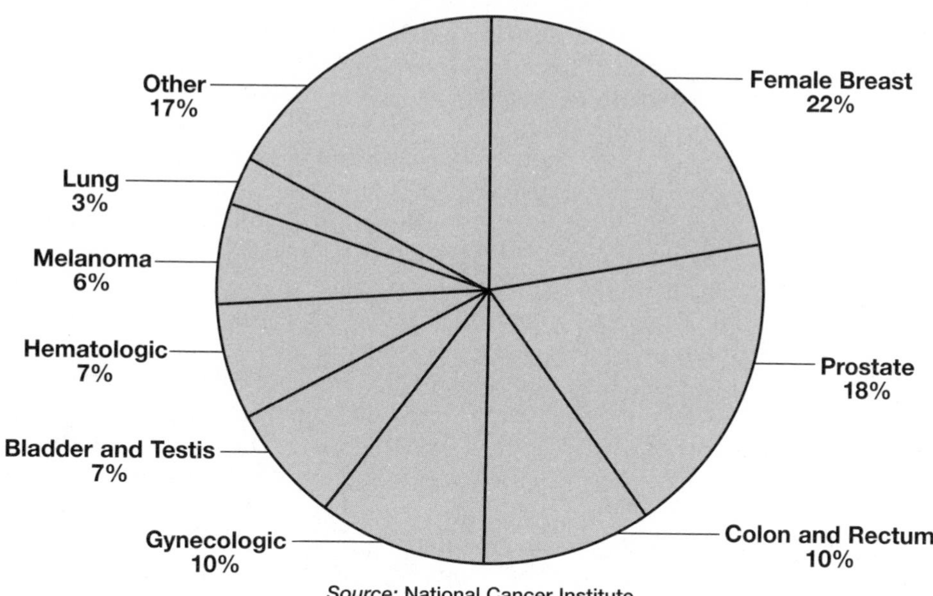

Source: National Cancer Institute.

mental distress, and help improve cognitive brain functioning. A recent intervention development study, Project Leading the Way in Exercise and Diet (LEAD), worked with breast and prostate cancer survivors (sixty-five years and older) for a period of six months and found that physical functioning improved over the course of the intervention, concluding that home-based diet and exercise interventions hold promise in improving lifestyle behaviors among older cancer survivors.[2]

Even after a patient has overcome one cancer, exercise is still important for decreasing the risk of recurrent or second cancers. In a report published in *Oncology Times* showing a correlation between physical activity and low levels of tumor-promoting prostaglandins, Dr. David Alberts, director of the Arizona Cancer Center, stated, "Exercise is possibly the single most important component of health style change associated with good physical health, not only during cancer treatment but as a way to reduce the risk of second cancers."[3]

Cancer survivors who stay fit see big dividends. A daily routine of exercise

- Helps prevent falls and injuries and improves quality of life
- Improves coordination and balance
- Shortens reaction time
- Improves confidence
- Helps control weight and contributes to weight loss and diabetic control
- Improves heart and lung function
- Helps control blood pressure and cholesterol
- Decreases anxiety and depression and can help improve cognitive and memory functioning
- Improves ability to perform daily tasks and builds muscle group strength
- Helps maintain independence (e.g., the ability to climb stairs)

The motivation to keep exercising grows as its physical and emotional advantages are realized. Thirty-minute walks and gym exercise provide good benefits; survivors can also use everyday activities to improve muscle tone and balance, such as intermittent bursts of activities like housecleaning, laundry, or cooking, taking care to stay inside their safety zone to prevent falls or injuries. If needed, patients can use safety aids such as canes, walkers, or banisters.

Nationwide exercise rates are low: Only about 26 percent of Americans engage in adequate amounts of physical activity according to a national survey by the Centers for Disease Control and Prevention (CDC).[4] Unfortunately, physical education in schools has been reduced to as little as one class per week, if any, although one hour daily is suggested. This change denies American youth the opportunity to build exercise habits needed for a lifetime of health.

About 27 percent of survivors increase their physical activity levels; 10 percent do less than they had before diagnosis and treatment. The American College of Sports Medicine recommends exercise thirty minutes a day three times per week. Good benefits can be achieved by walking three to five hours a week. As we age, we lose muscle mass and strength over time. Although walking is a great starter for an exercise program, it does not increase muscle mass. Building muscle mass requires weight-bearing resistence activity (e.g., lifting weights) and strength training.

Exercise is now commonly measured in "metabolic equivalent tasks (METs)." The average person at rest burns about 70 calories an hour, and this amount equals 1 MET. For example, dancing is a good exercise and expends about 4.5 METs per hour. Housework expends about 4 METs per hour, or 245–280 calories per hour. Thus, thirty minutes of sweeping, vacuuming, and cleaning is a useful routine. Other good activities are jogging in place while watching television or using an exercise bike or treadmill.

Over a thirty-minute period, if one expends 3–6 METs at least five days a week, one will gain significant health benefits. Making exercise part of the daily routine is vital. Try to enjoy your daily workout. Make a commitment and follow through.

The reasons survivors cite for failing to maintain their exercise programs are:

- Lack of free time
- Nonspecific treatment side effects, making exercise more difficult
- Fatigue

These factors contribute to the 70–80 percent of survivors who do not exercise routinely.

Moderate or vigorous physical exercise (about one-half to one hour a day) has been estimated to reduce cancer risk by about 18 percent. For those with diabetes, heart disease, and colon cancer, the risk reduction is even greater. Two recent studies showed that posttreatment physical activities may reduce the risk of cancer recurrence and death from Stage I–III nonmetastic colorectal cancer by 40–50 percent compared with patients who exercised little or not at all.[5]

Many studies have convincingly shown that aerobic fitness is more effective in reducing fatigue and improving physical well-being. Also, home-based aerobic exercise programs have been shown to be acceptable, safe, and potentially effective in improving physical function, even in sedentary and older patients.

Tai chi not only has been shown to improve quality of life, balance, and self-esteem but also could increase longevity. Tai chi also promotes psychosocial support.[6] A pilot study on the influence of tai chi on the immune function was presented as a poster at the 2006 Multinational Association of Supportive Care in Cancer meeting. Researchers reported that immune function dysregulation is a consequence of cancer treatment leading to an imbalance of pro-inflammatory and anti-inflammatory cytokines (chemicals), resulting in debilitating side effects. A tai chi program promoting cardio-fitness exercises reversed the trend in pro-inflammatory cytokines among breast cancer survivors. This appears to regulate immune function and reduce side effects of cancer therapy.[7]

Yoga is a popular exercise program that promotes better health. Classes are available for beginners to advanced practitioners. Commercially available DVDs offer a variety of programs. Lorenzo Cohen of the M. D. Anderson Cancer Center studied women with breast cancer in a pilot test to determine the acceptance and feasibility of teaching yoga to patients with breast cancer undergoing radiation therapy. Those involved in the yoga program saw improvement in quality of life and improved objective physiological outcomes such as a reduction in fatigue, reduced depression, and fewer sleep disturbances.[8]

Not all studies agree on the benefits of exercise for cancer patients. For example, a study on men who underwent hormonal ablation therapy for prostate cancer did not show improvements in quality of life or survival from exercise. The men participating in the study were advanced in age and frail, and this study may not have been an adequate comparison. One of the barriers to quantifying the benefits of exercise is the difficulty in separating the effects of exercise from the effects of overweight and obesity. Also, the exercise studies available have used different amounts, types, and forms of activity, making their results difficult to compare for overall beneficial effects.

Exercise Effects on Specific Cancers

A recent study[9] examined physical activity and its role in prevention of specific cancers:

- The breast cancer evidence was reasonably clear that thirty to sixty minutes per day of moderate to vigorous physical activity provided a 20–30 percent lower risk of breast cancer compared with that of inactive women.
- For prostate cancer, data were not conclusive.
- Physically active men and women have about a 30–40 percent lower risk of developing colon cancer than inactive people. Thirty to sixty minutes of moderate to vigorous daily exercise is needed to decrease the risk.
- The findings of one lung cancer prevention study suggested that physical activity contributed to a lower risk of lung cancer, but it was difficult to assess the effects of cigarette smoking.

Exercise and Breast Cancer

It is believed that exercise can reduce breast cancer risk. Many studies have been done associating physical activity with decreased risk of recurrent cancer. The Nurses' Health Study, involving 573 participants, demonstrated that exercise could reduce mortality from breast cancer, showing a reduction in a woman's risk of dying from breast cancer of up to 50 percent. Interestingly, the amount of exercise done before the cancer diagnosis did not affect the treatment outcome. Other studies have confirmed that physically active breast cancer survivors had superior survival rates compared with those who were sedentary.[10] There is also a relationship between sex hormones and exercise in postmenopausal women. Women who exercise regularly have 25–50 percent lower circulating estrone and androgen concentrations than sedentary women.[11]

The Nurses' Health Study, evaluating leisure activity two years after diagnosis of breast cancer, found that both lean and overweight women with higher activity levels showed a lower risk of recurrence or death. Unfortunately, as shown in the HEAL study (following 800 patients with breast cancer one year after diagnosis), only 50 percent of patients had resumed their level of prediagnosis physical activity. This finding was more pronounced in overweight patients.[12]

A randomized study of seventy-seven women with early-stage breast cancer, who either followed a moderate-intensity walking program or were in a control group while undergoing radiation or chemotherapy, showed a favorable impact for those in the walking group in both sleep enhancement and fatigue reduction.[13] Another study, by Karen Basen-Engquist at the M. D. Anderson Cancer Center, showed that sixty breast cancer survivors who added thirty minutes of moderate exercise (which could be divided into shorter segments as desired) to their schedule five days a week had less pain, felt healthier, and had better quality of life than a standard care control group who did not exercise. Their exercise capacity in a six-minute walking test was better than that of controls.

The New York Breast Cancer Study Group[14] assessed women with BRCA1 and BRCA2 gene mutations, with a high lifetime risk for breast and ovarian cancers. Those who adopted a program limiting weight and increasing exercise, including sports and walking, delayed the onset of cancer. The study recommended that women with these gene mutations achieve and maintain a healthy body weight.

In looking at the physiological effects of exercise on breast cancer, one study determined that physical activity is a modifiable breast cancer risk factor, presumably because it regulates estrogen metabolism. This study examined the effect of physical activity on breast cancer incidence based on estrogen receptor (ER) and progesterone receptor (PR) status and histological subtype of breast cancer. The study included 41,837 women, and physical activity was self-reported on three levels: high, medium, and low. The study concluded that higher physical activity was associated with lower risk, mainly in PR-negative tumors (especially ER-positive and PR-negative) and more aggressive histologic types. Physical activity was reported to be associated with a 10 percent lower risk of breast cancer, mainly in the PR-negative tumors.[15]

For active women, strenuous physical activity (e.g., training for competitive marathon races) has been shown to lower hormone levels and thereby reduce the risk of breast cancer growth. Michelle Holmes of Harvard Medical School notes that forty-five minutes per day of strenuous exercise five days a week can lower estrogen levels in sedentary, overweight, postmenopausal women.[10] It can also improve quality of life and self-image for women who've had breast cancer and prevent weight gain.

Exercise and Prostate Cancer

Exercise is helpful in cancer prevention, and it also appears to improve cancer detection, coping, rehabilitation, and survival after diagnosis. Obesity, a high-fat diet, and a sedentary lifestyle may predispose men to prostate cancer through effects on serum factors such as hormones. American men who gain weight are at greater risk for prostate cancer, the leading cause of cancer morbidity and mortality in men. In 2007, over 218,800 new cases were diagnosed and there were over 27,000 deaths. Fortunately, 86 percent of men diagnosed with prostate cancer have local or regional disease, with about a 100 percent five-year survival.[16]

In a review of literature that examines the association between exercise and prostate cancer risk, Torti and Matheson found that between 1989 and 2001, thirteen cohort studies were conducted in the United States and internationally. Of these, nine showed an association between exercise and decreased prostate cancer risk. Five of 11 case control studies conducted between 1988 and 2002 reported an association between decreased risk of prostate cancer and high activity levels. Of all studies performed between 1976 and 2002, sixteen of twenty-seven studies reported lower risk in the men who were most active; in nine of sixteen studies the reduction in risk was statistically significant. Average risk reduction ranged from 10 to 30 percent. In aggregate, this evidence suggests a probable link between increased physical exercise and decreased prostate cancer risk. The abilities of exercise to modulate hormone levels, prevent obesity, improve immune function, and reduce oxidative stress have all been postulated as mechanisms that may underlie the protective effect of exercise. Exercise may also be of benefit in men undergoing treatment for prostate cancer.[17]

A series of studies by the Program in Human Biology at Stanford examined the association between exercise and prostate cancer risk.[18] In a twelve-year study of thirteen cohorts, nine of thirteen cohorts showed an association between exercise and decreased prostate cancer risk. Sixteen of twenty-seven studies reported a lower risk of prostate cancer in men who were most active.

In another study, the goal was to examine whether physical activity reduced prostate cancer incidence or progression.[19] Although the mechanisms were not all understood, the findings suggest that regular, vigorous activity can slow the progression of prostate cancer and might be recommended to reduce mortality from prostate cancer, particularly given the many other documented benefits of exercise. Exercise may also reduce the side effects of cancer therapy. In one study, men who followed advice to rest and take things easy if they became fatigued demonstrated a slight deterioration in physical functioning and a significant increase in fatigue at the end of radiotherapy. Home-based, moderate-intensity walking produced a significant improvement in physical functioning with no significant increase in fatigue. Improved physical functioning may be necessary to combat radiation fatigue.[20]

A significant inverse trend between occupational physical activity and prostate cancer risk has been shown in two studies.[21] It was hypothesized that the perceived trend could reflect favorable hormonal correlates of physical activity. The inverse trend was for physical activity at work associated with a lower prostate cancer risk. In another study, occupational physical activity in a job held during the longest period was inversely associated with prostate cancer.[22] The results of this study suggest that physical activity at work could reduce the occurrence of prostate cancer.

The risk reduction has also been suggested by a laboratory study in which the exercise group had lower serum insulin and insulin-like growth factor-1 (IGF-1) than controls.[23] The researchers concluded that a low-fat diet or intense exercise results in a change in serum hormones and growth factors in vivo that can reduce growth and induce apoptosis (cell death) of in vitro prostate tumor cells. Thus, regular activity may help reduce the risk of prostate cancer. Another study found that exercise training alters serum factors in vivo that increase cellular p53 protein content and is associated with reduced growth and induced apoptosis in prostate cancer cells in vitro.[24]

Not all the studies were positive. For example, in one study a higher risk of prostate cancer was found for men who were physically active for more than one hour per day in obese men and men with high baseline energy (calorie) intake. These results did not support the hypothesis that physical activity protects against prostate cancer.[25]

Exercise and Colon Cancer

Physical activity has consistently been shown to decrease the incidence of colorectal cancer.[26] The mechanism is not known, but it is believed by some that colon cancer risk is related to sedentary lifestyle and hyperinsulinemia. Insulin and the IGF family have been associated with enhanced tumor growth and antiapoptosis.[27]

Two recent studies by Jeffrey Meyerhardt at Dana-Farber Cancer Institute in Boston demonstrated that physical activity in patients with colorectal cancer Stage I–III (nonmetastatic) had a lower risk of developing recurrence and had a prolonged survival if they increased physical activity. They found that recreational physical activity after diagnosis decreased colon cancer recurrence and improved overall survival mortality.[28] Meyerhardt's study on Stage III (nonmetastatic) colon cancer patients undergoing adjuvant chemotherapy compared those performing 3 MET-hours per week of exercise with those engaging in 18–27 MET-hours activity per week and showed that higher levels of physical activity were associated with significantly lower cancer recurrence and cancer mortality than standard therapies.[29]

In their analysis, women who were more physically active after a diagnosis of nonmetastatic colorectal cancer had a significantly lower risk of colorectal cancer–specific death and of death from any cause. According to the authors of the study, "Colorectal cancer patients who increased their activity from their level before diagnosis had an approximately 50% reduction in both colorectal cancer-specific and all-cause mortality."

Physical activity has recently been shown to improve the outcome of patients with colorectal cancer, breast cancer, and prostate cancer.[30] The study's conclusions support the hypothesis that the beneficial effects of physical activity in reducing colorectal cancer mortality may result from interactions with IGF access. A study of 17,000 Harvard alumni aged thirty to seventy-nine who were being followed prospectively for colon cancer showed that greater activity levels reduced the risk of colon cancer by 50 percent.[26]

The Motivation to Exercise

Physical fitness is good for everyone, of course, but is essential for all cancer patients. The medical literature shows causal relationships between both exercise and prevention and between exercise and quantity and quality of life. The key to setting up and engaging patients in an exercise program is motivation. The patient must be convinced that although it is hard to find the energy to exercise when you are sick, the benefits of staying active are too great to ignore.

Exercise Benefits

- Improved prognosis. When you are in better physical condition, you are better able to tolerate aggressive cancer treatments, which can improve your chances of survival and cure.
- Prevention of muscle wasting during cancer treatments, surgeries, and even prolonged periods of bed rest.
- Faster recovery after treatment if you exercise even when you are sick or bedridden. Exercise helps prevent some of the dangers of bed rest, such as blood clots and bedsores.
- Better physical fitness, which promotes better health.

Motivational Tricks

- Use a simple program.
- Set up groups or have the patient exercise with friend or family.
- Use guided videotapes or DVDs with encouraging professionals leading exercises.
- Stress that any amount of exercise is better than none. Use charts to monitor progress or increased activity.
- Make up an exercise kit with weights, rubber stretchers (resistance bands), and balls that will help challenge muscles.
- Develop a program for various stages of exercise to correlate with wellness status, which can be used throughout treatment.
- Purchase some exercise equipment for home or join a gym. A stationary bicycle, rowing machine, treadmill, and stepping machine are just a few options. Patients can also walk briskly, swim, play tennis, or engage in some other sport.

When to Start

Become physically active as soon as possible during and after treatment. It is now general practice to get out of bed within one day of surgery and at least sit in a chair. Even this minimal activity helps reduce the loss of muscle mass, increase strength, and prevent pneumonia by moving air in and out of the lungs.

Pain can limit physical exercise after a mastectomy, bowel surgery, or other major operation. You may be depressed by a change in your body image and not feel like doing anything. You may need help to get going, but with appropriate timing, you should turn your attention to rehabilitation.

You should begin at least a gentle exercise program while you are still in the hospital. This may involve simple muscle tightening while you lie in bed or passive muscle exercises. As your strength returns, different forms of physical activity—isometric and isotonic exercises and rhythmic repeated movements for various muscles—will get you on the path to improved fitness. Massage therapy can complement these activities, helping you relax your mind and body and improving your circulation.

You might think all this will involve too much effort while you're still in the hospital. You will feel more confident when you go home if you have already started to regain your strength. You will also be less likely to fall, have an accident, or have a bone fracture that might result from a weakened condition.

Rules and Precautions

- Vital signs (pulse, blood pressure, and oxygen saturation) should be monitored during exercise for patients severely disabled by their illness.
- A Karnofsky performance scale is used to determine the patient's level of physical fitness and how much exercise is needed to maintain physical performance, and to grade restoration of body strength and promote muscle strength through exercise. A Karnofsky rating of less than 70 is a good indicator of severe disability. Patients can progress slowly, with close monitoring during multiple chemotherapy regimes or in the presence of shunt catheters or pulmonary or cardiac abnormalities relating to treatments.

Karnofsky Scale

100 percent	No evidence of disease
90 percent	Normal activity with minor signs of disease
80 percent	Normal activity with effort; signs of disease
70 percent	Cannot do normal activity but cares for self
60 percent	Requires occasional assistance
50 percent	Requires considerable assistance and frequent medical care
40 percent	Disabled; requires special care
30 percent	Severely disabled; hospitalization may be indicated
20 percent	Very sick; hospitalization necessary for supportive treatment
10 percent	Moribund

- Do not exercise if blood tests indicate any of the following:
  - Abnormal levels of sodium and potassium (electrolytes)
  - Abnormal low albumin
  - Low blood counts (hemoglobin, white counts, platelet counts)
- If numbness in legs or peripheral neuropathies occur (vincristine, vinblastine, cisplatin, oxaliplatin, docetaxel, paclitaxel, or vinorelbine):
  - Alternately contract and relax limbs.
  - Avoid excessive weight-bearing activity. Alternate walking with cycling. Avoid uneven surfaces. If balance is affected, work on a mat or bed in fully supported positions.
- If infection, anemia, low blood pressure, and bleeding (possibly caused by abnormal platelet counts and plasma volume and chemo drugs) are present:
  - Identify white count nadir period (seven to twelve days after chemotherapy) and avoid swimming during this time.
  - Check lab values with doctor or nurse:

    1. Bone density scans with a dual-energy x-ray absorptiometry DEXAscan test. A t-1 score shows osteopenia (weak

bones), and patients must advance slowly with weights and exercise in carefully supported positions.

2. White blood cell counts of less than 1,000/dl. Patients should wait for counts to come up.

3. Blood platelet counts of less than 30,000 cells/mm^3. Patients should avoid resistive exercise until the count comes up to 75–100,000 cells/mm^3.

- Drink lots of fluids.

- If cardiac problems are suspected (doxorubicin, idarubicin, mitoxantrone, epirubicin):
  - Monitor electrocardiogram and blood pressure initially and if not stable.
  - Watch for swollen ankles and shortness of breath and consult a physician for these symptoms.
- If bone weakening is suspected (long-term prednisone):
  - Do strength training with resistance bands, and do not use heavy weights.
  - Be careful when walking.
- Patients with metastatic bone cancer with greater than 50 percent bone cortex involved should not do any weight-bearing exercise or use weights with the involved limb.
- In patients with pulmonary tumors, watch for shortness of breath. Monitor oxygen saturations during exercise.
- Neck or back pain should be evaluated for spinal cord compression or bowel obstruction.
- Watch nutritional status. Make sure you are eating enough to exercise. Check for weight loss.

Rules for Exercising

- If you have never exercised before, it is important to know how to stretch before you begin. Use warm-up exercises.
- Pace yourself and build up both the number of repetitions and the amount of resistance gradually. It is not necessary to exercise until your muscles are aching or sore. Begin with no load and only five repetitions and advance slowly in repetitions and then add a load. Stop when tired and rest a few minutes or try to do more later.
- Breathe properly throughout exercise. Never hold your breath during your workout. Breathe in or out with any movement. You can also use breathing for relaxation and recovery between exercises or after an exercise routine.

The Medi-Gym

A few simple items of exercise equipment will help you increase your muscle strength by making you work against slight resistance. These items may be purchased together in the Medi-Gym kit described in this section, or you can make your own kit using the substitutions suggested.

- *Elastic sheets:* Items such as Thera-Band come in different strengths and colors. Some exercises using this elastic band are described in the next section.
- *Breathing incentive spirometer:* A breathing appliance with a mouthpiece. Used to increase lung capacity and to avoid pulmonary complications in bed-bound people. You can substitute a soft balloon or surgical glove with a mouthpiece.
- *Exercise putty (Theraplast):* Elastic putty. Used by bed-bound patients to strengthen and coordinate hands and fingers. You can substitute clay or Silly Putty.
- *Sponge ball:* A lightweight sponge ball, about 4 inches (10 cm) in diameter. Used by bed-bound patients for general limbering, strengthening, and coordination exercises. You can substitute a small Nerf ball, available in toy stores.
- *Clothespin:* An ordinary wooden clothespin. Used by bed-bound patients to coordinate hands and fingers. For added resistance, wrap a rubber band around the clothespin's tip.

- *Ankle weight:* A 3-pound (1-kg) ankle weight with Velcro closure, used for added resistance in general strengthening exercises. You can either purchase ankle weights at sporting goods stores or use moderately heavy household products in a bag or purse.
- *Exercise stretcher:* An elastic rope with looped handles. Used for stretching and strengthening the large muscles. You can construct a stretcher from elastic cord. Also called an Iso-Band bungee cord. Make loops at the ends by tying knots. Or you can substitute a piece of surgical rubber Penrose drain.
- *Jump rope:* Any type of rope will suffice. If you are bed-bound you can tie the rope to the foot of the bed and use it to pull yourself up to a sitting position. Also used in jump-rope exercises for postmastectomy patients. You can substitute a piece of rope or clothesline.
- *Weights (usually 1–3 pounds):* Begin with one set of ten repetitions. Work up to three sets of ten repetitions. Advance weights so that no discomfort or strain is experienced up to the desired intensity of the workout.

For Beginners

The Warm-Up

Begin each exercise session with a warm-up. The idea of the warm-up is to start moving slowly and gradually increase the blood flow to the muscles to prepare them for further work. Begin by taking a resting heart rate. If your heart rate is above 100 beats per minute, do not exercise unless you check with your doctor. The warm-up should be sustained for two to three minutes with an elevated heart rate ten to twenty beats above resting. Three to five minutes of stretching should follow.

Suggested movements include the following:

- Shoulder shrugs
- Alternate shoulder rolls
- Wrist rolls
- Alternate opening and closing of the hands
- Arm lifts to the side, front, and back
- Elbow bends, which bring hands up to the shoulder (bicep curls)
- Alternate arms to ceiling
- Double arm reaches to ceiling followed by pulldowns
- Add toe taps, heel touches, small knee lifts, marching, side stepping

Progressive Staged Program

For detailed picture demonstrations of most of these exercises by Jack LaLanne, see *Everyone's Guide to Cancer Supportive Care* (Andrews McMeel Publishing, 2005).

Stage I: In Bed, Beginning to Move

This exercise program is for patients who are too ill to get out of bed. It is just range-of-motion exercise for all four limbs and does not have any resistance other than gravity.

- *Straight arm lifts:* Lying on your back, place arms by sides, elbows straight. Lift arms up and over your head, then bring them back down.
- *Side arm lifts:* Lying on your back, place arms down by sides, elbows straight. Bring arms out to the sides and then over your head until hands touch, then return to sides.
- *Elbow touches:* Lying on your back, place hands behind head, elbows flat on bed. Bring elbows together in front of body, then lower elbows back to the bed.
- *Straight arm crosses:* Lying on your back, put right arm out straight to the side at a right angle to body, elbow straight. Bring arm across chest to the left side; repeat with left arm, then crisscross both.
- *Wrist bends:* Lying on your back, place arms down by sides, make a fist. Bend wrist up and down.

- *Wrist rotation:* Lying on your back, make a fist. Move hands in circles, then change direction.
- *Knee-to-chest lifts:* Lying on your back, place legs together flat on bed, bend left leg, and bring knee up toward chest. Straighten knee while lowering leg slowly to the bed. Repeat with right leg.
- *Straight leg lifts:* Lying on back, place legs together flat on bed, keeping your knees straight. Lift left leg as high as possible, rest, and then repeat with right leg.
- *Knee touches:* Lying on your back, bend both knees, keeping feet flat on bed. Relax and let knees fall slowly outward as far as they can comfortably go. Bring knees back up together.
- *Ankle relaxation:* Lying on your back, lift right heel a little off the bed and make small inward circles with foot; reverse direction. Repeat with other foot.
- *Side-to-side rolls:* Lying on your back, put both hands on the overhead trapeze. Lift buttocks off the bed.

Stage II: Bed or Chair with Resistance

This exercise program is designed for patients who are out of bed part of the day, walking around at home and, in a limited capacity, in the community. It incorporates the use of weights and other devices such as surgical tubing.

- *Straight arm cane twist:* Loop weight around the middle of a cane or broom handle. Lying on your back, take the cane in both hands. Keeping elbows straight, hold cane up overhead and twist cane side to side.
- *Straight leg lifts:* Strap weight around right ankle. Lying on your back, keep knee straight and lift leg straight up as far as possible. Repeat with other leg.
- *Backward leg lifts:* Strap weight around right ankle. Lie on stomach with abdomen on bed and feet touching floor. Keeping right knee straight, lift leg up off the floor backwards. Repeat with other leg.
- *Sideways leg lifts:* Strap weight around left ankle. Lying on your right side and keeping knee straight, lift left leg up and slightly back. Slowly lower the leg, and repeat with the other side.
- *Stand-up exercises:* Sitting on the edge of a chair, stand up and sit down slowly. Repeat five to ten times.
- *Crunches:* Lying on your back, raise head and reach for knees with both hands.
- *Oblique crunches:* Lying on your back, raise head and reach for the opposite knee. Alternate arms.

Stage III: Up and Around

These are general exercises for patients who have recovered enough to go out into the community. They can be used to regain full function or just to maintain a healthier way of life after recovery.

- *Side-to-side head leans:* Standing up with arms relaxed at sides, lean head toward left shoulder and then to right.
- *Head twists:* Standing up with arms relaxed at sides and keeping body still, twist head to look over left shoulder, then over the right.
- *Head circles:* Standing up with arms relaxed at sides, rotate head in a circle. Reverse direction.
- *Arm circles:* Hold arms out straight to the side, palms down, elbows straight. Move arms in small circles toward front. Reverse direction.
- *Arm lifts:* Standing up, hold arms straight down at sides, elbows straight. Lift arms up sideways and touch back of hands together overhead with elbows straight. Lower arms to sides.
- *Alternate elbow bends with resistance:* Standing up, hold right arm straight down at side, palm facing front. Grasp right wrist with left hand and bend right arm up to chest while resisting with left arm. Straighten right arm and repeat with left arm.

- *Side-to-side resistance:* Standing up, bend elbows and clasp palms together in front of chest. Push left elbow out to the side while resisting with right arm. Push right elbow out to the side while resisting with left arm.
- *Chair push-ups:* Put chair against wall. Sit on edge of chair and stretch legs out in front of you. Grasp edge of seat with hands and lower buttocks to the floor. Raise buttocks back to edge of seat.
- *Side stretches:* Standing up, legs together, bend left elbow and place left hand behind head. Step out to the right and stretch to touch the back of right knee with right hand. Stand up straight, pull legs in. Repeat on other side.
- *Knee to chest:* Sit in chair and stretch legs out in front of you. Bring knees alternately to chest. If you can, bring both knees up to your chest together.
- *Backward leg lifts:* Standing up, brace yourself against the back of a chair. Alternate lifting legs up backwards, keeping knees straight.
- *Leg lunges:* Standing up, hold onto back of a chair with left hand. Lunge forward with left knee. Return upright, and repeat with right leg.
- *Heel lifts:* Place a chair a couple feet away from you and lean over while holding onto back of chair. Lift heels and then drop heels back to floor.
- *Foot rolls:* Stand with feet slightly apart. Hold back of chair and bring knees together by rolling onto the inside of feet. Bring knees apart by rolling onto the outside of feet. Weight should be advanced, beginning with one set of ten repetitions. Work up to three sets of ten reps. Advance weights so that no discomfort or strain is experienced up to desired intensity of workout.

DVDs of these exercises are available at www.cancersupportivecare.com or for downloading from the Stanford Library Web site for exercise and other video programs at www.med.stanford.edu/healthlibrary/resources/videos.html#CancerSupportiveAnchor.

Aerobic Exercise

Aerobic exercise is exercise that rhythmically uses the large muscles of the legs and arms to elevate the heart rate within a certain range. Examples are brisk walking, jogging, swimming, bicycling, gardening, dancing, playing actively with children, and sexual activity.

Recommendations for Aerobic Programs

- Those with Karnofsky scores of 70–100 percent can begin with ten to fifteen minutes of gentle conditioning exercises and increase the time by one to two minutes each session until a total of thirty to forty minutes per session is achieved. Try to exercise five days per week. The conditioning portion of the exercise session should be intense enough to elevate the heart rate between 60 and 80 percent of the maximal heart rate (MHR), as estimated by a treadmill test. For those who have not had a treadmill test, use the following formula to predict your maximal heart rate: 220 minus your age. Begin your program working at the low end of your MHR (60 percent), and as you become more fit, increase the intensity of exercise by walking faster, gardening more vigorously, moving your arms more, and so on, until you are working at 80 percent of your MHR. The time it takes to become conditioned enough to be comfortable exercising for thirty to forty minutes at a higher heart rate varies with each person, but a reasonable goal is eight weeks.
- Those with a Karnofsky score of 50–70 percent can begin with five minutes of exercise at 55 percent of MHR three times per day, adding one minute to each interval time until ten-minute intervals

are achieved. Follow this program six to seven days per week, and then reduce the number of intervals to two, adding one minute each time until fifteen minutes are achieved. At that time, exercise once a day, adding on a minute each day and following the program prescribed for Karnofsky 70–100 percent as explained at the beginning of this section.

Note: Those who are taking certain blood pressure medicines may not be able to elevate their heart rate for determining appropriate work levels. Check with your physician to find out whether your exercise program is acceptable and whether your medications slow your heart rate.

Dynamic Resistive and Isometric Exercises

Dynamic resistive exercise is performed with weights or resistive tubing of some type. The joints are moved through excursion of the various ranges of motion. The force applied is sufficient to result in increased fiber thickness of the muscle belly. Isometric exercises are performed with the same types of resistance but do not involve joint movement or can just consist of contraction (squeezing) of the muscles without any movement of the limb. Examples are holding in your stomach, tightening your buttocks, and holding your legs straight. These squeezes are held for six seconds and then released.

13 Alcohol

Jack Gordon, M.D., and
Ernest H. Rosenbaum, M.D., F.A.C.P.

Alcohol in Survivors

In about fifty studies, alcohol consumption has been shown to be a small to modest cancer risk factor, where one drink a day increases the risk 8–10 percent and two drinks a day increases the risk about 25 percent. The recommended alcohol consumption is no more than two drinks for men and one drink for women per day. Women have a lower suggested allowance because of their lower weight and higher body fat ratio and because they metabolize alcohol less efficiently (more slowly) than men.[1]

The majority of habitual alcohol drinkers do not eat a nutritious diet, resulting in an additional health deficit. The alcohol abstinence rate for head and neck cancer survivors is about 50 percent; for breast and lung cancer survivors the abstinence rate is 8–16 percent.

Regular consumption of alcohol appears to increase the risk of breast cancer.[2] A large review study reported that data from many well-designed studies consistently show a small rise in breast cancer risk with increasing consumption of alcohol.[3] More recently, Terry and colleagues observed that the risk of breast cancer increases by 30–50 percent with moderate alcohol intake of one to two drinks per day.[4] Research reviewing fifty epidemiologic investigations of the role of alcohol in breast cancer suggests a modest positive association between alcohol and breast cancer ("an approximate 25 percent increase in risk with daily intake of the equivalent of two drinks") and a dose–response relationship.[5] The causality, they thought, was not fully established, so they suggested further research.

Additionally, a recent study found that as little as a half a glass of wine a day increased a woman's risk of developing breast cancer by 6 percent (and by 18 percent in postmenopausal women).[6] Furthermore, the consumption of one or two drinks a day increased risk by 21 percent, and two or more drinks a day increased risk by 37 percent. This effect appears to be greater in postmenopausal women with estrogen receptor–positive tumors.[7] How and why is unknown exactly, but it appears to raise estrogen levels. In 2006, Dr. Marsha E. Reichman at the National Cancer Institute showed that premenopausal women given the equivalent of two drinks a day had a shift in estrogen levels that could be the mechanism behind the rise of breast cancer associated with alcohol. Breast tissue is actively sensitive to estrogen, and certain types of estrogen are known to stimulate the growth of breast cancer cells.

Alcohol also increases the need for folic acid, so 400 mcg per day is suggested for those who consume alcohol. It has been observed that women with low folate and high alcohol consumption had a 43 percent greater risk of breast cancer than nondrinkers with adequate folate intake.[8] Breast cancer survivors are advised to avoid or limit alcohol. Alcohol is a major contributor to the development of oral (head and neck) cancer. Most alcohol consumers also smoke or chew tobacco, which are the major contributors for at least 75 percent of oral cancers.

If you drink *and* smoke, you multiply the carcinogenic effect of each substance and greatly increase your risk of oral and throat cancer (about tenfold). This deadly combination is responsible for about 75 percent of oral cancers.

New studies involving brain imaging techniques (positron emission tomography, or PET) have led to the view that alcoholism involves a genetic predisposition. This growing body of evidence suggests that D_2 dopamine receptors and dopamine (a chemical found in the brain circuitry) play an important role in alcoholism. People who have a high level of D2 dopamine receptors have an adverse response to stimulant drugs.[9]

Alcohol Effects

A majority of American adults use alcohol. In small amounts, that is to say one or two standard drinks per day, it appears to be harmless. In fact, through its favorable effect on cholesterol fractions, it probably contributes to some reduction of coronary heart disease. Unfortunately, an estimated 8 million adults in the United States are alcohol dependent.[10]

What is a "standard drink"? This means 1 ounce of spirits, such as whiskey, gin, scotch, vodka, or brandy, which contain 40–50 percent alcohol; 2 ounces of fortified wine, such as sherry; 4 ounces of regular table wine; or 12 ounces of beer. All these are equivalent to 1 ounce of spirits.

Drinking as a part of normal social activities, such as eating, family gatherings, or social events, can be a harmless practice that contributes to general well-being and all-around happiness. In fact, if we use alcohol sensibly, it can add years to our lives. However, when alcohol is used inappropriately, it is one of the major hazards in American society. What do we mean by inappropriate use of alcohol? We mean the abuse of alcohol or alcoholism. The abuse of alcohol can be defined as the use of alcohol in inappropriate amounts, times, or places.

Alcohol should never be used in the following circumstances:

- During pregnancy. Even a small amount of alcohol taken at the wrong moment during the development of the fetus can result in significant fetal damage. Regular use of alcohol during pregnancy results in lower birth weight.
- When one is engaged in work that entails fine coordination or careful concentration or when running dangerous machinery. Many industrial accidents occur under these circumstances. Serious business mistakes may also occur in this way.
- When one is driving an automobile. In this instance, even a single drink can cause slight impairment. Even within the legal blood alcohol limit there can be slightly lowered attention and slightly altered judgment. This may result in an accident. A surprising number of small airplane accidents, as well as boating accidents, occur when alcohol is used.
- In diabetes. This disease, especially the insulin-dependent variety, is nearly impossible to regulate if alcohol is taken. Insulin-dependent diabetics must avoid alcohol entirely. In non–insulin-dependent diabetes, the use of alcohol is inadvisable

because weight loss usually is necessary. Alcohol seriously interferes with weight loss.

- Among older adults. A small amount of alcohol can be harmless, and probably beneficial, to older people, but great caution must be taken because of the possibility of falling. Older adults are more likely to fall and to sustain injuries in a fall, and alcohol can increase this tendency and result in serious fractures.
- In youth. Young people should use alcohol only in small amounts and should be supervised strictly. Alcohol intensifies the impulsive nature of young people and can result in accidents. Many tragedies occur on graduation nights this way. Unwanted pregnancy is often the result of alcohol abuse.
- When one is dieting. It is nearly impossible to consume alcohol and lose weight. Alcohol contains calories and reduces willpower. Most weight loss clinics today advise against alcohol in all forms.
- To relieve psychological symptoms, such as anxiety or depression. If alcohol gives even temporary relief to these symptoms, it may easily lead to excessive consumption. This response probably is a leading introduction to alcohol addiction.
- When one is taking other medications. Alcohol intensifies the sedative effects of many medications. It may alter the metabolism of others, especially anticoagulant drugs.

Alcoholism, the ultimate form of alcohol abuse, is characterized by increasing tolerance to alcohol, so that a person may have a high blood alcohol level without showing it. An alcoholic may drink a fifth of a gallon of spirits daily, and with this greater tolerance comes physiological dependence. Therefore, an alcoholic must continue to take spirits in order to avoid withdrawal symptoms such as shaking, sweating, palpitation, and other more serious symptoms, even convulsions. A withdrawal program under medical supervision is recommended.

What are the results of such excessive alcohol use?

- Damage to the vital organs. Excessive alcohol consumption causes liver disease (cirrhosis, hemochromatosis [iron overload], and liver cancer). For many this results in enlargement of the liver, which is serious and may be fatal. In fact, the entire gastrointestinal tract is damaged in some way. Gastritis, pancreatitis, and injury to the absorbing surfaces of the intestine are common.
- Malnutrition. Because alcohol contains 7 calories per gram, it tends to displace regular dietary intake. Because alcohol contains no proteins, vitamins, or other essential nutrients, this results in relative malnutrition. In addition, alcohol metabolism uses more vitamins than regular food metabolism. It injures the absorbing surfaces in the gut, so further malnutrition follows. Neurological diseases caused by alcohol occur in this way. Alcoholic people do not eat well, which promotes malnutrition.
- Alcohol heart disease. Excessive alcohol consumption results in changes in heart rhythm and palpitations. This may be the first sign of a condition that advances to dilation of the heart and finally intractable heart failure. This is called alcoholic cardiomyopathy.
- Contribution to head and neck (oral) cancer. At least 75 percent of oral cancers are related to tobacco smoking and chewing along with alcohol consumption. The effect of alcohol is additive, probably increasing the risk of developing an oral cancer tenfold. Perhaps the combined toxic effect of alcohol intensifies the toxic effects of the tobacco components. Malnutrition probably contributes.

Recent evidence confirms that alcohol increases the risk of breast cancer and contributes to the increased risk of mouth, oral, head, neck, and esophageal cancers. It is recommended that women have no more than one drink per day to minimize their risk.

Alcohol abuse could be approached as a matter of education and attitude. We must learn when, where, and how much to drink. Patients with chronic alcoholism have lost control of their alcohol consumption, and medical attention is urgently needed. Alcoholism should be considered a serious disease and treated actively. Certain blood tests can indicate whether a serious drinking problem is present. Hospitalization in a rehabilitation center is very common and can be life-saving. Alcoholics Anonymous has become nearly indispensable in alcohol dependency treatment and rehabilitation. This wonderful group has developed a philosophy of mutual help and support, which can be an invaluable assistance in recovery. It is a ready-made support group to promote sobriety.

Alcoholism is a major preventable dependency and a major cause of mortality and morbidity. In a recent study, participants received medical management with naltrexone or acamprosate either alone or in combination with behavioral interventions.[11] Both treatments had positive effects, but the group receiving naltrexone and behavioral intervention was most successful. Acamprosate was not effective. Additional studies are in progress.

14 Tobacco

Ernest H. Rosenbaum, M.D., F.A.C.P.

If they were real people, the Virginia Slims woman and the Marlboro man would be dead by now. Smoking is one of the leading causes of death in America, and its paths to the grave are many. The World Health Organization states that worldwide, tobacco is responsible for 5 million deaths every year, and this figure will double by 2020. Through heart disease, cancer, lung diseases, and strokes, more than 440,000 American tobacco users die every year. Another 50,000 people die annually from breathing secondhand smoke. Adults who smoke died an average of thirteen to fourteen years early. One hundred million people died of smoking-related diseases in the twentieth century. It is estimated that 1 billion people will die of smoking-related diseases in the twenty-first century.[1]

Smoking has been causally related to lung, bladder, head and neck, cervical, kidney, and esophageal cancer, cardiovascular disease, strokes, and chronic obstructive pulmonary disease (COPD). The only good news is that when smoking is stopped, the cancer risk is reduced even when smokers are over fifty years of age and after a cancer diagnosis.

Approximately 25 percent of cancer survivors continue to smoke. Quitting rates are about 40 percent for lung and head and neck cancer survivors and about 4 percent for breast cancer patients. The use of tobacco is diminishing: Fewer cigarettes were sold in 2005 than in 1951, more places are now designated as nonsmoking areas, and there are more nonsmokers than smokers. This is in part because of evidence from the U.S. surgeon general and leading medical researchers about the role cigarettes play in heart disease, cancer, stroke, and lung disease and improved public education. Secondhand smoke remains a major problem.

Unfortunately, more children in the eighth grade are now smoking. Approximately 35 percent of high school students are smokers, 14 percent use smokeless tobacco, and 25 percent smoke cigars. Unfortunately, younger cancer survivors continue to smoke more than older survivors.

Findings from a National Institutes of Health state-of-the-science panel that assessed the available scientific evidence on tobacco use prevention, cessation, and control were released in June 2006. The panel found that 70 percent of the 44.5 million adult smokers in the United States want to quit, but of the 40 percent who make attempts each year, less than 5 percent succeed.

They concluded that smoking cessation interventions and treatments, such as nicotine replacement therapy, telephone quit lines, and counseling, were individually effective and even more effective in combination. The panel also stated that use of these interventions could double or triple quit rates. Initiation to tobacco use was found to occur primarily in adolescence, with almost all adult daily smokers having tried cigarettes before age eighteen (statistics demonstrate that more than 20 percent of twelfth graders have smoked in the prior thirty days). The panel found that programs aimed at preventing tobacco use in youth are most effective when they use multiple approaches, such as mass media campaigns and price increases through taxes on tobacco products.[2] Cessation efforts are necessary for survivors. Five minutes of a physician's advice on how to stop smoking can be very successful.

U.S. Surgeon General Richard Carmona announced a report on June 26, 2006, on the significance of secondhand smoke. He estimated that 126,000 nonsmoking Americans were exposed to secondhand smoke, putting them at risk for cardiovascular disease, cancer, and COPD. Children are at greatest risk at home when exposed to secondhand smoke (increased rates of asthma, cardiovascular disease, heart attacks, vascular disease, and cancer and possibly even sudden infant death syndrome [SIDS]). According to the surgeon general, "You harm your children if you smoke around them." Secondhand smoke exposure can be controlled only by making indoor spaces smoke-free. The surgeon general also notes that indisputable scientific evidence shows that the health effects of secondhand smoke exposure are more pervasive than previously thought.

Currently nicotine replacement therapy for nicotine dependence is the mainstay of therapy (chewing gum, tablets, skin patches, inhalers, and nasal sprays); they reduce withdrawal symptoms by replacing nicotine in the blood. New therapeutic approaches include two new drugs, varenicline tartrate and cytisine. A vaccine is also under development by the National Cancer Institute, NicVAX.[3]

More money is spent yearly on promoting cigarettes than is spent on all cancer research, cancer education, and cancer programs combined. The Centers for Disease Control estimate that tobacco costs the U.S. economy $157 billion a year in healthcare costs and

In 2006

1 in 5	Number of Americans who die from smoking in a lifetime		50 percent of smokers will die of smoking-related diseases
>444,000	Number of Americans who die from smoking each year		
		>90,000	Deaths from cardiovascular disease
		162,000	Deaths from lung cancer
		127,000	Deaths from respiratory disease
		>65,000	Other diagnoses, stroke, and other cancers
96,000	Lung cancers in men caused by smoking		
81,770	Lung cancers in women caused by smoking		

lost productivity.[4] The Tobacco Institute spends $1 million a year in direct advertising and promotional campaigns to merchants for rewards and discounts to get good shelf space.

Every time you light up a cigarette, you're exposing yourself to more than 7,000 different chemicals, more than 4,000 of which are pharmacologically active, toxic, radioactive, or mutagenic. Forty-three of them are known carcinogens, including nicotine and tar. Nicotine, the most active agent in tobacco, poisons the body and narrows the blood vessels, producing high blood pressure and a higher heart rate. The particles that make up the tar are the main contributors to cancer, heart disease, and chronic lung disorders. Many other carcinogens make their way into cigarettes during production, including pesticides, fertilizers, and other chemicals and impurities.

Cigarette smoke also contains harmful chemicals known as oxidants, which reduce the lungs' ability to cleanse themselves. As a result, resistance to germs is lowered, and the smoker's lungs are more vulnerable to illness. Other compounds found in cigarette smoke include carbon monoxide, benzene, formaldehyde, vinyl chloride, arsenic, and hydrogen cyanide.

No Cigarette Is Safe

After fourteen years and many millions of dollars of government-funded research on tobacco, studies have concluded that there is no such thing as a "safe" cigarette or a "safe" level of smoking. Don't be fooled by the tobacco industry's advertising. All smoking is hazardous to your health, regardless of fancy filters or reduced tars. In fact, in the past few years cigarette companies have increased the nicotine content in cigarettes an average of 10 percent, making them more addictive. Furthermore, smokeless tobacco, which has become increasingly popular in the past two decades, carries a major risk for mouth cancer.

Quitting

The U.S. Public Health Service calls smoking "the most deadly form of drug dependence." More and more, the habit is viewed as an antisocial behavior because many nonsmokers don't like having their air polluted. But it's a tough addiction to break because smokers develop both a physiological and a psychological dependence on nicotine. Attempting to quit can trigger severe withdrawal symptoms: tobacco craving, insomnia, increased appetite, difficulty concentrating, irritability, drowsiness, anxiety, and headaches. But it can be done. Ninety-five percent of the ex-smokers in the United States today kicked the habit on their own. Last year alone, one in every eight smokers stopped lighting up.

The best approach for smoking cessation combines pharmacologic and behavioral methods with counseling, stress reduction, and supportive treatments.

The following agencies offer antismoking activities:

- The National Cancer Institute
- The American Cancer Society
- The Centers for Disease Control and Prevention
- The World Health Organization
- Other organizations, such as the Robert Wood Johnson Foundation

Preparing to Quit

- Designate your "quit" day a week in advance.
- Buy one pack of cigarettes at a time.
- Keep a daily record of each cigarette smoked.
- Smoke only when you strongly crave a cigarette.
- Wait five minutes after an urge occurs before lighting up.
- Don't smoke the last third of a cigarette; it's the most toxic part.
- Give up your cigarette lighters, cases, and holders. Get rid of ashtrays in the home, office, and car.

The Chemical Anatomy of a Cigarette: Toxic Gas and Particulate Phases of Cigarette Smoke

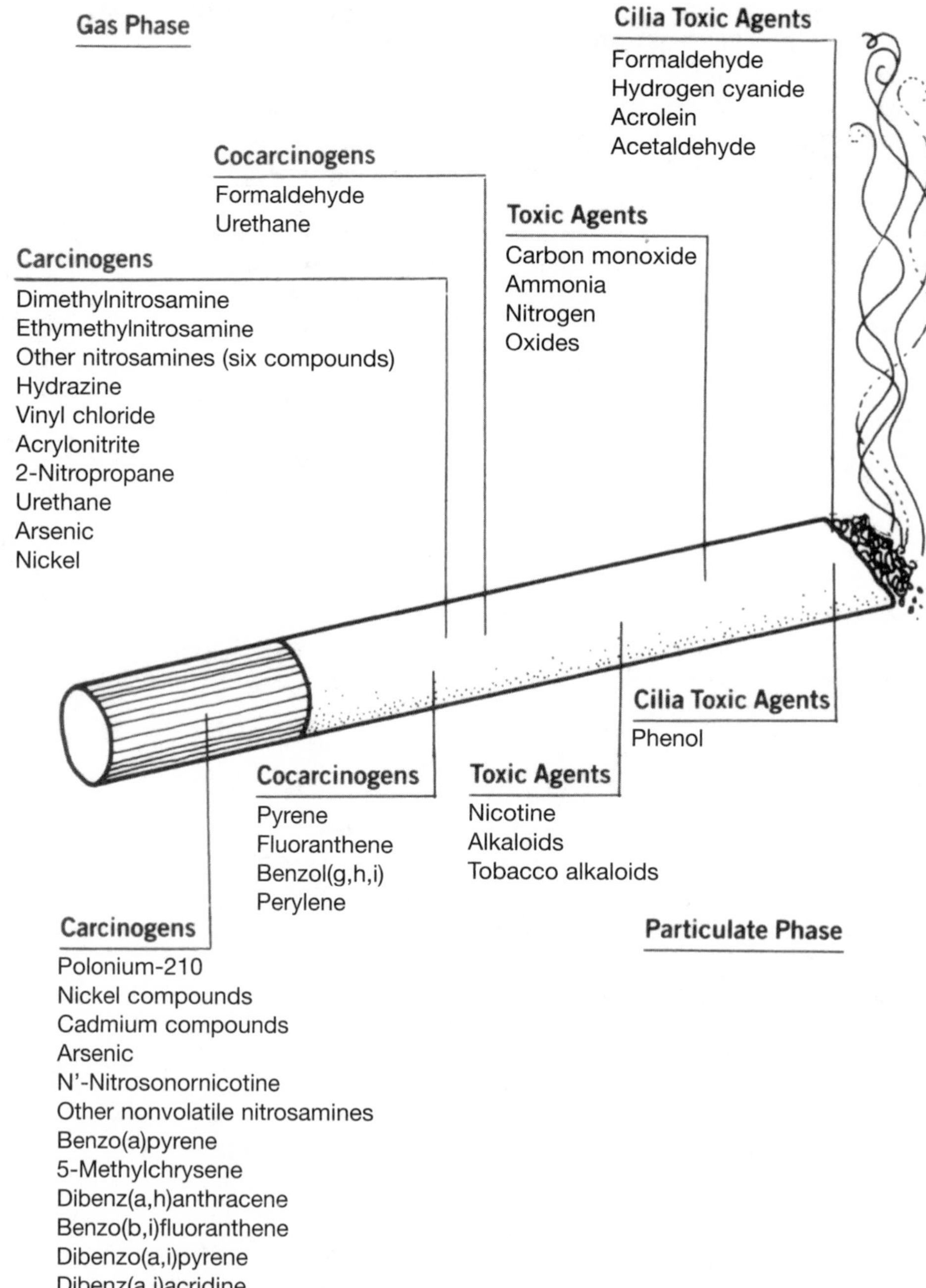

- Stay away from other smokers.
- Reduce intake of caffeinated beverages and alcohol.
- Reduce stressful situations and learn relaxation techniques.
- Use nicotine substitutes instead of cigarettes.

Information about cigarette substitutes is available at www.quitnet.org and at www.mayo.edu. The most popular substitute materials, listed here, are available in drugstores. Pharmaceutical supports for quitting are available by prescription from your physician.

- Nicotine replacement therapy (NRT):
  - Nicorette
  - Nicorette Patch
  - Nicorette Gum
  - Nicorette Lozenge
  - Nicorette Inhaler
  - Nicorette Nasal Spray
- Commit Stop Smoking Lozenges.
- Bupropion (Zyban or Wellbutrin), an FDA-approved antidepressant drug that has been found effective in reducing nicotine dependence. Bupropion appears to double the smoking cessation rate when compared with placebo.[5]

These substitutes have side effects, including dry mouth, insomnia, and nausea. There are nicotine toxic effects if one smokes while using a nicotine patch. NRT should not be used by those who have had a recent heart attack or have persistent high blood pressure. NRT should not be used during pregnancy. Nicotine gum is unpalatable to some, and its absorption is poor in those who drink acidic beverages. Nicotine withdrawal symptoms may persist with treatment, and a rebound phenomenon can occur with abrupt cessation.[3]

Currently, NRT (chewing gum, tablets, skin patches, inhalers, and nasal sprays) is the mainstay of therapy for nicotine dependence. An evaluation of various forms of NRT found a continuous abstinence success rate of 20 percent for nicotine gum, 21 percent for patches, 24 percent for sprays, and 24 percent for inhalers. Addiction was noted with inhalers in nonsmokers who after one year were still using them.[3]

New Therapeutic Approaches

New therapeutic approaches to quitting smoking include two new drugs: varenicline tartrate (Chantix) and cytisine.

Varenicline is a novel medication approved by the U.S. Food and Drug Administration. It is a selective alpha4, beta2 nicotine receptor partial agonist that mimics the agonist effect of nicotine. That is, it blocks the nicotine receptors in the body in order to decrease the desire for nicotine. In a double-blind, randomized, placebo-controlled trial the continuous quit rate was 49 percent, compared with 11.6 percent in the placebo group.[6]

Cytisine is a plant agonist of the nicotine receptor that binds with the alpha4, beta2 nicotinic receptors. It has been used for forty years in Europe for tobacco dependence. A literature review of ten studies of the effectiveness of cytisine on smoking cessation revealed that these studies were not of the best quality but suggested that cytisine had an effective role in smoking cessation.[7]

15 Psychological Support

David Spiegel, M.D.

Plato said that courage is knowing when to be afraid. There are many stories of courageous people who become very ill or face some other crisis yet count themselves fortunate. In the face of a dismal diagnosis or harsh circumstances, they can take stock of their resources and find strength and love.

Many people have faced sickness but were not overtaken by it. Although one part of them became ill, they did not give up. Their bodies may have suffered, but their spirits remained strong. Indeed, serious illness is a reminder that we are not immortal. Those who respond creatively to a life-threatening illness hear it as a wake-up call, a reminder of how time is short and life is precious. They do what matters most while they can, experience the joys of living and loving, and let the people around them know how much they are loved and appreciated. They trivialize the trivial, drop useless commitments, eliminate relationships that are taxing and not worth the trouble, and "just say no" to what they think they should do rather than what they want to.

The tradition of writing "ethical wills" to pass on a person's spiritual legacy to family and friends provides a codification of what that person has learned in life about what has meaning and value. This underscores the importance of feeling embedded in the world of people, using the contemplation of the end of one's life not to deny death but to reaffirm the values of life.

People often talk about and illustrate the will to live in a realistic and meaningful way. They do not demonstrate some artificial determination to prolong life no matter what. They assess life's resources, goals, and values. They take stock and see how fortunate they are to have people who care about them and whom they care about. Mind may not always triumph over matter, but mind does matter.

Years ago, a clever graduate student taking a statistics course was wandering through a cemetery and realized there were two types of data on the headstones: birth dates and death dates. She wondered whether they bore any relationship to each other. Theoretically, they shouldn't. When you die, you die, period. That was not what she found. People tended to die after their birthdays, not before. The difference was not large, usually several weeks, but was significant. People seem to hang on until after their birthdays or some other special event. This doesn't mean you can make yourself live indefinitely through mental calisthenics but rather that meaning makes a difference in the course of disease.

Another crucial theme is the power of social connection: No man or woman is an island. Prisoners of World War II on Bataan kept themselves alive by giving one another lectures, playing together, and caring for one another. They developed a special relationship with each other and their God.

We have found that women with breast cancer help one another enormously through support groups in which they can vent their darkest fears and learn how deeply they can still care about each other.[1] To feel part of a network of caring at a time of serious illness is deeply reassuring. The will to live is not the denial of death. Rather, it is the intensification of life experience that comes when you realize how finite life is.

Be willing to make compromises, find the joy in life, find good support groups, and be partners with your doctors. Cancer patient stories make it clear that we are not simply happy or sad and that pleasure is not simply the absence of pain. Illness teaches us that we can be both happy and sad and that even the threat of progressive disease and death can provide a context in which life can be sweeter. One woman with advanced breast cancer once said, "All my life I had wanted to go to the summer opera in Santa Fe. This year I went. I brought my cancer with me, and it sat in the seat next to me. I loved it."

Creative Expression to Improve Quality of Life

Ernest H. Rosenbaum, M.D.,
and Isadora R. Rosenbaum, M.A.

Both activities and attitude can promote better health. Courage, hope, faith, sympathy, and love promote health and prolong life. Enhancing and enriching one's quality of life heightens emotional experiences and reduces depression. Attitude depends in part on what we expect from life and how good we think our lives have been. Health depends on the interaction between mind and body, joys and sadness, and on the sense of security and being loved and appreciated.

To achieve a better quality of life, survivors need to involve themselves in a positive living program to promote a healthy mind. Quality of life can be enhanced by the spiritual uplift and relaxation provided by interests and hobbies such as art, music, writing, and humor, enriching life through positive experiences. People achieve a special satisfaction through things that they create themselves. This improves feelings of self-worth, decreases depression, and promotes well-being.

The Role of the Mind in Health

Good health is one of the greatest assets we have in life, for without it one's future is uncertain. If health is impaired, through an accident or illness, life may become compromised by subsequent debilitation. Some of the new problems survivors may face are economic, social, emotional, and psychological.

Recently there has been a shift in the philosophy of healthcare to a more "holistic" type of medical care, as suggested by Plato a few thousand years ago. The mind plays a key role in promoting good health. We can't separate the mental from the physical because they are related as part of the whole body. Being a healthcare provider is like being a juggler trying to balance many balls—the medical, physical, environmental, psychological, and nutritional—in an attempt to keep the heart, brain, and body healthy.

Many authorities think that 50–80 percent of illnesses are stress related, including high blood pressure, colds, depression, and certain skin diseases. Research at the University of Utah evaluated the role of stress during a recent economic depression. There were more fatal strokes and heart attacks than were predicted. Continuing studies are looking at how stress relates to a decrease in the function of the immune system. If a direct link is found, an immune defect could precede many diseases. There is a relationship between anger, stress, and disease. One of the secrets of good health and longevity is knowing how to control stress.

It is an accepted fact that attitude and the will to live can determine one's future. How one accepts and deals with adversity, or controls stress and anger, determines one's coping skills. Norman Cousins coped with his incapacitating spinal arthritis by watching funny Marx Brothers and Three Stooges movies and used his inner strength not only to fight his way back to good health but also to increase his longevity through humor.

Survivors can help themselves and others live better if they:

- Live in the present and in the future, not in the past.
- Set reasonable goals as to what can be accomplished.
- Accept new problems and attempt to solve them through understanding and increased awareness.
- Try to resolve depression and negative emotions.
- Actively do things to help themselves and others.
- Learn techniques to relax and practice mind control by using simple methods to calm down, such as yoga, tai chi, self-hypnosis, biofeedback, or visualization.

PART IV

Survival with Disease Prevention and Control

16 Prevention of Cardiovascular Disease and Strokes

Gary F. Milechman, M.D., F.A.C.C., and
Jay S. Luxenberg, M.D.

Cardiovascular (heart) disease is the number-one reason people don't live as long and as well as they would like. The two most common causes of early death and debility are heart attacks and heart failure. Strokes are the third leading cause of death in the United States. There are approximately 700,000 strokes in the United States each year and about 160,000 deaths.[1] Perhaps because of the large number afflicted, there has been a tremendous amount of research seeking ways to prevent and treat cardiovascular disease. Coronary atherosclerosis is the number-one killer in America, and 2.5–3 million Americans have heart failure, a disease with a mortality rate higher than most cancers. Congestive heart failure is the number-one diagnosis for hospitalized patients over the age of sixty-five. The good news is that these diseases are very preventable. You have the power to lower your odds of being afflicted with heart disease.

The Causes and the Cures

Cardiovascular problems can interfere with your health as you age in a variety of ways. Of course, the first thing that comes to mind for most people is a heart attack. We'll discuss preventing heart attacks, but first we'll discuss another way in which our heart can betray us, a heart disease that can be prevented in many cases.

The heart is a pump. Its job is to pump the blood that carries oxygen from your lungs to the rest of your body—brain, muscles, kidneys, intestines, and so on. It also pumps back the blood from these organs, helping to eliminate waste products. When the pump fails, major trouble results. The waste products build up, and the vital tissues are starved for food and oxygen. The failing pump causes a buildup of salty fluid in the body, resulting in swollen ankles and often fluid in the lungs, which causes shortness of breath. When the heart fails to pump blood adequately, we call it congestive heart failure. It is one of the major causes of death in older people, and it impairs functions by leaving its victims constantly tired, weak, and with no energy. When people with congestive heart failure attempt physical work (e.g., lifting groceries or doing housework) they become short of breath and fatigued.

A common cause of congestive heart failure in older people is damage to the heart from heart attacks. The other common cause of heart failure is long-standing high blood pressure. If you lifted heavy weights on a regular basis you would expect that your arm muscles would get thick and bulkier. Exactly the same thing happens to the heart if it must pump blood with very high pressure. The thick and bulky heart gets so stiff that it doesn't fill well between heartbeats, and congestive heart failure results. Even though the thick and stiff heart is very strong, the high pressure needed to fill it doesn't allow it to work efficiently. If you keep the filling pressure high, fluid backs up into the lungs, and you become short of breath. If you lower the filling pressure so the lungs are clear, the heart does not fill, thus pumping only a small amount of blood, and you become fatigued and your kidneys and muscles don't function well. Often, after this thick and stiff and strong phase, the heart muscle "burns out," becoming weak and dilated. The reason for this "burnout" is unclear.

Congestive heart failure is a disabling and often fatal form of heart disease. Fortunately, we have a variety of ways of preventing and treating high blood pressure. Avoiding obesity, smoking, and alcohol will help prevent high blood pressure. Physical exercise will also help. If high blood pressure does develop, then avoiding excess sodium in the diet will help control it. If these measures fail, then adding one of the many safe and tolerable blood pressure medications will allow control of the blood pressure elevation, preventing heart failure down the road.

Another potentially preventable form of cardiovascular disease is coronary artery atherosclerosis. This is the process that leads to heart attacks, chest pain with activity (called angina), and even sudden death. *Atherosclerosis* refers to fatty deposits in the walls of blood vessels. If these deposits occur in the fairly small blood vessels that supply the heart muscle, we call this coronary artery disease (CAD). If the blood flow in these blood vessels is only partially blocked, then under conditions of low energy usage such as resting or minimal physical activity, all is well. When you try to perform more activity, such as walking or lifting, the heart muscle doesn't get enough blood flow, and pain or angina may result. This disorder can be so severe that you can lose the ability to work or perform the activities that provide pleasure in life.

If the blockage in the arteries supplying the heart muscle becomes more severe, then all blood flow to a portion of the heart may stop. The heart muscle without blood supply dies. This is what is generally called a heart attack, and in about 25 percent of cases the person dies before reaching the hospital. If all goes well and the initial period is survived, then the dead heart muscle tissue slowly turns into a scar. If enough of the heart muscle is damaged, the heart can't pump well, and congestive heart failure develops.

We have a number of very effective high-tech treatments for blocked coronary arteries. Angioplasty is a technique that opens up an artery nonsurgically, with a balloon. A stent is a slotted metal tube, sometimes impregnated with medication, mounted on a balloon and placed in the narrowed 2.5- to 5-mm diameter coronary artery. Then the balloon is expanded, the stent expands, and the balloon is deflated and removed, leaving the stent to hold the artery open. Bypass surgery places new conduits or pipes around the blockages, bringing fresh blood to starved myocardial tissue. These procedures can be very useful and lifesaving, but they do not address the underlying pathologic process.

Our goal is to prevent these serious heart problems from ever developing. Fortunately, in the last few decades we have learned much about what causes these problems and how we can prevent them. A major clue was the fact that heart disease is very uncommon in developing societies, where diets are much higher in fiber, fruits, and vegetables and much lower in animal fats. Physical activity is greater, and in most cases certain types of emotional stress are much less than in developed societies. By changing our dietary habits and increasing physical activity, we can lower our own risk of developing heart disease.

The atherosclerotic process is the predominant cause of heart attacks, strokes, and peripheral vascular disease. If cholesterol deposition occurs in an artery supplying the heart muscle, angina or myocardial infarction (heart attack) may ensue. If the same process occurs in an artery supplying the brain, a transient ischemic attack or stroke may occur.

A stroke is a highly treatable brain attack like a heart attack. One must immediately get to a stroke center or hospital for early treatment as, unfortunately, due to delays, many patients are left with major physical debilities that totally change their lives. Signs of a stroke include the sudden onset of dizziness; unsteadiness or a sudden fall; visual dimness, especially in one eye; difficulty speaking or trouble understanding speech; numbness and weakness in face, arms, or legs (especially on one side of the body); or a severe headache not experienced before. Once a person is in the recovery phase, an active rehabilitation program may take from six months to a year.

Peripheral vascular disease is caused by blockage of the arteries supplying blood to the legs. This can cause pain in the legs (usually the calves) with exertion (called claudication) or, when more severe, can lead to amputations. Obviously, one wants to stay as far away from the atherosclerotic process as one can.

Risk factors associated with atherosclerosis have been known for years. These are cigarette smoking, high blood pressure, high cholesterol, diabetes, age, being male, family history, lack of exercise, overweight and obesity, and probably stress and Type A behavior.

African Americans, Hispanics, and Asian Americans have a higher rate of strokes than non-Hispanic whites, and one in six people who survive ischemic (arteriosclerotic) strokes are at greater risk of another stroke within two years. People who have transient ischemic attacks (TIAs), or ministrokes, are at about a ten times greater risk of having a major stroke. It has been estimated that about 80 percent of the risk of a stroke is related to high blood pressure. When the blood pressure is controlled, the stroke risk may decreases about 40 percent, and that also reduces the heart attack rate by about 27 percent and heart failure by 54 percent. About two-thirds of Americans over age sixty-five have elevated blood pressure, making the brain arteries stiffer and more fragile, which puts them at risk of a possible bleed, especially if there is hypertension.[1]

Much has been learned recently about significant modifications we can make to retard or even reverse atherosclerosis. Stopping smoking is the most critical and very obvious first step. Treating high blood pressure will help. It probably does not matter how the blood pressure is normalized, as long as it is. Common-sense ways, such as lowering salt intake, maintaining a reasonable weight, reducing stress, and exercising, should be first alternatives.

Cholesterol has received much well-deserved attention in both the media and the scientific community. Total cholesterol is divided into good (high-density lipoprotein [HDL]) and bad (low-density lipoprotein [LDL]) cholesterol. HDL acts as a scavenger to remove cholesterol deposits from vessel walls, whereas LDL encourages cholesterol deposition. High HDL is protective, and low HDL is associated with a significant risk for coronary disease. Your HDL level is largely hereditary, although exercise can increase your level. Eating foods high in monounsaturated fats (e.g., olive, canola, and nut oils, plant sterols, avocados, and walnuts) and low in saturated fats can significantly raise your HDL. Partially hydrogenated oils (often found in packaged and processed foods) are highly atherogenic and should be avoided, so read the labels. Red wine (in moderation) and the vitamin niacin, or nicotinic acid, in pharmacological dosages (which have potentially significant side effects and should not be taken except under medical supervision) are two other ways of increasing your good cholesterol.

Your bad cholesterol (LDL) level is somewhat hereditary as well, but it is much more responsive to simple interventions. A low-fat diet by its nature (fat has twice the calories of carbohydrate or protein per ounce) is low in calories and the best way to get you to a healthy weight. There is increasing evidence that simple carbs (sugars or starches that are quickly broken down by the body) promote diabetes, weight gain, and the atherosclerotic process. Avoiding sugars and simple starches such as white bread, potatoes, and white rice while eating high-fiber brown breads and brown rice will help you lose weight, prevent diabetes, and improve your lipid profile.

It had been thought that atherosclerosis was an inevitable part of aging. Some recent studies show that this is not the case. Aggressive treatment of high cholesterol levels in patients with documented and quantified coronary narrowing (stenosis) has shown that many people can reverse the atherosclerotic process, and plaque can melt away (regression). Many medications are very effective and safe in lowering high LDL levels that do not respond to diet alone.

A group of medicines called statins (atorvastatin [Lipitor], simvastatin [Zocor], rosuvastatin [Crestor], fluvastatin [Lescol], and pravastatin [Pravachol]) can dramatically lower LDL levels and promote regression and have been proven to prevent progression, heart attacks, and strokes. Side effects, such as muscle aches and liver problems, are quite rare. Lower LDL is better. LDL levels as low as 60 mg/dl seem to be optimal for people with established disease or risk factors such as diabetes. Most people cannot get their cholesterol levels that low with lifestyle modifications only. Niacin, fibrates, or ezetimibe (Zetia) can be added to a statin to optimize your lipids and lessen the chance of progressive atherosclerosis causing big problems.

An intriguing study was performed by Dr. Dean Ornish in his Lifestyle Heart Trial. He showed that people with severe coronary stenosis can reverse atherosclerosis, and it can be done with lifestyle changes alone. The people in his trial were on a rigorous regimen of exercise, stress reduction, group support, and a superb diet with less than 10 percent of total calories coming from fat, with no animal fat at all.

Normally, LDL is oxidized and then sticks to the vessel wall. It was once hoped that antioxidant medications and vitamins (e.g., vitamin E) would slow or prevent cholesterol buildup in the vessels. Large-scale studies have not shown benefit from these supplements, and they may actually cause harm.

People who eat more fish tend to have fewer coronary events. Certain fats in fish are felt to be protective, although the exact mechanism is not clear. However, recent evidence shows that the mercury in larger fish (e.g., tuna, shark, sea bass, and tilefish) can cause a variety of illnesses, including coronary disease and neurological problems. So stick with sardines, herring, and wild salmon as your main fish sources.

In the past, it was thought that hormone replacement therapy (HRT) for women going through menopause would protect them against coronary disease. The female hormones do seem to increase HDL (the protective lipoprotein), and premenopausal women are at a much lower risk of CAD than men of a similar age. HRT also keeps a woman's bones stronger. Recently, however, the role of hormonal therapy has become limited because it appears to increase the risk of heart disease, stroke, blood clots, and breast and uterine cancer. Although HRT increases HDL, it makes the blood clot more easily (blood clots in the arteries can cause heart attacks or strokes), so overall it is not protective. HRT is no longer recommended to help prevent heart disease.

There is evidence from the Women's Health Initiative study that estrogens used near menopause may reduce CAD. Women treated for severe vasomotor symptoms (hot flashes) may have a delay in atherosclerosis. The greatest risk is seen with estrogen combined with progesterone therapy. The Women's Health Initiative estrogen-alone trial was stopped in February 2004 because it showed increased risk of stroke and no benefit for heart disease.[1] Women who have had a hysterectomy can safely take estrogen without increasing breast cancer risk.

Estrogen should be used in the lowest dosage for women with a uterus or in alternative forms such as gels, creams, vaginal pills, and patches (because there is less body absorption of estrogen) for vaginal dryness, decreased mucus, burning, or irritation associated with menopause. Alternative nonestrogen treatments for menopausal symptoms include patches, vaginal rings, antidepressants, and topical gels and creams. Avoiding spicy foods and alcohol and dressing in layers can be helpful.

One of the exciting implications of Dr. Ornish's Lifestyle Heart Trial and other human trials attempting to prevent and regress atherosclerosis is that some of the biggest improvements were found in patients with the most severe fatty deposits in the walls of their blood vessels. In other words, it may never be too late to make lifestyle changes and, if needed, take cholesterol-lowering medication to decrease your chances of having a heart attack or stroke.

Another encouraging finding of Dr. Ornish's study was that women seemed to respond even more dramatically than men to the lifestyle changes. Because many early research studies excluded women, we often don't have strong data to make recommendations for women. For example, many of the early studies of treating high blood pressure were done entirely on men, and the ones that included women had an inadequate number to make any strong recommendations. For regression of fatty deposits in blood vessels with improvement in diet, exercise, and stress reduction, we can confidently say that both men and women will benefit. Another important finding is that even moderate decreases in the amount of fatty deposits seem to produce a substantial decrease in the number of deaths and heart attacks.

Summary

In summary, there is overwhelming evidence that we are not limited by our heredity. By taking charge of our health we can eliminate much of the death and disability caused by cardiovascular disease.

The ways to prevent cardiovascular disease and improve the quality and enjoyment in your life are apparent:

- Get regular aerobic exercise. Walking thirty to forty minutes three or four times a week is all that is needed.
- Exercise lowers blood pressure and reduces blood clots, and can cut the stroke rate in half. Those who are overweight or obese have at least a 30–50 percent higher risk for a stroke respectively compared to normal-weight men. Exercise helps maintain a healthy weight and blood pressure and also treats diabetes actively.
- Get your blood pressure within the normal range.
- Stop smoking.
- Eat nutritious food. Stay away from red meat, chicken skin, dark meat poultry, eggs, fried foods, tropical oils, and hydrogenated oils. Don't be fooled by foods that advertise "no cholesterol" because they may be filled with hydrogenated vegetable oil. Try to calculate the percentage of calories from fat in what you consider buying, and if it's over 30 percent, strongly

consider not buying it. Eating fish two or three times a week provides omega-3 fatty acids that may help lower stroke and heart attack rates. Those eating salmon, tuna (baked or broiled), or herring four times a week were seen to have a 27 percent lower risk of stroke than those who ate it once a month. Those eating fried fish or fish burgers more than once a week had a 40 percent higher risk of stroke. Eat plenty of the right kinds of fish, white meat chicken or turkey, high-fiber bread, brown rice, beans, vegetables, and fruit.

- If you have strong risk factors for coronary disease such as family history, high cholesterol, or a history of smoking, and your cholesterol is not in a good range despite a good diet (this happens often), strongly consider medications to get your total cholesterol down under 200 and increase your HDL while lowering your LDL.
- Talk to your doctor to see if daily aspirin would be beneficial for you.
- Consider stress reduction. Stress reduction may be in the form of a support group, yoga, running, swimming, Type A behavior modification, changes in your work environment or schedule, or more time with your family.

17 Prevention of Osteoporosis

Felix O. Kolb, M.D., and
Ernest H. Rosenbaum,
M.D., F.A.C.P.

Most people consider it natural and inevitable that our bones grow weak with age. A long-term diet and exercise program designed to promote and maintain bone strength may offset the increased bone tissue breakdown that begins in middle age. Without such preventive measures, bones can become porous, brittle, and ultimately subject to spontaneous fracture. These problems, which result from a gradual bone loss with acceleration after menopause, are called osteoporosis.

How Common Is Osteoporosis and Who Is at Risk?

Osteoporosis is responsible for more than 1.5 million fractures annually, mostly of the hip, spine, and wrist. Ten million Americans already have osteoporosis, and 34 million more have low bone mass, placing them at higher risk (osteopenia) for this disease. Eighty percent of those affected by osteoporosis are women. It is called a silent disease because it takes many years to develop, and most sufferers do not learn that they have the disease until middle age or later. The most common form afflicts women after menopause. Senile osteoporosis occurs much later in life and affects both sexes.

One in every two women and one in four men over fifty will have an osteoporosis-related fracture in their lifetime. Five percent of women over eighty fracture a hip each year, and 20 percent of these women die within a year. Forty thousand people die each year of complications from osteoporosis-associated fractures. Based on figures from hospitals and nursing homes, the annual medical costs associated with osteoporosis are between $14 and $18 billion and will increase as the baby boomer generation enters their sixties.

In addition to increasing age, risk factors include:

- Being female and postmenopausal
- Being chronically underweight
- Being Caucasian or Asian
- A history of infrequent periods or prolonged absence of periods (amenorrhea)
- A family history of osteoporosis
- A poor diet lacking minerals, especially calcium
- A sedentary lifestyle
- Lack of weight-bearing exercise

The Shrinking Woman

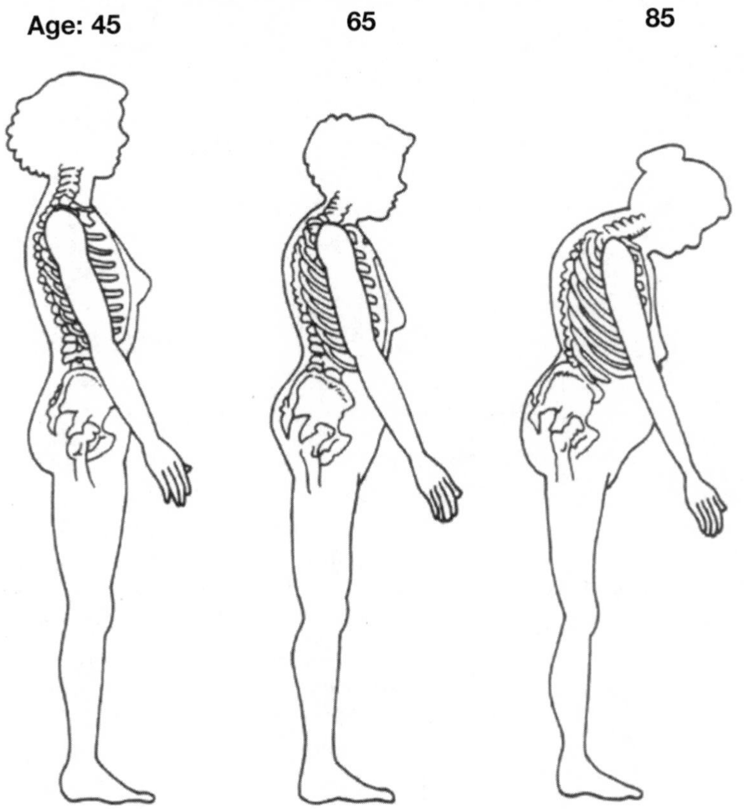

- Smoking, drinking alcohol in excess, taking excess caffeine, and certain drugs such as cortisone, thyroid hormone, and anticonvulsants

Osteoporosis in Cancer Survivors

Osteopenia (bone weakening) and osteoporosis (significant bone weakening) are common problems associated with age and cancer survivorship. In most cases, breast and prostate cancer patients have good skeletons before treatment, which then become osteoporotic with therapy (ovarian failure and hormone ablation). A study by Twiss showed that 80 percent of older breast cancer patients had osteopenia at their initial visit.[1]

How Do You Discover Osteoporosis?

Routine x-rays and blood and urine tests are not adequate in uncovering osteoporosis. Loss of height and development of so-called dowager's hump are late developments. It is now possible to discover mineral loss early by the use of dual energy x-ray absorptiometry (DEXA), which can measure bone mineral content at the wrist, the spine, and the hip (the most common sites of fracture) accurately with little discomfort, rapidly, and at reasonable cost with minimal exposure to x-rays. People at risk should have baseline measurements. Repeat measurements annually will show progression of bone loss or stability and response to and compliance with treatment. Medicare has approved repeat bone density scans every two years.

How Do You Prevent and Treat Osteoporosis?[2]

Although little can be done about hereditary factors (being female and of a small frame size), a program started in childhood and continued throughout life will help prevent or delay the onset of osteoporosis. The more bone you build in early life (called peak bone mass), the better you will be able to withstand bone loss later.

The two essential ingredients in a long-term preventive program to promote bone strength for a lifetime are:

- A well-balanced diet
- An exercise program emphasizing weight-bearing activities

Giving up smoking and heavy alcohol intake is also mandatory.

The diet must contain specific kinds of food in proper balance. Adequate amounts of calcium in balance with phosphorus and protein, with vitamin D to help in its absorption, are most important. A lifetime of inadequate calcium intake is common and contributes to the development of osteoporosis. It is often difficult to obtain enough calcium from food products. Supplementation with calcium carbonate or calcium citrate to achieve the recommended daily allowance of 1,000–1,200 mg (in divided doses twice a day) usually is necessary. Vitamin D at a dosage of 800–1,000 IU usually is necessary for maintenance. Vitamin D promotes calcium absorption, which diminishes in later years.

Weight-bearing exercise should be a part of your daily life. Sporadic exercises won't do it. The best exercises are walking, cycling, dancing, and weight lifting. Jogging in moderation is helpful, but excessive running leads to weight loss and cessation of menstrual periods, which can lead to bone loss. The combination of adequate calcium and regular exercise will stimulate and maintain bone mineral content.

Calcium and Vitamin D Therapy

Older adults need supplementation with vitamin D and calcium. Ten databases, conference abstracts, bibliographies, and other studies were reviewed comparing vitamin D or a vitamin D analog alone or in combination with calcium versus no intervention in postmenopausal women or men over age sixty-five. People taking corticosteroids were excluded.[3] This study showed that in postmenopausal women and older men, vitamin D alone did not reduce the risk of fractures more than a placebo, but vitamin D with calcium reduced the risk of hip and nonvertebral fractures more than placebo or no treatment. This is especially important for frail people, often living in institutions, who are at risk for falls.

In general, it is recommended that between 800–1,000 IU of vitamin D and 1,000–1,200 mg of calcium be taken daily to help protect bones from fractures during falls or injury. Calcium-rich foods are also recommended as part of a prudent diet.

Patients with bowel disorders, anorexia, or liver impairment may not derive the benefits of the nonactive vitamin D and should receive either larger than physiologic dosages or one of the soluble activated vitamin D analogs, such as calcifediol or calcitriol, monitoring the serum calcium carefully to avoid hypercalcemia and renal impairment.

Patients with renal impairment should receive calcitriol, the most active form of vitamin D, to help calcium absorption and avoid the development of secondary hyperparathyroidism detrimental to their bones.[3]

Dairy and Nondairy Sources of Calcium

Food	Serving Size	Calcium (mg)
Dairy		
Milk		
Evaporated	1 can	1,034
Skim or nonfat	1 cup	298
Low-fat	1 cup	297
Buttermilk	1 cup	296
Whole	1 cup	288
Chocolate	1 cup	284
Yogurt, low-fat or nonfat	1 cup	415
Cheese		
Parmesan	1 oz.	390
Ricotta, part-skim	1/2 cup	337
Swiss	1 oz.	272
Cheddar	1 oz.	211
Muenster	1 oz.	203
Mozzarella	1 oz.	183
American	1 oz.	174
Camembert	1 oz.	110
Cottage cheese, low-fat	4 oz.	77
Brie	1 oz.	52
Nondairy		
Fish		
Sardines with bones	3 oz.	372
Salmon with bones	3 oz.	167
Oysters	3 oz.	113
Shrimp, canned	3 oz.	98
Vegetables (cooked)		
Collard greens	1 cup	289
Bok choy	1 cup	250
Kale	1 cup	206
Spinach*	1 cup	200
Mustard greens	1 cup	193
Broccoli	1 med. stalk	158
Muffins		
Bran*	1 medium	142
Corn	1 medium	105
Almonds, whole	1/2 cup	166
Tofu, processed with calcium sulfate	4 oz.	145
Blackstrap molasses	1 tbsp.	137
Tortilla, corn or flour, unrefined	2 6-inch	120
Orange	1 medium	54

*Contains substances that block calcium absorption.

Hormone Therapy

More specific measures can be taken to offset the risk of osteoporosis or to treat advancing disease. When premature menopause occurs—especially after oophorectomy or hysterectomy—estrogen therapy is necessary to help prevent osteoporosis. Estrogen treatment of the natural menopause likewise slows the accelerated bone loss in women past fifty. Low-dose estrogen, often combined with cycling progesterone, is the most effective means of preventing and treating advancing postmenopausal osteoporosis. If breast or uterine (endometrial) cancer is a problem, hormone therapy should be discussed with your doctor.

Hormone treatment used to be the gold standard of therapy for postmenopausal osteoporosis, but recent evidence shows that it does not protect against CAD, as was claimed in the past, but may actually increase the risk of heart attacks, strokes, and venous blood clots. It is therefore no longer the first choice for all women with osteoporosis.[4] For most women, and for those in whom estrogens are contraindicated (e.g., women past the age of seventy-five or with history of breast or uterine cancer), other drugs such as nasal calcitonin; the bisphosphonate drugs alendronate (Fosamax), risedronate (Actonel), ibandronate (Boniva); and the intravenous bisphosphonates (zoledronic acid and pamidronate) are now used under medical supervision. They have shown progressive increases in bone mass, with reduction of fracture rates similar to or greater than those of estrogens, for periods up to ten years.[5]

An alternative to an estrogen and progesterone program is the use of raloxifene (Evista, a selective estrogen receptor modulator), which has effects on bone similar to those of natural estrogen but has no stimulatory effect on the breasts or uterus.[6]

Parathyroid Hormone Therapy

A surprising newcomer to the treatment of osteoporosis in postmenopausal women and in men with osteoporosis is recombinant human parathyroid hormone (PTH; both full-length 1–84 [Preos] and fragment 1–34 [Forteo] teriparatide). Although continuous administration of PTH causes bone loss, intermittent use appears to increase bone mass far more than the other modalities, which appear to be mainly antiresorptive. The drug has few side effects, but it must be given as a daily injection (like insulin) and it is costly. Recent studies have shown that PTH can normalize severely osteoporotic bone with restoration of architecture. It is the treatment of choice for severe osteoporosis in both sexes.[7]

Combination Therapy

Attempts to combine therapies for osteoporosis have been reported. The combination of nasal calcitonin and estrogen may be indicated in patients with recent fractures because calcitonin has a nonspecific analgesic (pain-relieving) effect. The combination of estrogen and bisphosphonates (both antiresorptive agents) has been tried and seems to show somewhat greater increases in bone mineral density (BMD) than either agent alone. However, it may be wise to start with one therapy, and if a significant rise in bone density is not seen, the second agent can be added. The addition of bisphosphonates to PTH has shown partial inhibition of the beneficial effects of PTH and should be avoided.[8]

Potential Agents

Androgens

These hormones are not superior to estrogens (to which they are metabolized) for the treatment of postmenopausal osteoporosis, and they have undesirable virilizing side effects. They may be of value in hypopituitary patients.

Growth Hormones

Growth hormone and insulinlike growth factor increase bone density in patients with growth hormone deficiency. Their use in postmenopausal women with osteoporosis is ineffective, is expensive, and has significant side effects.[9]

Thiazide Diuretics and Potassium Bicarbonate

These drugs reduce urinary calcium losses and may help in the treatment of postmenopausal women with osteoporosis and hypertension.

Isoflavones

These phytoestrogens have mild estrogenic actions. Their effect in postmenopausal osteoporosis is not certain, but they may be of value in helping stabilize low BMD.

Statins

These cholesterol-lowering agents were thought to be of benefit to bone on theoretical grounds, but a large study over four years showed no benefit in terms of increase in BMD or fracture rates.[10]

Folate and Vitamin B_{12}

These agents may lower the fracture risk after a stroke.

Newer Potential Agents Not Yet Available in the United States

Tibolone

This synthetic steroid has been reported to increase bone density in the spine and to reduce vasomotor symptoms in postmenopausal women, but its safety regarding uterine and breast cancer is not certain, and there are no convincing reports of reduction in fracture risk.

Strontium Ranelate

This orally effective drug, which appears to be well tolerated, has been shown to both increase BMD in the spine and hip and reduce the relative risk of spine and hip fractures significantly.[11]

Denosumab

This humanized monoclonal antibody against the receptor activator of NFkappaB ligand (RANKL), the potent antiresorptive agent considered to initiate osteoporosis, given by subcutaneous injection every three to six months, has been shown to increase BMD in the spine and hip as much as or slightly more than the bisphosphonate alendronate. However, there have been no long-term studies of fracture risk and potential side effects because RANKL also functions in the immune system, causing concern about potential infectious complications.[12]

Osteoporosis and Breast Cancer Endocrine Therapy

The original treatment for metastatic breast cancer (1898) was surgical oophorectomy or, in the 1900s, radiation ablation of the ovaries to stop estrogen production. This can also be accomplished chemically through treatment with luteinizing hormone–releasing hormone (LHRH) analog injections such as leuprolide (Lupron) or goserelin (Zoladex). These estrogen hormonal blockers can be reversed by stopping the LHRH agonist injections.

Adjuvant and therapeutic chemotherapy, radiotherapy, or hormonal ablation can also reduce or stop ovarian function and thereby reduce or stop estrogen production. Amenorrhea (loss of menstrual periods) commonly results from ovarian failure in premenopausal woman, especially those under age forty. This can result in premature bone loss and osteopenia (weakened bones) or osteoporosis.

The Zoladex Early Breast Cancer Research Association study of premenopausal patients assigned to adjuvant cyclophosphamide, methotrexate, and fluorouracil (CMF) chemotherapy or goserelin showed amenorrhea for more than 95 percent of patients, which was permanent in most cases. BMD decreased in both groups in the first two years, more so with goserelin injections. Within three years after goserelin treatment was stopped, there was a partial recovery of BMD, but bone loss persisted in the CMF group.

The National Surgical Adjuvant Breast Program showed that adjuvant tamoxifen therapy gave a five-year benefit, with not only improved overall survival and disease-free survival but also a protective effect on bone density in postmenopausal women, with less osteoporosis and bone weakening.[13] Fisher also showed that using tamoxifen for five years reduced the risk of not only invasive and noninvasive breast cancers but also hip, radius, and spinal fractures. This effect was greater in postmenopausal than in premenopausal women.[14] In another study, Richard Love and associates showed that tamoxifen increased BMD by 0.61 percent, compared with controls, in whom there was an approximately 2 percent loss of BMD over two years.[15]

Cancer, Osteoporosis, and Bone Density Treatment for Metastases[7]

Bone metastases from breast cancer are common. When activated, bone osteoclast cells accelerate bone resorption, causing osteopenia (bone weakening) or osteoporosis (extensive bone weakening). Bone resorption is accelerated in breast cancer, leading to an increased vertebral and bone fracture rate. The relative risk of vertebral fracture increases more than fourfold, and if there are soft tissue metastases, the risk can increase as much as twentyfold.

For hormonally sensitive estrogen receptor–positive breast cancers, one of the treatment goals is estrogen deprivation to reduce the risk of progressive breast cancer. Unfortunately, this increases the risk of osteoporosis. Postmenopausal women have a lower estrogen level, which can increase the rate of osteoporosis and bone fractures. For women with undetectable serum estradiol (less than 5 pg/ml), the relative risk of hip fracture is 2.5 when compared with controls with positive estradiol levels.[16] These patients must undergo intensive drug therapy to help restore their destroyed bones. A new alternative approach is the injection of plastic material into collapsed vertebral bodies to restore their height and relieve bone pain.

Osteoporosis and the Aromatase Inhibitors

The aromatase inhibitors are a new class of drugs that block estrogen production from the ovaries and adrenal glands. In many instances, aromatase inhibitors have become the first drug used for a hormonal approach in postmenopausal patients as adjuvant and metastatic breast cancer therapy. Aromatase inhibitors interfere with estrogen production by inhibiting conversion of angiogenic precursors to estrogens by peripheral aromatization. The three types of aromatase inhibitor drugs—anastrozole and letrozole (nonsteroidal drugs) and exemestane (a steroidal drug)—are irreversible inhibitors of aromatase. *These three drugs reduce serum estrogens in postmenopausal women to nearly undetectable levels but also increase bone resorption.*

Tamoxifen has a different set of side effects, including a low incidence of endometrial cancer and ischemic cerebrovascular and venous thrombotic disease, whereas the aromatase inhibitors have side effects of joint stiffness, arthralgias, and an 11 percent six- to eight-month fracture incidence, compared with 7.7 percent for tamoxifen. In the Arimidex [anastrozole], Tamoxifen, Alone or in Combination trial, there was a higher fracture rate with anastrozole. The recurrence rate of estrogen receptor–positive breast cancer was 17 percent lower with anastrozole than with tamoxifen, but there was no significant difference in overall survival.

Another trial comparing letrozole with tamoxifen over five years showed a lower rate of distant metastases in postmenopausal women with letrozole, but there was a significant incidence of hot flashes, arthralgias, and myalgias in the letrozole group. Similar results were also found with exemestane.

An alternative to tamoxifen is the selective estrogen receptor modulator raloxifene, which acts as an estrogen antagonist against hormone receptor–positive breast cancer, reducing the risk of invasive breast cancer. It also reduces the risk of osteoporosis, with increased bone density in the spine, vertebrae, and femoral neck, with a reduction in spine fractures but not in hip fractures, but may cause endometrial hyperplasia or cancer. Like estrogens, however, it increases the risk of venous thromboembolic and fatal strokes.[17]

Bisphosphonate Therapy

Oral and intravenous bisphosphonates have been found to be potent inhibitors of osteoclastic activity in bone resorption. In trials, premenopausal women whose breast cancers were estrogen receptor and progesterone receptor positive were randomized to tamoxifen, tamoxifen with zoledronic acid or anastrozole, or anastrozole with zoledronic acid.

DEXA bone density studies on the spines and hips of three hundred patients showed that anastrozole produced a steady reduction in BMD in the spine and hips of approximately 10 percent over one year. There was less BMD reduction with tamoxifen. The addition of zoledronic acid to either anastrozole or tamoxifen helped prevent lumbar spine bone loss. The adjuvant use of vitamin D and calcium also helped to prevent osteoporotic fractures in older people.

In prostate cancer osteopenia and osteoporosis develop after hormone ablation therapy LHRH agonists (leuprolide or goserelin), which block testosterone production. This results in control of advanced metastatic prostate cancer in a way similar to the way breast cancer is controlled. Treatment for osteopenia and osteoporosis is the same as for breast cancer, with vitamin D, calcium, and bisphosphonates (alendronate, risedronate, ibandronate, zoledronic acid, or pamidronate) as indicated.

The most potent bisphosphonates, zoledronic acid and pamidronate, rarely have caused jaw necrosis, usually associated with poor dentition or recent tooth extractions. This problem merits special attention from a dentist for a teeth and jaw bone evaluation before taking a biphosphonate.

Osteoporosis and Prostate Cancer

Osteoporosis is a potential problem for men whose treatment has included androgen deprivation therapy (ADT) through orchiectomy (castration) or LHRH agonist therapy.

Fasting plasma glucose levels higher than 110 mg/dl, elevated serum triglycerides, a high-density lipoprotein level below 40 mg/dl, high waist circumference, and blood pressures greater than 130/85 all can occur with androgen deprivation therapy (ADT) and, in combination, are known as the metabolic syndrome.

Osteoporosis and osteopenia are well recognized in hypogonadal (low testosterone) patients. Of note is that 63 percent of men have low BMD on DEXA scans even before they start ADT. Low vitamin D and calcium intake is also a contributing factor. Follow-up DEXA scans are recommended for prevention and treatment of osteoporosis in men on ADT.

Progression of bone loss increases while patients are on ADT. The decrease in serum testosterone through ADT can result in osteoporosis in as short a period as 6 months to two years after treatment, increasing the risk of fractures.[18] In one study, loss of BMD with ADT for prostate cancer was well recognized, with significant loss of BMD occurring within twelve months of the beginning of therapy. With ADT, annual loss of BMD is about 2–8 percent at the lumbar spine and 1.8–6.5 percent at the hip; the loss appears to continue indefinitely while treatment continues, and there is no recovery after therapy ends. In men surviving at least five years after a diagnosis of prostate cancer, 19.4 percent have a fracture if treated with ADT, compared with 12.6 percent of men not treated with ADT. Vitamin D deficiency exacerbates the development of osteoporosis, so vitamin D status should be evaluated before ADT begins in men with prostate cancer. Treatment with bisphosphonates (zoledronate, pamidronate, and alendronate) in men treated with ADT has been shown to prevent bone loss in prospective studies and to increase BMD in one randomized controlled trial.[19]

Older treatments used estrogen, which was discontinued because of cardiac complications. Now men undergoing ADT can be treated with bisphosphonates, calcium, and vitamin D. Treatment for osteoporosis with bisphosphonates could include pamidronate 60 mg every twelve weeks for one year. Zoledronic acid 4 mg intravenously every three months was similarly effective in reducing osteoporosis.

An alternative is the use of raloxifene (Evista) 60 mg per day in men receiving gonadotropin-releasing hormone agonists, also resulting in a significant decrease in bone turnover and an increase in hip BMD. Current studies testing bisphosphonates and raloxifene appear to be positive.

Summary

Aside from the prevention and treatment modalities described in this chapter, measures for managing osteoporosis include avoidance of falls, proper back support, assistance in walking with a cane or walker, and pain relief. A novel experimental approach for patients with severe compression fractures of the spine is the injection of plastic material into the vertebrae to restore their height and prevent bone pain.

Osteoporosis is a major public health problem in the United States that can and must be reduced. Diet, exercise, and, in many patients, hormonal and other drug therapy can result in major improvements in bone mineral status in our population. Bone measurements to detect osteoporosis and assess response to treatment are generally available.

It is easier to prevent osteoporosis early than to treat advanced disease when fractures have occurred. Eat a balanced diet, exercise regularly, and discuss with your physician the possible need for hormonal replacement and bone mass. Although the ultimate culprit in postmenopausal and senile osteoporosis has not yet been clearly identified, the pharmacological measures available to us now make it possible to prevent bone loss and to reverse it once it has progressed. We are close to a cure for all types of osteoporosis.

18 Prevention of Diabetes

Robert J. Rushakoff, M.D., F.A.C.P.

Diabetes is a common, chronic disease. It can lead to retinal (eye) damage, kidney disease, and nerve damage and is a risk factor for cardiovascular disease. Most people with diabetes are overweight and have type 2 diabetes, or non–insulin-dependent diabetes mellitus. Although excellent control of blood sugar levels can decrease the risk of complications, prevention of this type of diabetes through lifelong diet modification and exercise remains the best option for a healthy life.

Diabetes Mellitus

Diabetes mellitus is a chronic disease that can affect the entire body. Two major problems occur with diabetes. First, the body is not able to store and use glucose (sugar) appropriately, and this leads to hyperglycemia, or high levels of glucose in the blood. Second, as a result of the hyperglycemia, complications of diabetes may occur: eye damage, kidney disease, nerve damage, atherosclerosis or heart disease, and strokes. Diabetes is a common cause of kidney failure, blindness, and amputations and is a major cause of heart disease and stroke. Efforts are being made to better control major risk factors such as hypertension, dyslipidemia, and hyperglycemia (elevated blood sugars).

In the past decade, large studies in both the United States and Europe have shown conclusively that with good control of the glucose levels in the blood (lowering the glucose level to nearly normal), the risk of developing the complications of diabetes may be reduced dramatically. In addition, these studies have also shown that lowering cholesterol and blood pressure levels can reduce the risk of heart disease and stroke.[1] More than ever before, it is clear that control of diabetes and its associated conditions is of primary importance and will lead to a healthier life.

The Scope of the Problem

Overall, approximately 7 percent of the U.S. population has diabetes. However, this percentage is misleading because the incidence of diabetes increases dramatically with age. For example, between the ages of twenty and forty-four, 2.1 percent have diabetes; between forty-five and fifty-four, 8.7 percent have diabetes; between fifty-five and sixty-four, 13.1 percent have diabetes; and between sixty-five and seventy-four, 17.9 percent have diabetes. It is estimated that by age eighty-five, 25 percent of people in the United States will have diabetes. These percentages are even higher in certain racial groups such as African Americans. Currently a Hispanic male born in the United States has more than a 50 percent chance of developing diabetes in his lifetime. Much of this increase is associated with the increase in obesity seen throughout the United States. Recent research shows that the average lifetime risk for a normal-weight eighteen-year-old man is 20 percent, compared with 30 percent, 50 percent, and 74 percent risk for overweight, obese, and very obese men, respectively. For eighteen-year-old women in these weight categories the risks are 17 percent, 35 percent, 55 percent, and 74 percent, respectively.

Because the signs and symptoms of diabetes may be subtle in older adults, it is estimated that half of the people with diabetes do not know that they have the disease. This point is extremely important. Although people with undiagnosed diabetes may feel good, they are at full risk for developing the complications of diabetes.

Diagnosis

How do you know whether you have diabetes? You may have symptoms of high blood sugar, including the following:

- Excessive thirst
- Frequent urination
- Fatigue
- Itching
- Numbness

By current criteria, if you have these symptoms and have a random blood sugar that is high (generally over 200 mg/dl), then you have diabetes. If you do not have any symptoms, and your fasting blood sugar is higher than 126 mg/dl on two different days, then you also have diabetes. The normal fasting blood sugar level is between 70 and 100 mg/dl. Other tests, such as oral glucose tolerance tests, may be performed, but these tests are rarely needed.

Types of Diabetes

There are two major types of diabetes: type 1 diabetes (previously called insulin-dependent diabetes mellitus or juvenile-onset diabetes) and type 2 diabetes (previously called non–insulin-dependent diabetes mellitus or maturity- or adult-onset diabetes).

In type 1 diabetes, the insulin-producing cells of the pancreas are slowly destroyed, and eventually not enough insulin can be made to maintain normal glucose levels. Therefore, lifelong insulin use is needed for survival. Although most people who develop this type of diabetes do so before age thirty, it can occur at any age. About 5 percent of all people with diabetes have type 1 diabetes.

Most people with type 2 diabetes develop it after the age of forty, although it also may occur at any age. In fact, there is now an epidemic of type 2 diabetes in teenagers. These people are genetically at risk for this type of diabetes but have developed the disease early, secondary to obesity. In type 2 diabetes, insulin initially is produced in large quantities, but the insulin does not work properly, and glucose levels increase. Most people with this type of diabetes are overweight. Although diet and exercise remain the basis of all treatment of type 2 diabetes, most people need multiple medications to control their glucose levels. In addition, as the disease progresses, insulin levels decrease, and to successfully treat type 2 diabetes, insulin generally is needed eventually.

Complications of Diabetes

With the treatment of diabetes, it is generally easy to control blood sugar levels in a range that will allow you to feel normal. Unfortunately, this degree of control is not good enough to decrease the risk of developing complications. Because about 50 percent of people with diabetes do not even know that they have the disease, it is not unusual for people to have advanced complications even before they realize they have the disease, hence the fallacy of saying one has "mild" diabetes or "a touch of sugar." These people are at as great a risk of developing complications as those with severe diabetes.

The eye disease in diabetes is *retinopathy,* or damage to the blood vessels on the retina (inside back wall) of the eye. These blood vessels can leak fluid or blood and lead to diminished vision or blindness.

Nephropathy is the kidney disease caused by diabetes. In people who develop this complication, initially increasing amounts of protein are leaked into the urine, then the ability of the kidneys to filter the blood decreases to the point that dialysis or a kidney transplant is needed.

In *neuropathy,* or nerve damage, occasionally severe burning pain can occur, especially in the feet. More commonly, there may be a tingling, numbness, or even complete loss of sensation in the feet and sometimes in the hands. The loss of sensation can be extremely dangerous because trauma to the feet goes unrecognized, and even a minor injury can lead to ulcer formation and amputation.

Diabetes also is associated with an elevated risk of cardiovascular disease such as heart attacks and strokes. Studies have shown that people with type 2 diabetes, with no known history of heart disease, have the same risk of a heart attack as a person without diabetes who has already had a heart attack. Another condition, claudication, is caused by blocked arteries in the legs. In this situation, walking or climbing stairs may lead to extreme calf pain that resolves when the movement is stopped.

Reducing the risk of complications has been the major goal in diabetes control. In the past there was controversy as to whether improving a patient's glucose levels would decrease the risk of complications. In 1993, results from the Diabetes Control and Complication Trial (DCCT) were released. In this study 1,400 people with type 1 diabetes were followed for nine years. Half of the people had their glucoses maintained close to normal. The other half had their glucoses controlled to eliminate symptoms but not to approach normal glucose control. The group with excellent glucose control had a 50–70 percent lower risk of developing the complications of diabetes and a similar reduction in progression of complications if early problems were already present.

A few years later the United Kingdom Prospective Diabetes Study (UKPDS) looked specifically at type 2 diabetes, and the results were similar to those of the DCCT. Recent studies have shown that tight blood glucose control in type 1 diabetics can cut the risk of heart disease and stroke in half.[1] Thus far, this has not been determined for type 2 diabetics, but research is ongoing in the Veterans Affairs Diabetes Trial.

Based on the results of the DCCT and UKPDS, the goal for all people with diabetes is to maintain glucose levels as close to normal as possible. The method to obtain this control is described briefly in this chapter.

The UKPDS and other studies have shown that when people with diabetes aggressively control their blood pressure and cholesterol levels, the risk of cardiovascular disease also decreases dramatically.

Prevention

Type 1 diabetes is an autoimmune disease. This means that if people at risk can be identified, then bone marrow stem cell transplants to restore the immune system may be able to prevent destruction of the insulin-producing cells of the pancreas. This type of treatment remains under intense investigation.

Because 95 percent of people who develop diabetes have type 2 diabetes, prevention of this type of diabetes certainly will have a major impact. In a study of physicians, it was shown that those who had exercised during their lives had a much lower chance of developing diabetes than those who did not exercise.

Proper diet can also help prevent the onset of type 2 diabetes. Numerous studies have shown that when the standard American diet is adopted by people who were previously isolated from modernization, the incidence of diabetes increases dramatically. One possible explanation for this is the thrifty gene theory. Our ancestors had to deal with times of both feast and famine. Those who were able to store food most efficiently during times of feast (by storing fat) would be best able to survive during famine. Because we are now in a time of constant feast, the previously beneficial thrifty gene leads to obesity and elevated risk of diabetes.

Recently a very large study in the United States, the Diabetes Prevention Program, followed more than 3,200 people who were at high risk for developing diabetes. Participants in the lifestyle intervention group—those receiving intensive counseling on effective diet, exercise, and behavior modification—reduced their risk of developing diabetes by 58 percent. This finding was true for all participating ethnic groups and for both men and women. Lifestyle changes worked particularly well for participants aged sixty and older, reducing their risk by 71 percent.

Thus, for type 2 diabetes, the current best treatment is prevention with improved diet, exercise, and medical treatment.

Treatment of Diabetes

In people with type 1 diabetes, the cornerstone of treatment remains insulin injections. Although many approaches are used to administer insulin, currently multiple-shot regimens (four or more shots of insulin per day) or insulin pumps generally are used to mimic the normal release of insulin as closely as possible. Inhaled insulin is used by a small group of people at this point.

In type 2 diabetes, some people initially obtain control of blood sugar with diet modification and exercise. The diet is similar to the healthy diet described in detail in Chapter 10. The main difference is that highly concentrated sugars are avoided (e.g., fruit juices, large quantities of fruit). Exercise is of equal importance. The exercise must be almost daily for at least thirty minutes in order to achieve significant lowering of glucose levels.

Unfortunately, many people are unable to meet the dietary and exercise recommendations. Diet often is difficult to modify as we age. In addition, exercise may be difficult in patients with other medical conditions such as osteoarthritis and heart disease. In addition, the natural history of type 2 diabetes shows that less insulin is made over time. Thus, for most patients, medications are generally needed early, and often multiple medications with different mechanisms of action are used.

Several oral medications are used to treat type 2 diabetes. Some of these medications increase the ability of the pancreas to produce insulin; others help the insulin work more effectively. For most people the weak link is insulin production, and we now understand that no matter what treatment is being used, there is a slow decrease in insulin production. So for most people with type 2 diabetes, insulin treatment is needed at some point. The major mistake people make is thinking that starting to take insulin means that they have a worse type of diabetes and that because they take insulin they will be at greater risk for complications. In fact, the insulin is needed to control the glucose and prevent complications that will be more likely to occur if the insulin is not taken.

Summary

Diabetes is a common, chronic disease. It can lead to eye damage, kidney disease, and nerve damage and is a risk factor for cardiovascular disease. Most people with diabetes are overweight and have type 2 diabetes. Although excellent control of blood sugar levels can decrease the risk of complications, prevention of this type of diabetes through lifelong diet modification and exercise remains the best option for a healthy life.

19 Prevention of Skin Cancer

Bernard Gordon, M.D.,
and Ernest H. Rosenbaum,
M.D., F.A.C.P.

Excess sun exposure can damage the skin, causing premature aging and sometimes cancer. A skin protection program is vital for preventing skin cancer.

Because skin cancers are among the most common second cancers, especially for those treated with radiation therapy, survivors should take extra care to protect their skin from sun exposure. This includes regularly using sunscreen with a sun protection factor (SPF) of 15 or more, wearing protective clothing, avoiding outdoor activities from 10 a.m. to 2 p.m., when the sun's rays are most intense, and not tanning.

In addition to avoiding excessive sun exposure, be aware of changes in your skin. Any nonhealing sores and changes in skin lesions, moles, or freckles merit a physician examination.

The Dangers of Excessive Sun Exposure

The sun's radiation is made up of infrared, visible, and ultraviolet (UV) rays. It is the ultraviolet rays, UV-A and UV-B, that affect the skin. UV-B rays, in particular, penetrate your skin's top layer (epidermis) and are the primary cause of sunburn and skin cancer and also contribute to premature skin aging. They are the strongest and most potentially damaging rays and are most common between 10 a.m. and 3 p.m.

Recent studies have shown that UV-A rays penetrate the skin even more deeply, reaching into the underlying skin layers of connective tissue. They play a major role in aging and are strong all day long, all year long. When your skin absorbs UV rays, the exposure triggers the production of melanin, a natural sunscreen pigment. This creates what is known as a tan. People with light hair and complexions have less natural protection from melanin, so they burn quickly, but even a tan does not prevent long-term harm because the skin "remembers" each exposure. With each burn, it can grow weaker in its ability to protect itself. Over years, damage to the skin's basic structure from sunlight can lead to premature aging and possibly skin cancer.

Sun Protection

People have been flocking to beaches and tanning salons to try to gain a fashionable look with bronzed skin. Excess exposure increases the risk of chronic sunburn to achieve this fashionable glow, associated with a healthy body and lifestyle. In recent years, dermatologists have found not only that sun exposure is unhealthy and unbeneficial but that the sun can cause nearly 90 percent of the cosmetic changes associated with aging, such as wrinkling, a leathery appearance, irregular pigmentation, and age spots. It may also lead to photodamage, which can evolve into several forms of skin cancer; the most deadly one is malignant melanoma. It has been estimated that using sunscreen on a regular basis during the first eighteen years of life could reduce the incidence of skin cancer by up to 70 percent.

Precancerous Skin Lesions

Excess sun exposure can lead to the growth of actinic keratoses or solar keratoses: rough, scaly skin lesions that can be a precursor to cancer. These lesions are seen in teenagers and in people whose occupations require sun exposure, such as farmers and sailors, and they are usually seen on the face, lips, ears, back, forearms, and hands where there has been excessive sun exposure. People with such precancerous skin lesions are at risk for developing basal, squamous, or melanoma cancers. The lesions are scaly, rough, and slightly raised, often have sharp boundaries, and are often present at more than one site. The color can vary from flesh-colored to darkly pigmented or tan lesions. These lesions usually do not spread and can be treated effectively.

Types of Skin Cancer

Skin cancers are the most common form of cancer. Fortunately, 90–95 percent of people with this disorder can be cured. There are three basic types: basal cell, squamous cell, and melanoma. Basal cell and squamous cell carcinomas are called nonmelanoma skin cancers.

Nonmelanoma

Cancer of the skin (including melanoma and nonmelanoma skin cancer) is the most common of all cancers, probably accounting for more than 50 percent of all cancers.

Some people estimate that there are at least as many nonmelanoma skin cancer cases diagnosed each year as all other cancers combined (more than 1 million in 2006). Most of the cancers are basal cell: about 800,000–900,000 cases. Squamous cell cancer occurs less often, perhaps about 200,000–300,000 cases per year. Men are approximately twice as likely to develop these cancers as women. The number of these cancers has been increasing, probably because of a combination of increased detection and more sun exposure.

Although it is thought that 1,000–2,000 people die each year from nonmelanoma skin cancer, death is uncommon with these cancers. In fact, the death rate has dropped by almost 30 percent in the past thirty years. Most of those who die of this disease are elderly and were not treated soon enough. Other people likely to die of skin cancer are those whose immune system is suppressed, such as those who have received organ transplants.[1]

Basal Cell Carcinoma

Basal cell carcinoma is the most common form; it develops in sun-exposed areas of the face and body and looks like a pale, waxlike or pearly nodule (lump) that may ulcerate. It is linked to ultraviolet radiation exposure usually occurring on:

- Fair-skinned people, especially those who sunburn easily but tan poorly
- People who live in a warm, sunny region or who take frequent outdoor vacations

Most basal cell cancers are treated effectively with surgical removal, and fortunately most are removed before they grow large or are more aggressive and thus more difficult to cure. The cure rate is higher than 95 percent with early treatment. Long-term follow-up is necessary, and it is important to use sunscreen for protection and to prevent future lesions.

Squamous Cell Carcinoma

Squamous cell carcinoma occurs in the skin layer that produces protective keratin in the epidermis (top layer) and may occur anywhere on the skin—whether or not the areas have been overexposed to the sun—or on the mucous membranes. It appears as a red, scaly, raised lesion that arises on the sun-damaged skin or sites of previous burns, scars, or chronic sores. It can appear wartlike or cauliflowerlike in shape, especially on the hands, feet, and linings of the mouth or genitals.

Squamous cell cancer usually is related to too much ultraviolet light exposure, and people at risk usually are those who:

- Have fair skin and burn easily but tan poorly
- Develop precancerous lesions such as solar keratoses
- Have preexisting dermatologic problems, such as scars and ulcers

Fortunately, most new squamous tumors, when caught early, are effectively cured, but they may metastasize.

Melanoma

Although melanoma accounts for only about 4 percent of skin cancer cases, it causes most skin cancer deaths.

Melanoma tends to occur at a younger age than most cancers; half of all melanomas are found in people under age fifty-seven. Adolescents can have melanoma also. About 1 of every 30,000 girls aged fifteen to nineteen will develop melanoma. For boys of this age, the rate is about 1 of every 15,000.

The American Cancer Society estimates that more than 59,900 new melanomas will be diagnosed in the United States in 2007, a rate that is increasing in the United States. Among white men and women in the United States, incidence rates for melanoma increased sharply at about 6 percent per year from 1973 until the early 1980s. Since 1981, however, the rate of increase has slowed to less than 3 percent per year.

Almost 10,850 people in the United States were expected to die of melanomas in 2007. Since 1973, the mortality rate for melanoma has increased by 50 percent. Much of this increase has been in older people, mostly white men. More recently, the death rate from melanoma has leveled off for men and dropped slightly in women.[2]

Melanoma (meaning a black tumor) is a potentially deadly tumor. It is the most malignant type of skin cancer and one of the most lethal cancers of any kind. It often arises in pigmented cells (melanocytes) of the epidermis (upper layer of skin) and can spread quickly to any part of the body. It is rarely seen before puberty.

Risk Factors

- A family or personal history of melanoma
- A light complexion
- A tendency to freckle
- A tendency to sunburn
- Any moles or birthmarks
- Unusual moles or birthmarks
- High-dose radiation

Symptoms

Melanomas may develop in normal-looking skin or in dark or fleshy-colored moles. Pigmented spots usually are not melanoma. Several warning signals can help identify melanomas:

- A change in color, lightening or darkening of a reddish, bluish, or grayish tinge
- A growth or change in size, shape, or thickness
- Irregularity of the margins of the growth
- Itching, crusting, bleeding, erosion, or ulceration
- Personal or family history of melanoma or dysplastic nevi, usually moles that look like melanoma under the microscope

Melanoma patients often have a lower capacity to repair the DNA damage that results from UV-B exposure. A higher frequency of chromosomal DNA breaks has also been associated with a more than twofold elevated risk of both basal and squamous cell carcinomas.

Melanoma is a potentially deadly form of skin cancer, but when it is caught early and treated early, most patients do very well. Examine your skin regularly, especially for moles, as you become a responsible partner in your own healthcare.

Diagnosing and Treating Skin Cancer

In all three types of the disease, skin biopsies are necessary to confirm the diagnosis of cancer. The treatment is a wide excision, although the therapy varies depending on the patient, the type of tumor, and the doctor's skill. Long-term follow-up is essential to observe for potential recurrence, spread of the cancer, or development of new lesions.

Recommendations for Skin Screening

- Examine your skin periodically for changes. Pay special attention to moles. Ask a friend to check areas you can't see or use a mirror.
- Have your skin checked during your physical examination every three years if you are between the ages of twenty and forty and every year if older.
- If you are at a higher risk for cancer, ask your physician for specific recommendations.

Precautions to Avoid Excess Skin Damage

- Avoid the sun at midday (10:00 a.m.–3:00 p.m.), when UV-B rays are most intense. UV-A rays are responsible for premature skin aging and are strong all day, all year, so wear protective clothing whenever you are outside.
- Cover up. Light, long-sleeved shirts and long pants can help shield you against the sun's ultraviolet rays. Umbrellas may be needed to deflect strong, direct sunlight or light reflected off sand, snow, or water.
- Use sunscreens. Suntan lotions are designed to moisturize the skin and permit tanning without sun protection. A sunscreen, on the other hand, absorbs or reflects UV energy from the sun, protecting the skin from its harmful effects. Try a broad-spectrum sunblock: Unlike conventional sunscreens, which filter out only UV-B rays, broad-spectrum products screen out UV-B and UV-A rays. An SPF of 15 or higher offers protection. With an SPF of 15, a person who would normally begin to sunburn in ten minutes could remain in the sun for two to three hours before turning pink. Some people may be allergic to para-aminobenzoic acid (PABA), which is the active ingredient in sunscreens. PABA-free sunscreens are now available.
- Apply sunscreen once a day in the morning, and reapply after swimming or heavy exercising. You should begin using a sun protective agent in childhood, especially if you have fair skin.
- Avoid tanning salons. Getting a year-round suntan is appealing but dangerous. Tanning salons have serious effects on both skin and eyes, some of which are irreversible. The intensity of the UV-A rays received in a tanning parlor is twice what you get while sunbathing at noon on the beach in the summer. Not only might this increase your risk of skin cancer and cataracts, but it may also trigger photosensitive reactions if you are taking antibiotics, birth control pills, or other drugs.

Summary

Skin cancers are the most common form of cancer, and fortunately, 90–95 percent of people with this disorder can be cured. The best cure for skin cancer remains early detection, prompt treatment, and continuing prevention measures. Recognize warning signs of the disease through regular skin self-examination. Even more important, however, is to protect yourself from the sun's rays. By avoiding the peak hours of ultraviolet radiation and by wearing sunscreen and protective clothing, you can keep skin cancer from happening to you. The prevention of skin aging and cancer can lead to a healthier, longer life.

PART V

Survival with Side Effect Control

20 Pain and Pain Management

Wendye Robbins, M.D., Ernest H. Rosenbaum, M.D., F.A.C.P., and Richard Shapiro, M.D.

Ask any group of cancer patients to describe their greatest fear, and chances are that they will say, "Pain and suffering—not death." This is not an unreasonable response. Pain is terrifying and debilitating: It can lead to depression, loss of appetite, fitful sleep, irritability, and feelings of isolation that, in turn, can strain relations with family and friends and erode the will to live.

Pain has been rated by some as the most common symptom in cancer survivors, especially when bones are involved. Pain is often seen in advanced metastatic disease, although it can also be an early harbinger of a diagnosis of cancer. Palliative care is essential to pain control and will improve the quality of life. The debilitating effects of pain cause overall suffering that merits control.

It has been estimated that 50–80 percent of cancer survivors have some form of chronic pain. Unfortunately, thus far the American healthcare system has failed to meet their pain needs. Seventy percent of cancer survivors report that oncologists do not offer them adequate guidance in coping with pain, depression, and infertility.[1]

Pain can occur at any time in the course of some forms of cancer—during treatment that leads to remission or cure or in the terminal phase. However, 90–95 percent of pain problems can be controlled, according to the Committee on Pain of the World Health Organization (WHO). Yet many cancer patients are still not receiving adequate pain relief. Why?

Obstacles to giving and receiving appropriate pain medication include the following:

- Widespread misunderstanding about the effects of opioids
- Poor communication between patients and caregivers
- A lack of awareness by caregivers, friends, and families

The goal of pain management is to help decrease suffering, distress, and loss of function and to improve quality of life. In some instances, a neurological evaluation can be helpful in assessing neuropathic (nerve) and other types of pain. Constant pain may necessitate special, often neurosurgical procedures to relieve nerve pain. Many treatments are used, including narcotics, local radiation, and epidural spinal blocks. An additional mechanism is the use of patient-controlled analgesia, using infusion pumps or intravenous lines to administer narcotics for severe, uncontrollable pain.

Common Misunderstandings About the Use of Opioids for Pain Control

Opioids are drugs originally derived from the poppy plant; morphine is the best known member of this class. Many similar molecules (including oxycodone, hydromorphone, fentanyl, hydrocodone, and methadone) have been synthesized to produce effects similar to those of morphine, and these synthetic drugs are also called opioids.

Unfortunately, many people hold certain myths about the use of opioids for pain control, with the result that they take insufficient dosages or refuse to take them at all. Descriptions of the five most prevalent myths, and the actual facts, follow:

- *Myth 1: Opioids should be administered only as a last resort to the gravely ill or those near death.* In fact, opioids are highly effective at any time in the disease process when severe pain calls for strong medication.
- *Myth 2: The use of opioids for pain leads to addiction.* Addiction is a compulsive need to take a substance despite a known risk of harm. Opioids used for pain control do not function in this manner. Patients do not become drug crazed or switch to street drug abuse, and they do not misuse them. However, they can become physically dependent on opioids if they take them over a long period of time. When such people achieve a cure through therapy, they can reduce their opioid intake slowly to avoid withdrawal symptoms.
- *Myth 3: People who take opioid medications develop a tolerance for them, leading to a need for increasingly larger dosages.* If it occurs at all, tolerance does not develop suddenly. If it does occur, it is true that physicians will respond by increasing the dosage; however, when administered correctly, opioid medications are safe even at very high dosages.
- *Myth 4: Opioids are dangerous because they make it harder for terminally ill patients to breathe.* Morphine and other opioid drugs are not dangerous respiratory depressants in patients with advanced cancer and pain. Tolerance to the respiratory depressant effects of these drugs usually develops before tolerance to their pain-relieving effects. Other drugs—such as sedatives and antianxiety agents—present a greater risk of respiratory depression than opioids.
- *Myth 5: Patients should take opioids by injection because they are poorly absorbed when taken orally.* Most opioids are absorbed very well when taken orally. However, because a fair amount of an oral dose is lost to nontarget body tissues, oral dosages usually are three times larger than those given intravenously or intramuscularly.

Poor Communication Between Patients and Caregivers

Good communication between patients and caregivers is essential to achieving optimal pain relief. Many people think they should be able to tolerate pain and therefore are ashamed to discuss the extent of their suffering with their physicians. Not wanting to be perceived as weak, they do not receive adequate pain relief.

A reason for poor communication between patients and caregivers is that pain has its own vocabulary, making it difficult for many people to accurately describe its quality, texture, and intensity. Is it sharp? Dull? Electric? Sporadic? Insistent? Moreover, the memory of pain is inexact. Between attacks of pain, people tend to forget about the level of intensity and other specifics. To compound the problem, some caregivers may not be sufficiently experienced at eliciting such crucial information from their patients.

For example, pain can be somatic (originating in tissue, skin, extremities, muscles, joints, bones, or organs), neuropathic (resulting from damage to or pressure on nerves), or a combination of the two. Somatic pain is often described as "achy, dull, and localized" when it results from a broken bone associated with tumor involvement or as "crampy and diffuse" when it results from an obstruction in the intestine or urinary tract. Bone metastases often are associated with pain, both locally and generally, necessitating an active treatment program.

Neuropathic pain, on the other hand, usually is described as "sharp, burning, electrical, shooting, or buzzing." These sensations typically occur in areas served by the injured nerves, which can be either in the peripheral nerves or in the central nervous system. Such an injury can be caused by the direct spread of a tumor, such as that of colon cancer in the pelvis, where the nerves to the legs or pelvic structures reside. It can also be caused by pressure on nerves, as when spinal tumors pinch or press on nerves to the arms or legs. Other types of neuropathic dysfunction include hypersensitivity of the skin or an exaggerated, painful response to nerve stimuli (even a simple touch) and occasional motor changes such as weakness or atrophy of an affected muscle group. Surgery, various chemotherapeutic drugs, and radiation treatment can also produce temporary side effects of somatic or neuropathic pain or discomfort.

Pain can also occur in muscles and joints. As with bony metastases, one's body structure is affected and may put stress on areas not accustomed to altered activities. There can also be organ pain (caused by tumor expansion of organs such as the liver or spleen), intra-abdominal pressure, or neuropathic (nerve) pain, which can relate to the therapy (some chemotherapy drugs) or the cancer itself. Radicular radiating neuropathic pain from spinal metastases, caused by spinal (bone and spinal cord) nerve root tumor invasion, is common, as is visceral organ (internal) pain, which may also respond to chemotherapy or radiation therapy narcotic treatment. Other associated problems are anxiety, depression, and general suffering, which can be caused by the cancer at the pain site.

Progressive Pain Relief Measures

In recommending palliative measures for pain, physicians use guidelines set forth by the WHO, which include standard treatments for mild, moderate, and severe pain, sometimes given with adjuvant medications. For those who do not benefit from these standard procedures, physicians can try one of several means of direct intervention. To augment all of these options, patients can also experiment with any of several methods that enlist the mind and emotions to reduce the stress that exacerbates pain.

An expert committee convened by WHO's Cancer Unit developed a pain ladder on a scale of 1 to 10 to help physicians assess the source, quality, and intensity of pain and determine the most appropriate relief measures. The goal is to keep pain down to a level of less than 4 through continual reassessment of the cause of the problem and the effectiveness of the means of control. Effectiveness requires that a balance be maintained between the administration of any necessary increases in the strength of a medication and the production of toxic side effects such as delirium, confusion, constipation, nausea or vomiting, allergies, or skin rashes.

In order to effectively treat pain, one must first assess the level of pain, try to localize the areas of pain, and then work out appropriate individual treatments for either localized or generalized pain. Use of a combination of antidepressants, antianxiety and antipsychotic medications, and an anti-inflammatory agent with the pain medicine (nonnarcotic or narcotic medicine) may also be helpful to obtain optimal pain control.

1. Rate on a standard Likert scale of 0–10 the intensity and duration of pain and how it affects the patient's quality of life

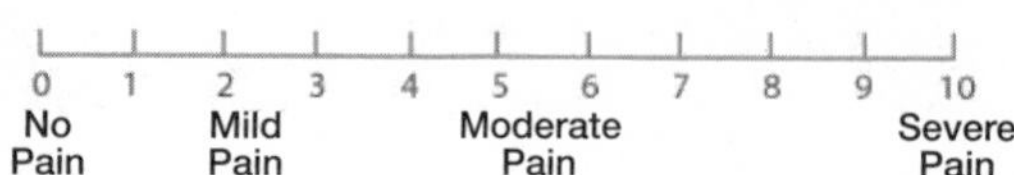

WHO Pain Scale

(0 = *no pain*, 10 = *severe pain*). The first thing is to ask the patient to describe his or her understanding and degree of pain: severity, time of onset, location, and duration.[2] One commonly uses the scale of 0 to 10 to help grade pain and make comparative assessments that can be used on future days or office visits to grade the change in intensity of the pain.

2. Rate the patient's response to his or her current pain medications. It should be reassessed on each visit.
3. After evaluating the patient, work out a written pain relief program.
4. Provide a backup relief program if the prescribed program is ineffective.
5. Consider adding a dual- or triple-drug program such as an anti-inflammatory agent (e.g., ibuprofen [Motrin or Advil]) and an antidepressant (e.g., nortriptyline [Pamelor] or amitriptyline [Elavil]) to pain medication and adding narcotics as indicated.
6. Increase the basic pain medication using the WHO's stepladder approach, using nonopioids such as acetaminophen (Tylenol) as the first step for mild to moderate pain control before progressing to the second step using short-acting opioids for moderate pain (e.g., codeine, hydrocodone, or oxycodone). If pain persists or increases, progress to the third step using short- and long-acting opioids for moderate to severe pain (e.g., morphine, hydromorphone, meperidine, methadone, or fentanyl patches) in addition to other supportive measures.
7. Be willing to modify the program when satisfactory pain relief has been achieved or when pain becomes progressive and breakthrough opioids are needed. It is estimated that 50–90 percent of patients experience breakthrough pain necessitating extra doses of rescue opioids. Use rescue doses when necessary to obtain adequate pain relief.
8. Supportive adjuvant antidepressant drugs that can be used to aid in pain control include amitriptyline (Elavil), nortriptyline (Pamelor), gabapentin (Neurontin), carbamazepine (Tegretol), dexamethasone (Decadron), prednisone, topical lidocaine, or lidocaine patches.
9. Often two or three adjuvants are used to obtain optimal pain control.

Primary Pain Relief Measures

The following medications are recommended for different levels of pain, as determined by the pain ladder scale:

- *Mild pain:* Nonnarcotic medications such as aspirin, acetaminophen (Tylenol), or other aspirinlike drugs, known as nonsteroidal anti-inflammatory drugs (NSAIDs), including ibuprofen (Motrin, Advil).
- *Moderate pain:* A combination of NSAIDs and weak narcotics, such as codeine, hydro-

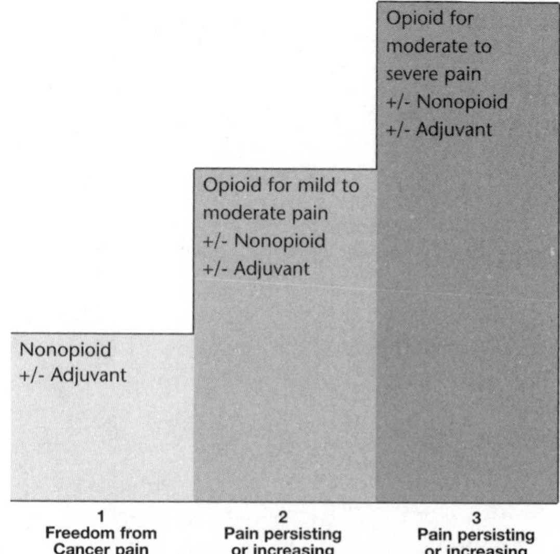

WHO Pain Relief Ladder

codone (Vicodin or Lortab), oxycodone (Percocet or Percodan), or propoxyphene (Darvon).

- *Severe pain:* Strong opioids such as morphine, meperidine (Demerol), hydromorphone (Dilaudid), fentanyl (Duragesic) patches, or methadone in combination with an NSAID. The use of longer-acting opioids such as morphine (MS-Contin or Kadian), fentanyl (Duragesic) patches, oxycodone (OxyContin), and methadone offer an additional array of drugs that can be very helpful.

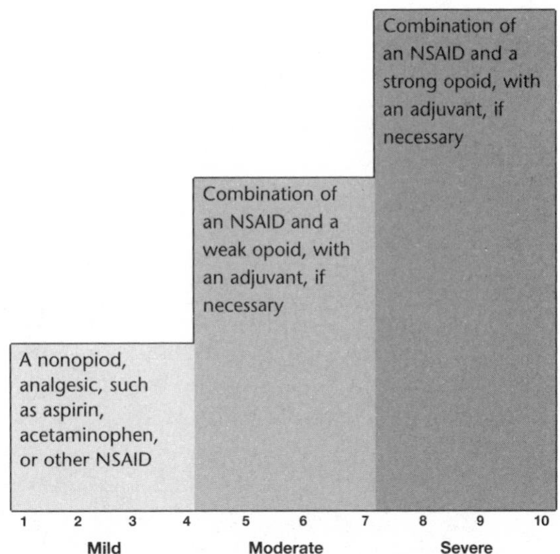

Progressive Pain Relief Measures

(Adapted from the World Health Organization's analgesic ladder for the management of cancer pain)

Adjuvant Medications

When the aforementioned medications do not achieve the desired results, the WHO guidelines suggest using an adjuvant (added) medication with either an opioid or non-opioid medication, as appropriate. In cases of mild to moderate pain in which larger or more frequent doses of aspirin, acetaminophen (with or without codeine), or ibuprofen have not succeeded, adjuvant medication can sometimes make the difference. Similarly, for pain that is not responsive to opioids, doctors have found that adjuvant medications such as steroids, anticonvulsant and antidepressant medications, antihistamines, and sedatives have been successful, although they are not usually labeled for relief of pain. A few examples of adjuvant medications are as follows:

- Steroids used in association with cyclo-oxygenase-2 inhibitors (selective anti-inflammatories such as celecoxib [Celebrex]) and opioids or other pain medications can reduce pain. Steroids can also help patients with metastases to the bone, spine, brain, and liver by reducing swelling and pain. They can be very useful in gaining control over bone pain, especially when there are expansile tumors in the limbs or vertebral metastases, and can be complemented by palliative radiation therapy. In addition, they can counteract the loss of appetite and decrease the nausea that often accompany chemotherapy.
- Another approach can be to add adjuvant NSAIDs to other pain relief agents to increase the efficacy of opioid medications.
- Bisphosphonates reduce bone pain from metastases by inhibiting osteoclasts (bone growth cells) from reabsorbing bone, and they delay progression of skeletal progressive cancer when there is a high risk of osteolytic (destructive) bone metastases. This is commonly treated in breast and prostate cancer patients with zoledronic acid (Zometa), pamidronate (Aredia), alendronate (Fosamax), or ibandronate (Boniva).
- Two tricyclic antidepressants—amitriptyline (Elavil) and nortriptyline (Pamelor)—can help reduce pain with hepatic and bone metastases and decrease the severity of headaches from cancer.
- Some selective serotonin and norepinephrine reuptake inhibitors (SSNRIs), such as

duloxetine (Cymbalta) and venlafaxine (Effexor), which help control depression and pain, are replacing the tricyclics. SSNRIs have fewer side effects than the tricyclics and can help counteract the sedative effects of opioids.

- Anticonvulsants such as carbamazepine (Tegretol), phenytoin (Dilantin), and pregabalin (Lyrica) can also play a role in pain relief. Carbamazepine can be helpful to patients with diabetic neuropathy or cancer neuritis, and 100 mg of pregabalin twice a day can ease pain and help restore normal sleep patterns, even for those on anti-inflammatory agents and physical modalities, such as heat, ultrasound, or massage.
- The benzodiazepines diazepam (Valium) and lorazepam (Ativan) decrease anxiety.

Radiation is also used for control of local pain, especially bone pain, and it has been noted that with metastatic disease, localized radiation therapy can relieve up to 50 percent of major pain symptoms. At low dosages, it can provide excellent palliative care for many lesions by shrinking them. Often five to eight treatments are all that is needed to achieve quick and, for many people, prolonged effects. Localized radiation often is combined with the use of low- to high-dose opiates. The use of multidrug chemotherapy can also aggravate pain by causing side effects such as nausea and vomiting or sedation.

External spinal catheters for epidural and intrathecal spinal space blocks can also provide great pain relief.

Other Pain Relief Options

For the 5–10 percent of patients who do not receive adequate pain control under WHO guidelines, there are other options. By means of direct intervention, pain specialists can prevent pain stimuli from reaching the central nervous system. Such interventions include the implementation of nerve blocks with a local anesthetic (bupivacaine [Marcaine] or lidocaine [Xylocaine]) or with nerve-destroying agents; the use of alternative delivery systems, such as the administration of opioids and other drugs subcutaneously or into the spine; or the use of a local spinal anesthetic. Transcutaneous electrical nerve stimulation is also effective, as is ultrasonic stimulation.

Many people find that the ancient arts of acupuncture and acupressure or the application of heat and cold compresses can relieve pain. Exercise helps maintain strength and flexibility, which actually changes muscle cells, making them less sensitive to pain.

Harnessing the Mind and Emotions to Aid in Pain Relief

Anxiety, fear, and loneliness increase stress and heighten the experience of pain. Therefore, any means by which patients can limit the power of these emotions also decreases the amount of drugs needed for pain control. Many people have been helped by biofeedback, psychotherapy, family counseling, and music.

- Biofeedback teaches patients how to manipulate unconscious bodily processes such as heartbeats or brain waves, thereby gaining control over the negative effects of stress.
- Psychotherapy can provide patients with a sounding board and insight into—and tools for dealing with—depression, anger, and fear.
- Family counseling (with a professional counselor or a member of the clergy) allows patients and family members to talk openly about the tensions of living with cancer.
- Listening to music not only provides relaxation and raises spirits but has proven to have an analgesic effect twice as strong as that of plain background sound.

Side Effects of Pain Control Medications

Constipation is a major problem with opiate use, and a stool softener (docusate [Colace, DOSS]), a stimulant laxative (Senokot), or lactulose should be used as needed.

Other side effects include nausea and vomiting, sedation, pruritus (itching or skin rash), confusion, delirium or hallucinations, and myoclonic jerking (muscle spasms or shaking). Various drug solutions are available to control these side effects.

Another potential problem is hypercalcemia (elevated serum calcium), which can occur in 10–15 percent of patients with bone metastases that release bone calcium into the bloodstream. It can cause decreased mental capacity, confusion, constipation, cardiac arrhythmias, or coma. Hypercalcemia can be treated with intravenous fluids, steroids, and bisphosphonates (zoledronic acid, pamidronate).

Pain can also be progressive, especially during cancer relapses, necessitating additional attention and treatment. One also needs to control nausea and vomiting secondary to the therapy and cancer pain medications and to consider additional treatments for bony metastases, such as the use of radiation therapy or bisphosphonates such as zoledronic acid (Zometa), and ibandronate (Boniva). Patients with lytic (bone destruction) lesions are at risk of fractures and may need orthopedic pinning to stabilize and help prevent fracture of the long bones.

Caution: Respiratory depression is seen with overdosing of narcotics.

Post–Breast Therapy Pain Syndrome

Robert Wascher, M.D., F.A.C.S., Ernest H. Rosenbaum, M.D., Alexandra Andrews, W.M., Charles M. Dollbaum, M.D., Ph.D., Francine Manuel, R.P.T., Jean Chan, B.A., M.A., S.Ed., and Richard Shapiro, M.D.

Post–breast therapy pain syndrome (PBTPS) is a complex constellation of symptoms. PBTPS can be defined as persistent neuropathic pain and is often associated with symptoms of numbness, dysesthesia, edema, and allodynia located in the chest wall, axilla, arm, or shoulder of the surgical side. The old term, *postmastectomy syndrome,* is not sufficiently descriptive with breast-preserving therapy. Recent research suggests that newer approaches to the surgical treatment and staging of breast cancer, such as sentinel lymph node biopsy, may significantly decrease the incidence of PBTPS.

PBTPS may result from neuropathic changes associated with surgery, chemotherapy, radiation therapy, and hormonal therapy. Chemotherapy drugs commonly associated with peripheral neuropathy include vincristine, vinblastine, vinorelbine, cisplatin, paclitaxel, docetaxel, carboplatin, oxaliplatin, cisplatin, etoposide, teniposide, thalidomide, bortezomib, and interferon. Any breast-associated surgery (e.g., mastectomy, lumpectomy, lymph node biopsy, breast implant placement, and breast augmentation or other types of breast reconstruction) may result in the development of PBTPS. Scar tissue that forms after surgery is not as elastic as healthy skin and may entrap nerve fibers as the incision heals. Any healing complications such as an infection may further increase the risk of PBTPS. Abnormalities in the healing of divided sensory nerve fibers (e.g., neuromas) may also lead to chronic pain in or near incisions.

Chronic upper extremity swelling, or lymphedema, may also adversely affect breast cancer survivors, with short-term or long-term discomfort, chronic pain, debility, and loss of function in the affected limb. Edema adds weight to the limb, causing a sensation of heaviness. In some cases, severe lymphedema may put pressure on major motor and sensory nerves, causing varying degrees of paresthesia and paralysis. Lymphedema, which may occur in 5–15 percent of patients after breast cancer surgery, is a chronic problem that may lead to distress, pain, loss of function, and anxiety and act as a daily reminder of a patient's prior treatment for cancer. Another specific area of PBTPS-related functional impairment is the inability to comfortably use a computer, which may result in significant professional and personal challenges to affected patients.

Complications of breast cancer therapy, lymphedema and PBTPS in particular, can have an adverse impact on quality of life for millions of breast cancer patients. Current standard clinical management approaches often are ad hoc in nature, in the absence of well-defined and evidence-based clinical practice guidelines. Chronic symptoms associated with breast cancer therapy often lead to daily challenges at home and at work, with attendant anxiety and depression for many patients.

In postsurgery follow-up visits, patients may report mild postoperative pain symptoms; however, the symptoms of PBTPS, when it does arise, may not manifest as a chronic problem until thirty to ninety days after surgery or, in some cases, many years later. More than 50 percent of patients diagnosed with PBTPS unexpectedly experience chronic pain and other serious sensory disturbances. They report pain with movement, leading to clinically significant arm and shoulder restriction of motion. PBTPS discomfort interferes with active daily living and sleep and impairs overall quality of life.

PBTPS often remains underreported, and when it occurs it may be a debilitating repercussion of breast cancer therapy. Because PBTPS is not well understood by many physicians, breast cancer patients often are not advised about this risk before surgery, or the risk may be minimized. Clinical standard management approaches are not well delineated, resulting in confusion and frustration for patients. Many patients are advised to seek psychiatric care by well-intentioned physicians who are unfamiliar with PBTPS. In some patients, PBTPS may leads to fears of cancer recurrence, resulting in additional anxiety and, for some patients, depression.

PBTPS is best treated as early as possible because it may become chronic and more resistant to effective treatment if diagnosis and initiation of therapy are delayed. The timely diagnosis and treatment of PBTPS requires that both physicians and patients have a clear understanding of this syndrome and that appropriate referrals to experienced pain management specialists are made in a timely fashion.

Patients undergoing therapy for breast cancer should be fully counseled, before treatment, as to the potential short-term and long-term risks associated with breast cancer therapy. Evidence-based treatment guidelines should be developed and integrated into breast cancer clinical pathway algorithms.

What to Expect After Treatment

The effects of cancer and its treatment endure long after medical treatment ends. Some changes may actually be positive (e.g., you may have a better appreciation of life, or you may become closer to your family and friends). Negative changes (e.g., lingering pain, scars, or lymphedema) may serve as constant reminders that you have been diagnosed with cancer.

When painful or uncomfortable symptoms persist, you may interact with others who seem to be lacking in compassion and empathy. Friends and family, and even healthcare personnel, may appear judgmental or skeptical regarding your concerns because posttreatment pain is not visible and can't be easily measured.

PBTPS is an uncommon diagnosis. This is especially so because healthcare professionals often have little experience in making this diagnosis and treating this syndrome. You may need to take a proactive approach to educate your healthcare team about this problem and to seek effective solutions from them. As previously noted, PBTBS is best treated as early as possible because it may become a chronic condition and more resistant to effective treatment when diagnosis and initiation of therapy are delayed.

It is normal to have tightness around the incision (and under your arm if you have had lymph nodes removed from the armpit region) in the first few months after surgery. Moreover, sensory nerves often are intentionally cut during surgery to remove the lymph nodes. This generally results in a tingling pins-and-needles sensation in the upper inner arm in the first few weeks after surgery as the brain attempts to compensate for the loss of innervation of this area. Later, numbness of the affected area usually ensues, but for most patients it is not unsettling or uncomfortable. However, severe burning, stabbing pain, or severe itching near incisions or in the upper inner arm months after surgery is unusual and may indicate the development of PBTPS. If pain interrupts your sleep or significantly impairs your daily life, or if wearing clothing is uncomfortable, then you should ask your physician to refer you to a physical therapist or pain management specialist.

Suggestions for Discussing PBTPS with Your Medical Team

- Keep a daily symptom diary and make three copies: one for you, one for your doctor or caregiver, and one to be placed in your medical records. Examples of noteworthy observations include the following:
  - Time of pain or other symptom occurrence
  - Type of pain (e.g., stabbing, burning)
  - Pain duration, whether chronic or sporadic
  - Pain triggers
  - Location of the pain
  - Things that help relieve the pain
- Address your needs for symptom management. Make sure that all members of your healthcare team are communicating with each other about your pain problem and that a plan of action is established. If your physician dismisses your complaints with statements such as, "It's just phantom pain" or "You're just anxious," you can consider referring your provider to this chapter. If he or she remains unresponsive to your complaints, seek a second opinion from an oncology physician who understands PBTPS. The best advice to anyone who has PBTPS is that the pain is real and can be treated.

Most importantly, remember the pain does not necessarily mean recurrence of your cancer.

Suggestions for Alleviating PBTPS

- *Medications:* Your healthcare provider may prescribe medications in an effort to reduce the severity or frequency of your symptoms, including NSAIDs such as ibuprofen or naproxen, low-dose antidepressants (and selective serotonin reuptake inhibitors in particular), and, in rare and severe cases, narcotic pain relievers.
- *Physical therapy:* Early restoration of range of motion in the shoulder and arm is important to prevent a "frozen shoulder" syndrome or to treat symptomatic muscle weakness associated with inadvertent injury to the nerves controlling shoulder muscles. These entities can cause pain separate from the neurogenic syndromes that can result from axillary lymph node dissections. Early restoration of upper extremity and shoulder mobility, and use of the arm, will also help reduce the severity of lymphedema.

- *Pain management specialists:* A referral to a pain management specialist who is certified by the American Board of Anesthesiology–Added Pain Qualification or the American Board of Pain Medicine should be made in patients who do not rapidly respond to the measures already outlined.
- *Supportive care approaches* may be useful, including guided imagery training, biofeedback, acupuncture, massage therapy, exercise (e.g., swimming, stretching), hypnosis, nutritional therapy, topical salves (e.g., calendula, capsaicin, and mentholated creams), placing a small pillow between you and the seatbelt, and wearing loose-fitting clothing made from soft, natural fibers.

Remember to consult with your physician or other primary healthcare provider when considering these interventions.

Summary

To achieve optimum pain control, patients need to be able to articulate the quality and intensity of their pain and to understand that doctors are not mind readers. Caregivers need to sharpen their assessment skills. And both patients and caregivers need to stay abreast of available treatments, their side effects, and appropriate use. Finally, successful pain control entails an individually tailored program of appropriate drugs, adjuvant or other therapies, and stress reduction techniques, consistently monitored and reevaluated by all concerned.

There is much to be known, and studies are under way to find better pain solutions for cancer survivors through national nursing initiatives and physician and psychosocial programs.

References for Additional Information on Pain

- American Chronic Pain Association: www.theacpa.org
- American Pain Foundation: www.painfoundation.org
- National Cancer Institute: www.cancer.gov/cancerinfo/understanding-cancer-pain

21 Toxic Side Effects of Chemotherapy and Radiation Therapy

Ernest H. Rosenbaum, M.D., F.A.C.P.

Cardiac Toxicity

Chemotherapy Related[1]

Many drugs cause cardiac toxicity. Cardiomyopathy (heart muscle damage and weakness affecting ventricular systole function or diastolic function) is most commonly caused by doxorubicin (Adriamycin), trastuzumab (Herceptin), and sometimes high-dose cyclophosphamide (Cytoxan). Paclitaxel is associated with arrhythmias (irregular heart rate) or bradycardia (slow heart rate). Rarely, fluorouracil can also cause arrhythmia. Trastuzumab (Herceptin) has shown the possibility of causing congestive heart failure in patients who have had mantle chest wall radiation for Hodgkin's disease or left chest wall radiotherapy for breast cancer, who have preexisting heart disease or other cardiac risk factors, or who have received drugs that could have additive or synergistic effects, such as cyclophosphamide (Cytoxan) or doxorubicin (Adriamycin).

The first data collected on doxorubicin-related congestive heart failure showed that heart failure started to occur at a total doxorubicin dosage of about 550 mg/m^2. Recently, prospective studies have shown that congestive heart failure can occur at a lower total dosage closer to 300 mg/m^2.

In women over sixty-five, combined doxorubicin, cyclophosphamide, and fluorouracil treatments were associated with a higher cumulative incidence of cardiomyopathy in patients who got adjuvant breast cancer therapy. Thus, even standard chemotherapy treatments can cause myocardial damage.

Using anthracycline analogs, such as epirubicin (Ellence), as a substitute for doxorubicin (i.e., combined cyclophosphamide, epirubicin, and fluorouracil) produces less cardiotoxicity. Other alternatives to reduce toxicity include dosing schedules, intravenous doxorubicin infusions, selective delivery systems, or liposomes such as Doxil (doxorubicin in lipid capsules). There are also blocking protective agents, such as dexrazoxane (Zinecard).

The following different types of cardiotoxicity have been described:

- Anthracyclines may cause cardiac problems. An evaluation of cardiac risk factors, including prior heart disease, hypertension, age, smoking, diabetes, obesity, increased cholesterol and cardiac lipids, left chest wall radiation, and an assessment of familial cardiac disease, is essential. Despite the known possible risk, premenopausal women frequently receive anthracycline combination therapy (with or without Herceptin). Postmenopausal women who could be at risk for future cardiac problems now have the option of omitting risky anthracycline drugs and substituting a combination of Taxol (or taxatere) with carboplatin with similar results for reducing the risk of recurrence and improving survival.
- Chemotherapy-related cardiac dysfunction, called Type I myocardial, is associated with myocardial damage and is defined as permanent irreversible heart damage. This heart dysfunction is cumulative and dose related. The results of heart damage (vacuoles, necrosis, and myofibrillar heart muscle disarray) can be seen using heart muscle examination electron microscopy or under the microscope with hematoxylin and eosin staining. There is a decreased left ventricular ejection fraction (LVEF). On rechallenge with more chemotherapy, progressive cardiomyopathy and sequential stress-related heart dysfunction will result.
- Only recently defined, Type II myocardial dysfunction involves the targeted agents (bevacizumab [Avastin], erlotinib [Tarceva], and cetuximab [Erbitux]) currently in use. Type II myocardial dysfunction is low-sequential stress-related cardiac dysfunction and is not dose related as far as we know but rather due to blocked signaling caused by trastuzumab (Herceptin). No electron microscope ultrastructural damage or microscopic abnormalities are evident on hematoxylin and eosin staining. There is a decreased LVEF, and it may be safe to rechallenge. For this type of toxicity, recovery usually occurs in two to four months.

In an analysis reported at the American Society of Clinical Oncologists June 2006 meeting, patients who received trastuzumab (Herceptin) concurrently with paclitaxel (Taxol) showed a very high disease-free survival benefit, but needed cardiac surveillance because of a possible decrease in LVEF. LVEF often decreases in patients given the standard treatment for breast cancer (doxorubicin and cyclophosphamide given over three months followed by paclitaxel and trastuzumab given for six months or longer depending on whether treatment is adjuvant or for metastatic disease). The addition of trastuzumab resulted in a 4.1 percent incidence of heart failure, compared with 0.8 percent in patients who did not receive the trastuzumab, representing a 3.3 percent increase in cardiac toxicity with heart failure. Most cardiac dysfunction was seen soon after the completion of treatment, although toxicity appeared later in some patients.

The National Surgery Adjuvant Breast Cancer Program, a national breast and colon treatment research organization, found that the greatest potential heart failure risk factor in breast cancer patients was age. The incidence of heart failure increased significantly in patients over sixty-five years of age.

Potential complicating toxic factors include the following:

- Smoking
- Prior left-sided heart irradiation for a left breast cancer, Hodgkin's, or non-Hodgkin's disease treatments
- Hypertensive medications (borderline associated, because of stress on the heart with hypertension)
- Diabetes
- Elevated cholesterol and lipids
- A family history of heart disease
- A baseline low normal LVEF, associated with a much higher incidence of heart

failure (14.5 percent) than in those who had a normal LVEF

- Patients over fifty years of age who had a low normal LVEF

There was a significant difference in LVEF when evaluations looked at declines in LVEF in patients who had a greater than 10 percent relative decline in LVEF. That is an important relative decline, often with symptoms of congestive heart failure. There was a decrease in all the patients who had symptomatic heart failure, but after eighteen months LVEF returned to normal in many of the patients.

Dr. Yuer from the M. D. Anderson Cancer Center recently published research demonstrating that trastuzumab-induced cardiotoxicity (cardiomyopathy) is potentially reversible, and patients can be treated through it with cardiac medications.[2]

There are currently no recommended patient monitoring schedules, but researchers suggest monitoring heart function (LVEF) every three months until nine months from treatment and again at eighteen months. If heart stability has been reached, further monitoring is unnecessary. For example, patients on long-term trastuzumab treatment who are stable after months of treatment probably don't need continued cardiac monitoring if they have metastatic disease. Here are some other suggestions:

- It is possible that treating with trastuzumab (Herceptin) first and then doxorubicin (Adriamycin) may reduce or eliminate this cardiotoxicity.
- Use of docetaxel (Taxotere), cyclophosphamide (Cytoxan), or carboplatin, or possibly a hormonal therapy alone is being tested in the metastatic setting. Infusions on weekly schedules could be used, or liposomal doxorubicin (Doxil) could be used as a substitute for doxorubicin (Adriamycin).
- Pharmacogenomics (heart genetic testing) could be helpful in determining which patients are susceptible to cardiac toxicity. Proteomics, or the study of the composition, structure, function, and interaction between proteins, could also prove useful to cancer research, as could microchip research technology to help predict the success or failure of a drug or drug combination.

The aromatase inhibitors have taken hold as first- or second-line breast cancer therapies. Studies of the effects of aromatase inhibitors on lipid profiles show that tamoxifen decreases cholesterol and increases high-density lipoprotein, whereas anastrozole (Arimidex), letrozole (Femara), and, to a lesser extent, exemestane (Aromasin) result in higher total cholesterol than tamoxifen (Nolvadex). Exemestane (Aromasin) seems to have a smaller effect.

Cardiac events are defined differently in all aromatase inhibitor trials. The aromatase inhibitors are associated with higher low-density lipoprotein (LDL) levels and less increase in high-density lipoprotein (HDL) levels. One study showed a greater risk of cardiac events with aromatase inhibitors.

Radiation Therapy Related

The overview data of mastectomy followed by left chest wall radiation demonstrated a higher incidence of mortality related to cardiovascular events, but recent data for breast-conserving therapy and radiation had lower all-cause mortality, suggesting that, at least at the fifteen-year follow-up, there is not an increase in cardiac events with chest wall irradiation.

For internal mammary lymph nodes (near the center of the chest, substernal), improved radiotherapy treatments where deep tangent radiation is chosen or superficially penetrating electrons and treatment planning with computed axial tomography (CAT) scans help minimize the heart exposure. A study of the Surveillance Epidemiology and End Results Medicare database of about 15,000 patients who had adjuvant radiation showed that with regard to cardiac disease up to ten years later, there was no difference in left- and right-sided radiation damage or toxicity.

Pulmonary Toxicity

Pulmonary toxicity after therapy with bleomycin (Blenoxane) or radiation is greater in cigarette smokers. Radiation has long-term side effects on other organs and tissues. The lungs can be affected by radiation to the chest and by treatment with bleomycin.

Chemotherapy can damage the endothelial (lung lining) cells, resulting in an inflammatory reaction or drug-induced pneumonia. This may be a part of an immunological mechanism (allergic reaction) damaging the lungs. There can be changes in the connective tissue with obliteration of the alveoli (lung air sacs) and dilation of air spaces. Bleomycin, used for many cancers including testicular and lymphoma, at dosages greater than 400 mg/m^2, has been implicated, as have other drugs including cytarabine (Cytosar), high-dose cyclophosphamide (Cytoxan), carmustine (BiCNU), mitomycin-C (Mutamycin), busulfan (Myleran), methotrexate (Amethopterin, Folex, Mexate), procarbazine (Matulane), liposomal doxorubicin (Doxil), docetaxel (Taxotere), and gemcitabine (Gemzar).

Pulmonary toxicity such as pneumonitis and fibrosis (scarring) can be a result of the radiation alone. This depends on the volume of irradiated lung and the dosage and daily radiation fractionation. Radiation destroys cells lining the alveoli (lung air sacs at the end of the bronchioli), and the alveoli become inflamed and accumulate fluid. This affects the passage of oxygen and carbon dioxide within the alveoli to the blood vessels.

When chemotherapy and radiation therapy are combined, the risk of cardiopulmonary toxicities increases.

Radiation recall (delayed radiation reaction) may occur with redness, blistering, and breakdown of the skin in the irradiated field. This is sometimes seen when radiation is given before or after anthracycline drugs.

Prevention of Cardiopulmonary Side Effects

There have been long-term survivors from many cancers, such as breast cancer, testicular cancer, Hodgkin's, and non-Hodgkin's lymphoma. Some of these patients have developed long-term cardiopulmonary toxicity because of cancer therapies.

Cyclic chemotherapy, with or without radiation, has been shown to lead to the development of subclinical and clinical abnormalities of heart ventricular function many years after treatment. Pulmonary fibrosis (lung scarring) and pneumonia hypersensitivity toxicities have occurred after radiation and chemotherapy. Valvular complications, myocardial infarctions (heart attacks), and restenosis (blocking of an artery) with coronary and carotid artery disease have also been observed after treatment.

Cardiopulmonary effects can occur soon after treatment or be delayed by many years. Significant cardiac changes often involve the LVEF showing electrocardiogram or echocardiogram changes indicating possible irreversible congestive heart muscle failure. Cardiac toxicity is most commonly seen with the use of anthracycline drugs such as doxorubicin (Adriamycin), epirubicin (Ellence), and mitoxantrone (Novantrone). There is damage to the heart muscle cells, resulting in loss of heart muscle fibers and cellular destruction with the cardiac muscle. Congestive cardiomyopathy (heart muscle abnormality) has been related to the dosage of anthracyclines and other drugs, such as high-dose cyclophosphamide (Cytoxan), fluorouracil (Adrucil, Efudex), paclitaxel (Taxol), ifosfamide (Ifex), and trastuzumab (Herceptin).

After radiation therapy to the left chest, cardiac toxicities have been reported in cases where large x-ray fields included the heart. This can occur years after treatment. Radiation-induced pericarditis (inflammation of the sac covering the heart) and blood vessel injury with thickening of the arterial walls leading to coronary or carotid artery disease have also been reported.

Fortunately, with new technology using computerized radiotherapy treatment (CAT scan) planning, the risk of radiation heart damage has been minimized. In recent years more sophisticated radiation therapy with better radiation dosing information and improved radiation delivery techniques have been used to help reduce potential toxicity. One needs to check for symptoms such as shortness of breath, chest heaviness or pain, and rapid heartbeat. A cardiopulmonary evaluation by a cardiologist and/or pulmonary specialist is essential. Other problems include swelling of the legs (from heart failure or possibly blood clots, which could lead to pulmonary emboli), fatigue, tiredness, and a low-grade fever.

A chest x-ray, CAT scan, electrocardiogram, echocardiogram, and physical examination are part of the standard assessment. The use of Doxil (doxorubicin within a fat capsule) may also be helpful because it is less cardiotoxic. Administering doxorubicin by prolonged intravenous infusions may help reduce the late toxicity, and newer drugs called radioprotectants (such as dexrazoxane) that have been developed for administration with the anthracyclines may help prevent or delay heart damage. Following a prudent, heart-healthy diet, exercising regularly, not using tobacco, and reducing stress are especially important for people who have had anthracyclines or left chest radiotherapy.

Renal Toxicity Side Effects

Patients treated with radiation therapy that included the kidneys or who received chemotherapy with any of the platinum compounds are at risk for kidney problems and possibly kidney failure. Platinum compounds (cisplatinum and carboplatin) can also result in some hearing loss, especially for high-frequency sounds rather than those in the speech range. Amifostine (Ethyol) has been effective in reducing platinum kidney toxicity.

Abdominal radiation can cause intestinal adhesions, malabsorption, chronic diarrhea, lactose intolerance, and subsequent discomfort and weight loss.

The Need for Long-Term Surveillance

After the completion of cancer therapy, patients who have received radiation or cardiopulmonary toxic chemotherapy drugs merit long-term follow-up. LVEF less than 45 percent, or a decrease of 5 percent or more from the resting level, is abnormal and merits careful assessment. Asymptomatic patients should have a baseline pretreatment echocardiogram and a yearly echocardiogram for the first five years and then periodic follow-up as indicated, at approximately three-year intervals, except for high-risk cases, which merit yearly echocardiograms.

A pulmonary consultation can also be very helpful. Pulmonary evaluations include chest x-ray, CAT scans of the chest, and pulmonary function tests to assess for any pulmonary toxicity. Careful follow-up is recommended.

Often oxygen combined with a special cardiac medication program can be very helpful in ameliorating cardiac or pulmonary symptoms.

22 Coping with the Side Effects of Chemotherapy and Radiation Therapy

Robert Ignoffo, Pharm.D., and Ernest H. Rosenbaum, M.D., F.A.C.P.

When you are ill, your overriding goal is to get well and return to an active life. If you are going to reach that goal, every part of your rehabilitation program is important: the psychological and social dimensions, nutrition, pain control, and all the others. But unless the side effects of treatment are ameliorated, you might not have the energy or even the desire to get back to a normal life. Side effects can be debilitating. They can sap your strength, weaken your resolve, and generally make life unpleasant. Some of the main problems include fatigue, nausea, vomiting, anorexia, loss of appetite, diarrhea, and constipation. Common solutions are provided in this chapter.

With support from the medical team, family, and friends, you can better manage these side effects and eventually overcome them. It may take quite an effort on your part, but the benefits will be well worth it.

Nausea and Vomiting

Nausea is a feeling of stomach distress or wooziness accompanied by a strong urge to vomit. Nausea and vomiting are temporary side effects of both chemotherapy and radiotherapy. They can also be brought on by an obstruction in the intestine, irritation of the gastrointestinal tract (gastritis), or a brain tumor.

Constant vomiting makes it impossible for you to eat or take fluids, so whatever can be done to reduce nausea should be done *before* vomiting starts. Paying attention to nausea's psychological causes and using antinausea drugs will help control what can be disturbing events.

Nausea and Chemotherapy Drugs

The goal of chemotherapy is to deliver a therapeutic amount of drugs with the fewest possible side effects. But each chemotherapy agent and each drug combination can cause nausea and vomiting. Getting three or four drugs at a time, which is often the case, can make the reaction even more severe. The dosage and the number of cycles to be given can also contribute to the reaction.

You, your family, and even your friends should talk with your doctor about the type of chemotherapy you'll be getting. For each drug, a program should be established so that you feel you have at least some control over the situation. With psychological factors playing such a big part, it is very important to be a participant in preventing nausea and vomiting.

Nausea Before and During Treatment

Fortunately, there are newer antinausea medications that greatly reduce side effects of chemotherapy. It is estimated that up to half of all people receiving chemotherapy will experience some nausea or vomiting not after they receive the drugs but before their treatment. This is known as anticipatory nausea and vomiting (ANV). ANV is the result of a conditioned reflex: If chemotherapy made you throw up once or twice, then you may feel nauseated whenever you take the treatment or even when something triggers the idea of treatment. This conditioned aversion often takes hold after two to four chemotherapy sessions and can last a long time. A standard joke among doctors is the one about the patient who met her oncologist on the street three years after therapy and threw up on the spot.

ANV usually makes nausea and vomiting even more severe when the chemotherapy is given. This can eventually become such a set psychological pattern that it affects the amount of chemotherapy that can be given. And once the psychological pattern of ANV is established, it is much harder to control nausea and vomiting before and after treatment. Fortunately, with newer antinausea medicine, ANV is greatly reduced and controlled.

Your anxiety state, how you feel about yourself and your cancer, and how you respond to stress and disease are all-important factors in setting up this psychological pattern. And once the pattern is established, all kinds of stimuli can trigger feelings of nausea: the colors or odors in the room where the chemotherapy is given, the smell of alcohol used to prepare you for the intravenous needle, or the sight of the nurse entering the room.

To deal with this problem, you will have to take steps to relax before your chemotherapy and to not inadvertently set up situations that become associated with nausea.

- Try to relax in a quiet, darkened room before your treatment sessions.
- Use behavioral techniques to help you relax and control any triggering stimuli: hypnosis, relaxation therapy, imagery, or listening to a tape of your favorite music or a relaxation tape.
- Perhaps try acupuncture or acupressure, which have been effective in controlling nausea or vomiting in some cases.
- The time of day when you get treatment can make a difference. If you have a problem with either the morning or the afternoon, try to change your appointment schedule.
- Avoid eating hot, spicy foods or other dishes that might upset your stomach or gastrointestinal tract.
- Eat slowly so you don't develop gas or heartburn.
- Try to avoid cooking odors that may bring on nausea by having friends or family prepare meals at their own homes and bring them over to you.
- Always avoid your favorite foods when you are getting chemotherapy. You might start to associate these foods with treatment, nausea, and vomiting and develop a strong aversion to them.

Nausea and Vomiting After Treatment

Nausea and vomiting are common side effects after chemotherapy or radiation therapy. They may begin one to three hours later or even as long as two to four days after treatment.

Like ANV, posttherapy nausea and vomiting can have significant therapeutic implications. You may start to fear therapy, a fear that can gnaw at you and make you want to avoid treatment. It may also make problems such as pain control and maintaining an overall good quality of life much harder to deal with.

Antinausea Medications

Two areas have been identified as being responsible for nausea and vomiting. Certain drugs and other methods can selectively block these areas. A wide variety of antinausea drugs have been developed, and some combination tailored to your specific needs usually will minimize or prevent the problem. Your doctor can work out a program to combat your nausea, although if one drug or drug combination doesn't work as well as you would both like, you may have to experiment with different programs. Generally, antivomiting drugs (antiemetics) should be taken thirty minutes before chemotherapy so that they have time to take effect.

- If vomiting has already started and you can't keep a pill down, antinausea suppositories such as prochlorperazine (Compazine) or trimethobenzamide (Tigan) may help.
- Long-acting prochlorperazine controlled-release capsules can be very helpful because they work for six hours.
- Lorazepam (Ativan) and dexamethasone (Decadron) may help block the brain's vomiting center. It is also a very powerful combination to block ANV. Lorazepam can be taken under the tongue for rapid absorption during severe nausea.
- Lorazepam is also an antidepressant and sleeping tablet that can cause amnesia, which might take the edge off any memory of vomiting once the episode is over.
- Some forms of marijuana—the natural delta-9-tetrahydrocannabinol (THC) and the synthetic form Marinol—may successfully control nausea and vomiting by working on the higher brain centers. But they can also cause drowsiness, dry mouth, dizziness, a rapid heartbeat, and sweating.
- 5-hydroxytryptamine antagonists such as ondansetron (Zofran), granisetron (Kytril), dolasetron (Anzemet), and palonosetron (Aloxi) are the most significant drugs used to control nausea and vomiting caused by intensive chemotherapy and radiotherapy. They work by linking to the 5-hydroxytryptamine receptor and preventing the release of serotonin, which stimulates the vomiting center. For delayed nausea and vomiting, aprepitant (Emend) has been very effective (used on days 1, 2, and 3), used in combination with ondansetron, granisetron, and palonosetron. These drugs may be needed when you are receiving chemotherapy drugs with the highest nausea potential or when you cannot get relief with other antinausea agents. They are often given with intravenous dexamethasone (Decadron) and lorazepam (Ativan). They suppress vomiting in 60–80 percent of patients and are even more effective in combination with other antinausea drugs.

Loss of Appetite

Loss of appetite, called anorexia, is one of the most common side effects of chemotherapy. It can also result from radiation therapy, stress and anxiety, depression, and the cancer itself.

For the sake of your health, your strength, and your ability to fight cancer, you have to get enough nutrition. But it's hard to keep your appetite when your mouth and tongue are sore or you have trouble swallowing. Fortunately, these side effects usually are short term, lasting only three to eight days. But even after they go away, you still might have trouble getting your normal appetite back.

You can talk to a dietitian, nurse, or doctor about ways to improve your appetite. If you don't seem to be making much progress, you might also ask your doctor about medications that can stimulate your appetite, such as the following:

- Prednisone, a corticosteroid hormone, in a short course at dosages of 10–20 mg a day.

Be aware that pneumonitis and greater susceptibility to infections have been seen in patients taking high-dose steroids.

- Megestrol acetate (Megace) 400 mg two or three times a day. It may take two to three weeks to observe an increase in weight.
- Marinol, a legally available synthetic form of marijuana in capsule form. It is usually used as an antinausea drug, but appetite stimulation is a positive side effect. Smoking or ingesting marijuana has also been effective.

Tips to Reduce Loss of Appetite

- Plan your meals in advance and arrange for help in preparing them. You might also better tolerate meals prepared by friends or family because cooking at home might produce offensive odors that will put you off food.
- Make your mealtimes a pleasant experience.
- Stimulate your appetite by exercising for five to ten minutes about thirty minutes before meals.
- Have an aperitif, such as a small glass of wine, before meals. It will help you relax and stimulate your taste buds.
- Relax for a few minutes before meals, using relaxation exercises.
- Eat frequent, small meals and have snacks between meals that appeal to your senses.
- Add extra protein to your diet. Fortify milk by adding 1 cup (250 mL) of nonfat dry milk to each quart (liter) of whole milk or milk recipe. Be creative with desserts. And use nutritional supplements (Carnation Instant Breakfast, Ensure, Scandishakes).

Taste Blindness

Many chemotherapy drugs can change your sense of taste and smell. What these changes are depends on the individual, but they are most common with foods that are either very sweet or very bitter. Oddly enough, sweet foods might taste sour and sour foods taste sweet. Chewed meat may have a bitter taste because of the release of proteins in your mouth. Sometimes there is a continuous metallic taste in your mouth after chemotherapy, which can affect what you eat and how you eat. Taste changes may not last long. But while you are experiencing them, you can do several things to lessen their effect:

- Brush your teeth several times a day and use mouth rinses such as diluted bicarbonate of soda.
- If foods and beverages taste bitter, add sweet fruits, honey, or NutraSweet.
- If meat tastes bitter, substitute bland chicken or fish, eggs, and mild cheeses or tofu. All of these might taste better if you use them in casseroles or stews.
- Marinate meats, chicken, or fish in pineapple juice, wine, Italian dressing, lemon juice, soy sauce, or sweet-and-sour sauce.
- Add whatever flavorings you enjoy, but avoid overdoing spicy, highly seasoned foods because this can cause oral and gastrointestinal discomfort.
- You might find that starchy foods such as bread, potatoes, and rice have a more acceptable taste if you eat them without butter or margarine.

Constipation and Impaction

Constipation means infrequent bowel movements. It also means a collection of dry, hard stools that get stuck in your rectum or colon. When you are constipated, you will often feel bloated and not have much of an appetite. If constipation persists, it may cause a stool impaction, a very large hard stool that you will have great difficulty passing.

It is important to try to prevent constipation and stool impaction, for both can cause great distress and pain. Patients with heart, respiratory, or gastrointestinal diseases can be especially aggravated by the discomfort and pressure of an impaction.

Causes

All kinds of things can make you constipated: lack of exercise, emotional stress, various drugs, or simply a lack of high-fiber or bulk-forming foods in your diet. Chemotherapy drugs such as vincristine, vinorelbine, and vinblastine often are constipating. So are narcotics such as morphine and codeine, gastrointestinal antispasmodics, antidepressants, diuretics, tranquilizers, sleeping pills, and calcium- and aluminum-based antacids. When prescribing these drugs, your doctor should anticipate the need for a stool softener (Colace or DOSS) or a mild laxative. Enemas or suppositories might also be needed.

Nutritional Hints to Prevent and Relieve Constipation

- Eat foods that are high in fiber and bulk. These include fresh fruits and vegetables (raw or cooked with skins and peels on), dried fruit, whole grain breads and cereals, and bran. Avoid raw fruits and vegetables, including lettuce, when your white blood cell count is lower than 1,800. *Note:* You should start a high-fiber diet before taking a chemotherapy drug that causes constipation.
- Drink plenty of fluids—eight to ten glasses a day. Avoid dehydration. Try to drink highly nutritious fluids (milkshakes, eggnogs, and juices) rather than water because liquids can be filling and may decrease your appetite.
- Add bran to your diet gradually. Start with 2 tsp (10 mL) per day and gradually work up to 4–6 tsp (20–30 mL) per day. Sprinkle bran on cereal or add it to meatloaf, stews, pancakes, baked goods, and other dishes. Dietary bran is helpful.
- Avoid refined foods such as white bread, starchy desserts, and candy. Also avoid chocolate, cheese, and eggs because these can be constipating.
- To make your bowel movements more regular, take prunes or a glass of prune juice in the morning or at night before bed. Prunes contain a natural laxative and fiber. Warmed prune juice and stewed prunes are the most effective.
- Eat a large breakfast with some type of hot beverage, such as tea, hot lemon water, or decaffeinated coffee.
- Get enough rest and eat at regular times in a relaxed atmosphere.
- Get some exercise to stimulate your intestinal reflexes and help restore normal elimination.

Laxatives and Stool Softeners

If you become constipated, talk to your doctor about a laxative program. It is essential to take laxatives, suppositories, and enemas only under your doctor's supervision. Don't try to diagnose and treat yourself because there may be more to the situation than you realize. For example, diarrhea can occasionally develop at the same time as a stool impaction, with the liquid stools moving around the impaction. If you decide to take antidiarrheal drugs, you can make the situation much worse.

There are many different ways to treat a wide variety of conditions, and your doctor may recommend several kinds of medications depending on your condition and other personal factors.

- Stool softeners help the stool retain water and keep it soft. Stool softeners such as docusate sodium (Colace or DOSS, 50–240 mg per day with a full glass of water, or Surfak) should be used early, before the stools become hard, especially because it can be days before any effect is noticeable.
- Mild laxatives help promote bowel activity. Examples are milk of magnesia, docusate, cascara sagrada, and mineral oil (a lubricant).
- Stronger laxatives include phosphosoda (Fleet), magnesium citrate, and senna (Senokot).
- Contact laxatives such as castor oil or bisacodyl (Dulcolax) suppositories or tablets increase bowel activity.

- Bulk laxatives include dietary fiber, bran, methyl cellulose (Cellothyl), and psyllium (Metamucil).
- Laxatives with magnesium should be avoided if you have kidney disease. Laxatives that contain magnesium can also cause diarrhea.
- Laxatives with sodium should be avoided if you have a heart problem.
- If you are taking narcotics, you should use stool softeners and mild laxatives rather than bulk-forming laxatives because the combination can cause high colon constipation.
- Nonstimulating bulk softeners such as docusate (Colace) help to soften the stool, and mineral oil or olive oil can be used to loosen the stool.
- Glycerin suppositories or bisacodyl (Dulcolax) suppositories may be used to stimulate bowel action as a contact laxative. Be aware that they can cause cramping.
- Bowel stimulants such as metoclopramide (Reglan) may be useful.
- Lactulose (Chronulac) is an acidifier that softens the stool and increases the number of bowel movements.

All laxatives should be used with care. If you use them continually, you might develop a gastrointestinal irritation that can make it difficult to regain your normal bowel habits once you stop taking them. Increasing dosages can also make your colon and rectum insensitive to the normal reflexes that stimulate a bowel movement.

Treating Stool Impaction

A stool impaction develops when all of a stool doesn't pass through the colon or rectum. The stool gradually gets harder and harder as water is absorbed by the bowel. Then the stool gets larger and larger. If you can't pass it, it may partially obstruct the bowel or cause irritation of the rectum or anus. If you do pass it, it may cause small tears or fissures in the anus.

The primary treatment is to get fluids into the bowel to soften the stool so it can be passed or removed. Using enemas—either oil-retention, tap water, or phosphate (Fleet)—may help accomplish this goal. Sometimes it might be necessary for a health professional to use a gloved finger in the rectum to break up a large bulky mass or to extract the stool.

Diarrhea

Diarrhea is a condition marked by abnormally frequent bowel movements that are more fluid than usual. It is sometimes accompanied by cramps.

You may get diarrhea because of chemotherapy, radiation therapy to the lower abdomen, malabsorption because of surgery to the bowel, or sometimes a bowel inflammation or infection. Some antibiotics, especially broad-spectrum antibiotics, can cause diarrhea, or it might develop because of intolerance to milk.

Treating Diarrhea

Effective treatment depends on finding the cause. A good general approach is to limit your diet solely to fluids to allow the bowel to rest. Drink plenty of mild liquids, such as fruit drinks (Kool-Aid and Gatorade), ginger ale, peach or apricot nectar, water, and weak tea. Hot and cold liquids and foods tend to increase intestinal muscle contractions and make the diarrhea worse, so they should be warm or at room temperature. Allow carbonated beverages to lose their fizz—stir with a spoon—before you drink them.

When you are feeling better, gradually add foods low in roughage and bulk—steamed rice, cream of rice, bananas, applesauce, mashed potatoes, dry toast, and crackers—eaten warm or at room temperature. As your diarrhea decreases, you may move on to a low-residue diet. Frequent small meals will be easier on your digestive tract. Low-residue nutritional supplements such as Precision

Low Residue, Vivonex, or Flexical, can also help.

Foods to Avoid

Many types of foods are likely to aggravate your diarrhea and should be avoided. These include the following:

- Fatty, greasy, and spicy foods
- Coffee, regular (nonherbal) teas, and carbonated beverages containing caffeine
- Citrus fruits such as oranges and grapefruit
- Foods high in bulk and fiber, such as bran, whole grain cereals and breads, popcorn, nuts, and raw vegetables and fruits (except apples)
- Beverages and foods generally that are served too hot or too cold

Replacing What Is Lost

Diarrhea can cause dehydration, so you will have to drink plenty of fluids. To replace the fluid, sugar, and salt you will lose, a good general formula is 1 quart (1 L) boiled water, 1 tsp (5 mL) salt, 1 tsp (5 mL) baking soda, 4 tsp (20 mL) sugar, and flavor to your taste. As with any specially prepared concoction, however, you should check with your dietitian or doctor to make sure you can tolerate the particular ingredients.

Potassium is also lost in diarrhea. It is a necessary mineral, and it must be replaced. Foods high in potassium include bananas, apricot and peach nectars, tomatoes, potatoes, broccoli, halibut, asparagus, citrus juices, Coca-Cola, and milk. Some patients may need supplementary potassium tablets.

Diarrhea Medications

- *Kaopectate:* Take 2–4 tbsp (25–50 mL) after each loose bowel movement.
- *Lomotil:* One or two tablets every four hours as needed. You can take Lomotil with Kaopectate or Imodium. Use a maximum of eight Lomotil tablets per day.
- *Imodium:* Two capsules initially, then one or two capsules every two to four hours. Use a maximum of sixteen capsules per day.
- *Paregoric:* Take 1 tsp (5 mL) four times a day. It may be used with Lomotil.
- *Questran:* A bile salt sequestering agent. Use one packet after each meal and at bedtime.
- *Donnatal or Robinul:* Anticholinergic, antispasmodic agents for bowel cramping. One to two tablets every four hours as needed.
- When all else fails, try Metamucil plus Kaopectate.

Milk Intolerance or Lactase Deficiency

Some people are born with lactose intolerance, and some develop it as they grow older. The intolerance results from a deficiency of lactase, an enzyme that digests milk sugar (lactose) in the intestine and is marked by cramping and diarrhea.

A lactase deficiency can sometimes develop after intestinal surgery, radiation therapy to the lower abdomen, or chemotherapy. Because you can no longer digest milk sugar properly, you feel bloated and experience cramping and diarrhea.

- If your diarrhea is caused by milk intolerance, you should avoid milk and milk products such as ice cream, cottage cheese, and cheese. Depending on how sensitive you are to milk, you may also have to avoid butter, cream, and sour cream.
- If you are very sensitive, look for lactose-free nonfat milk solids. You can even make your own lactose-free milk by adding Lactaid, a tablet containing lactase (an enzyme that digests milk), to your milk and keeping it in the refrigerator for twenty-four hours before using it.
- You can use buttermilk or yogurt because the lactose in them has already been processed and is digested. You might also tolerate some processed cheeses.

- You might try Mocha-Mix, Dairy Rich, and other soy products, or some lactose substitutes such as Imo (an imitation sour cream), Cool Whip, or Party Whip.

Oral Mucositis

Sol Silverman, D.D.S., and
Ernest H. Rosenbaum, M.D., F.A.C.P.

Oral mucositis, or mouth irritation, inflammation, sores, and pain, is a common and often severe effect of cancer radiation therapy and to cytotoxic chemotherapeutic agents administered singly or in combination. Mucositis manifests as varying degrees of inflammation (erythema), ulceration, and associated pain. The responses to these cancer treatments vary, depending on the agents used, dosages, and other factors such as immune competence, age, medical status, medications, and social habits.

When radiation is used as the only treatment modality, only the stratified squamous epithelium that lines the mouth and oropharynx is involved. The severity is influenced by the daily total dosages and duration of treatment.

When chemotherapeutic agents are administered, again the response depends on the drugs used and whether this is solo cycling, combined with head and neck radiation, or used as myelosuppression and tumor killing used with stem cell or marrow implantation to reconstitute blood cell elements. Chemotherapy-induced oral mucositis is a complex biologic response involving the entire mucosa (epithelium and connective tissue), immune competence, and oral microbial flora (mouth bacterium). These events are simultaneous and can be extremely severe and debilitating.

Grading of Oral Mucositis

There are several systems to grade the severity of the redness and ulcerations of oral mucositis. The most common is the five-grade World Health Organization system (0–4), with grades 3 and 4 being the most severe. In managing oral mucositis, the aim of intervention is to preclude or minimize grades 3 (unable to swallow solid foods) and 4 (unable to swallow any food). If successful, this leads to better patient compliance and attitudes, increases nutritional intake, reduces pain medication, avoids interruptions in therapy, shortens hospital stays, and lowers costs associated with treatment. In anticipation of a deficient dietary intake, tube feeding (nasogastric tube, gastrostomy) is a consideration. Intravenous protein, vitamin, and mineral supplements and liquids are critically important in minimizing complications of treatment.

Adverse Effects

The main adverse effect of mucositis is the pain that often precludes food and liquid intake. Dysphagia (difficulty swallowing) results in weight loss, dehydration, and depression. In addition to the mucositis, nausea and anorexia (loss of appetite) further complicate patient care. A common complaint of partial or complete loss of taste (dysgeusia or ageusia) is caused by alteration of the taste buds. Taste abnormalities often are accompanied by a decrease in saliva output. This leads to dry mouth (xerostomia). Xerostomia can result from radiation therapy or chemotherapy; however, with chemotherapy the symptoms are more transient.

Local infections are common with oral mucositis. Because of the ulcerations, bacterial infections from usually normal oral flora or opportunistic organisms can create pain and delay healing. When chemotherapeutic agents are used and leucopenia (a low white cell count) ensues, there is a risk of systemic infections and fever. There is often an overgrowth of fungi, usually candidal organisms, that can cause uncomfortable red or white mucosal changes. Lack of saliva contributes to fungal overgrowth. With chemotherapy, herpes viruses, usually stored asymptomatically in regional nerve ganglia, can migrate to the oral mucosa and lips and cause painful recurrent herpetic lesions. Herpetic lesions usually are manifested as ulcerations and associated redness (erythema).

Management

Optimal pretreatment and follow-up hygiene (office and home care) are essential in minimizing treatment sequelae. Also, managing any periodontal or tooth problems before treatment also minimizes the chances of an acute dental infection interfering with treatment or increasing pain.

If dryness is anticipated, applying fluoride topically by mouth rinses, toothbrushing, or gel applications will minimize tooth decalcification and dental decay. After radiation, healing after an invasive oral procedure may be delayed because of a permanent compromise in the blood supply to the mouth and jaw bones. When chemotherapy is involved, dental treatment should be delayed until the white cell count nears normal, except in emergencies. Dental x-rays for diagnosis are safe.

Agents used to prevent oral mucositis or accelerate healing if it occurs have been tested for many years. Unfortunately, meta-analyses following rigid criteria indicate that no single intervention is completely effective. Therefore, combination approaches are needed for optimal management.

Mouth rinses start with bland warm water–baking soda flushes. Antiseptic (antimicrobial) rinses have not been successful. Chlorhexidine is now made in a nonalcohol base and may be helpful, but there are no studies to support its use at present. Benzydamine is a nonsteroidal analgesic rinse that is not approved by the U.S. Food and Drug Administration (FDA) but has shown some benefits in preliminary studies. L-glutamine, an amino acid important in cell healing, has shown some promise and is awaiting FDA approval.

Amifostine is a scavenger for cellular free radicals. It is given subcutaneously. It has shown some near-term benefits in aiding saliva production but has questionable benefits for oral mucositis. The same holds true for intensity-modulated radiation therapy, used to maximize radiation energy to the tumor and spare adjacent normal tissues.

Palifermin (Kepivance) is a keratinocyte growth factor and has been shown to reduce grade 3 and 4 mucositis in patients with hematologic malignancies undergoing myelosuppressive stem cell transplant therapy. It plays an important role in the repair of damaged epithelial tissues. It is expensive and must be delivered intravenously. Toxicities have been rare, with skin rash being the most common.

Pain medications and corticosteroids have been helpful in reducing inflammation and pain and accelerating healing. Antibacterial, antifungal, and antiviral agents delivered systemically can often moderate but not prevent the signs and symptoms of mucositis. When there is immunosuppression (low white cell counts), increasing white cells to near normal values is essential.

Cryotherapy (using mouth ice chips) under certain conditions in administering cytotoxic drugs (e.g., bolus fluorouracil) may be helpful. The effectiveness and practicality of the soft laser warrant more study. There is insufficient evidence to support the effectiveness of either mucosal coating agents (e.g., sucralfate) or antimicrobial lozenges.

Newer agents to control malignancies are being developed to minimize the complications of cancer treatments. These are mainly targeted therapies. Cetuximab (Erbitux), a monoclonal antibody, is targeted for cellular epithelial growth factor receptors, but it has shown some activity even when receptors cannot be demonstrated. Cetuximab has shown effectiveness in improving control of head and neck cancers with apparent low toxicity. However, when cetuximab is combined with radiation, mucositis does occur, as do skin rashes.

With myelosuppression and lowering of blood platelets, bleeding from oral ulcerations or diseased gums can be of concern. Optimal hygiene is helpful here, and the use of soft bristle or foam toothbrushes will help prevent gingival abrasion.

Acute or chronic graft versus host disease, manifested by a mucosal reaction of inflammation, can cause oral discomfort and markedly affect the quality of life. Management involves the use of topical and systemic anti-inflammatory agents.

23 Fatigue

Ernest H. Rosenbaum, M.D., F.A.C.P.

Fatigue is the feeling of being tired after rest or a good sleep. It is one of the most common symptoms, affecting up to 90 percent of cancer patients, especially those under treatment. This commonly occurs after surgery, radiation therapy, chemotherapy, or immunotherapy with targeted agents. It can occur on the same day, for several days, or for long periods of time during and after therapy. Fatigue affects quality of life, the ability to function, and the capacity to live a productive, satisfactory life.

Fatigue is one of the most common problems during and after therapy, and an active fatigue reduction program may be needed. Both rest and exercise help in controlling debility and fatigue problems. In addition to treatment effects, fatigue can also be caused by emotional stress, anxiety, depression, pain, insomnia, hormonal problems such as hypothyroidism (low thyroid function), or anemia caused by cancer or its treatment.

Anemia is a reduction in the number of red blood cells (hemoglobin) that carry oxygen from the lungs and return carbon dioxide for elimination via the lungs. It is commonly diagnosed with a very simple blood test (hemoglobin or hematocrit) with instruments that measure the level of hemoglobin or count the number of red cells.

The bone marrow produces white cells, red cells, and platelets. When red blood cell production is reduced because of cancer, cancer chemotherapy, or radiation therapy, the level of functioning red cells in the body is deficient. This deficiency of red cells to carry oxygen can be one of the causes of fatigue.

Symptoms of anemia are tiredness, weakness, shortness of breath, dizziness, and possibly a decrease in heart function. Fatigue is common when a person has any type of chronic disease, including cancer, and can result from therapy, as when a patient has excess bleeding from surgery or reduced bone marrow function from radiation therapy or chemotherapy. Lack of iron, vitamin B_{12}, and folic acid can also cause anemia and can be detected easily. Fortunately, there are drugs that can help correct the anemia.

It is believed that pro-inflammatory mediators (immunological chemical cytokines, such as tumor necrosis factor) are triggered by malignant diseases, chemotherapy, immunotherapy, and radiotherapy, thereby causing fatigue. In a new approach, agents that block cytokine (chemical) production are used in clinical research trials to reduce fatigue and its symptoms. In progress are pilot research studies that use cytokine blockers of tumor necrosis factor alpha to reduce fatigue from chemotherapy.[1] A tumor necrosis factor, alpha antagonist infliximab, is being tested in clinical research to help reduce fatigue in breast cancer survivors.[2]

Modafinil (Provigil), a drug for treating sleep disorders, has been shown to improve cognitive function (concentration and attention) and mood and to reduce fatigue in patients with brain cancer. Memory and attention span improved by 21 percent, mood improved by 35 percent, and fatigue levels were reduced by 47 percent, thus improving quality of life.

Modafinil (Provigil) was reported at the 2006 Multinational Associated Supportive Cancer Care meeting to significantly reduce cancer-related fatigue in a one-month trial. It was effective in women with breast cancer who had fatigue up to two years after treatment.[3]

Managing Fatigue

Fatigue is one of the most common problems seen in cancer patients. The two basic rules for combating fatigue are rest and exercise. When you find that you are not able to function well because of fatigue, getting extra rest is important. At the same time, a daily exercise program can be very beneficial in helping to maintain and build up muscles that will help you in your daily life functions. You may need an aid such as a cane or walker, and if you're unable to do your housework, for example, you may need assistance for cleaning, cooking, and helping your family with transportation to their daily activities.

M. D. Anderson Cancer Center has developed a Brief Fatigue Inventory index using a scale of 0 to 10 (0 = *no fatigue,* 10 = *severe fatigue*) to rate the level of fatigue. This gives a general assessment of the level of fatigue. This index can be found at www.mdanderson.org/topics/fatigue.

Tips on managing fatigue include the following:

- Eat frequent small meals and high-protein foods.
- Nutritional supplements can be of some help, such as Ensure, Boost, and Scandishake.
- Maintain good fluid replacement with liquids and electrolyte-positive drinks.
- Plan your day's activities so that you do heavy activities at times of greatest strength.

Do not be shy; accepting help during this period is important. Fortunately, most people recover their strength, and as you regain strength, fatigue should subside, making the normal activities of daily life easier to achieve.

Try to schedule necessary tasks for times when you have less fatigue. Save your energy by being more organized; for example, plan your shopping trips with a list that is coordinated with the aisles in the store you use, or use a shopping service that delivers to your home. Accept help in carrying shopping bags to the car and from your family and friends when you get home. Shopping online is another option. Cooking is often a chore when you have fatigue. Cooking in larger quantities and freezing portions can allow you to save your strength for other activities. Accept help in cooking and housekeeping as needed.

You may be unable to do a full day's work, so planning and scheduling shorter but more productive hours may help you maintain a satisfactory workload.

Try to enjoy activities, both at home and outside, such as movies, music, and art, and spend leisure time with family and friends.

Use relaxation techniques, such as biofeedback, meditation, and other ways to relax that not only save energy but also promote happiness.

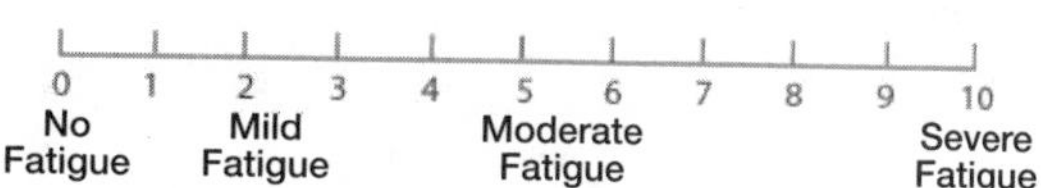

Fatigue Scale

Cancer-Related Fatigue and Sleep

There appears to be an association between cancer-related fatigue and disturbance in sleep patterns. A survey by Sarvaes and colleagues found that 40 percent of breast cancer survivors had fatigue problems after therapy, but most of them returned to a normal state with time.[4] Psychological factors such as depression and anxiety were also noted as contributing to fatigue, in addition to physical symptoms and sleep disturbances. Those who received chemotherapy had more significant symptoms and greater sleep difficulties. There is also a relationship between fatigue and psychological, social, cognitive, and behavioral factors.

Research is being performed to further elucidate the relationship between cancer-related fatigue and sleep disturbances, assessing a symptom cluster including pain, anxiety, and depression. The consequences of this combination of cancer-related fatigue (CRF), cardiorespiratory disturbances, and sleep disturbances include lack of concentration, difficulty making decisions, and irritability, all of which can affect family, school, work, and social life.

Ongoing research to define the causes of cancer-related fatigue, such as cytokine (cell chemical products) and hormonal imbalances, should lead to less debilitating cancer treatments. Also under assessment are efforts to establish the balance of exercise, work, and other activities, which may reduce fatigue and improve sleep patterns. Ways of better controlling pain, anxiety, and depression are being developed with improved treatment plans and symptom management.

Sleep Problems Specific to Cancer

Cancer patients may develop insomnia, caused by symptoms of the cancer itself, psychiatric problems, difficulty adapting to their new situation or condition, and drugs used to treat the cancer or its symptoms. Patients may not get adequate sleep if they are anxious in anticipation of a doctor visit or treatment. Patients awaiting surgery, chemotherapy, or radiation treatment tend to suffer from insomnia. Chemotherapy has also been shown to disrupt brain chemistry and some cognitive functioning, which in turn interferes with sleep. Pain may be caused by the underlying cancer, surgery, radiation treatment, or other treatments. Pain can make it more difficult to get to sleep or more difficult to stay asleep, or it may reduce sleep quality. Effective relief and control of pain may improve all of these problems.

Cancer patients often have breathing problems. Breathing may be more difficult because of the underlying cancer or other conditions such as asthma, emphysema, or congestive heart failure. Treatment focused on improving breathing should improve sleep quality and help a cancer patient feel more rested.

Anxiety and depression can seriously disturb sleep, especially for cancer patients. Fear of dying during sleep also prevents many cancer patients from getting adequate sleep. Anxiety and depression can be treated with medications, but changes in sleeping habits may improve sleep without a need for medications.

Finally, medication side effects can disturb sleep, particularly when cancer patients are treated with multiple medications. For example, pain medicines can cause daytime drowsiness, and antidepressants can cause insomnia. Caffeine and alcohol may also reduce sleep quality. Medications such as dexamethasone (a synthetic cortisone that can act as a stimulant) and tamoxifen (which can act as an antidepressant) change brain chemistry and often interfere with sleep patterns. A detailed review of medications and potential side effects is often of value. Talk to your pharmacist, doctor, or nurse.

24 The Role of Sleep in Health, Disease, and Therapy

David Claman, M.D.

Our knowledge about sleep and sleep disorders has increased dramatically since the 1950s, which is when rapid eye movement (REM) sleep was first described in the medical literature. Sleep is now viewed as an active state, with highly regulated physiological processes. Compared with a century ago, the average person today probably sleeps about one hour less per night, which makes sleep deprivation a common problem. Many people have disrupted sleep schedules, work drastically changing schedules, or simply do not spend enough hours sleeping. Many medical conditions may cause pain or discomfort that can disturb sleep.

Cancer patients have many potential physical and psychological problems. The sleep of cancer patients may be disturbed not only by physical pain or discomfort but also by psychological problems such as depression or anxiety over their condition or prognosis.

Stages of Sleep

A normal sleep pattern consists of the various REM and non-REM stages of sleep. People go through wakefulness (stages 1, 2, 3, and 4 of non-REM sleep) and then REM sleep. When you go to bed, you are awake for a few minutes and then go through the non-REM stages. The deepest sleep is in stages 3 and 4 of non-REM sleep, and the longest period of stages 3 and 4 occurs during the first one to two hours of sleep. This is when young children are likely to have night terrors and sleepwalking. During this period of deep sleep, the first period of dreaming or REM sleep occurs. At one- to two-hour intervals or more, REM periods occur throughout the night, so that in the early morning, most people have four to six separate dreaming periods. People usually remember the dreaming episodes only if they wake up immediately afterward.

A review article in the *New England Journal of Medicine* about sleep in older adults showed the normal patterns of sleep as the population ages. In the first few years of life, we sleep many more hours per day, and this amount slowly decreases through the age of twenty, by which time most people have settled into a stable pattern of sleep hours and sleep stages.

The amount of REM sleep as a percentage of sleep time remains fairly constant for many decades and may decrease only slightly in older adults. The total time in bed increases around sixty to seventy years of age, which is when many people retire from work. People have more time to go to bed earlier and tend to be in bed awake for longer periods of time, although they do not spend more time asleep. Sleep stages stay fairly constant over time, and sleep duration does not change significantly in later years.

The More Common Sleep Disorders

Purposeful Sleep Deprivation

Many of us undervalue sleep and take shortcuts when we go to bed and when we get up, so that we're not getting a full eight hours of sleep per night. The most common cause of sleepiness during the daytime is purposeful sleep deprivation.

Insomnia

Insomnia is by far the most common sleep disorder. From a survey done for the National Sleep Foundation in the early 1990s that studied how frequently insomnia was reported, we know that approximately 36 percent of the U.S. population has experienced either occasional insomnia or chronic insomnia. Nine percent of people currently report chronic insomnia.

Insomnia is a very subjective complaint. The first step in evaluating insomnia is asking whether the trouble is getting to sleep at bedtime, waking up frequently as the night goes on, or waking up too early and not being able to get back to sleep. The insomnia complaint can be a combination of these different problems. If you can't get to sleep at bedtime, it may be that caffeine is keeping you awake. Or perhaps you're worried or tense about different problems related to work, family, or your health that usually come up at bedtime. If you're waking up frequently at night, there may be physical or emotional reasons behind this. Waking up early in the morning could be related to stress or depression. Emotional causes are less common than physical problems, but they depend on the individual person, the problems involved, and the medications being prescribed.

There are four main categories of causes of insomnia: medical, psychiatric, situational, and pharmacologic. The more medical problems a person has, the more likely he or she is to complain of insomnia. This is an important area to focus on in patients who wake up with shortness of breath from lung problems, with ulcer pain, or with chronic arthritis in the hips, knees, or hands. Treating these medical problems should improve the sleep-related problems. Psychiatric problems are common causes of insomnia, especially in patients with depression, anxiety, or schizophrenia. It is estimated that about one-third of patients with chronic insomnia have some problem with depression or anxiety disorders. Situational concerns, such as tests, lectures, and job changes, can also cause insomnia. Most people in stressful situations that cause insomnia don't seek medical attention for it and hope that when the situation resolves, their sleeping will improve. Finally, many medications, both prescription and nonprescription, have sleep-related side effects. The two most common ones are caffeine and alcohol. If you drink caffeine in the evening, it may keep you awake at bedtime and be a cause of insomnia. If you drink alcohol at bedtime to get to sleep, and the alcohol wears off two or three hours later, you may find yourself waking up in the middle of the night and not being able to get back to sleep. Prescription drugs also have sleep-related side effects.

Important Factors in Insomnia

The factors that affect the development of insomnia can be classified as predisposing factors, precipitating factors, and perpetuating factors. Predisposing factors include personality type, sleep–wake cycle, and age. As the population ages, insomnia is a common subjective complaint. All of us struggle with occasional precipitating factors, such as changes in situation or environment, medical or psychiatric illnesses, or new prescription or nonprescription medication. Most people struggle with some amount of predisposing and precipitating factors, have a brief episode of insomnia, but slowly improve over time; they do not necessarily develop chronic insomnia or need to see a doctor about the problem. Most people who have chronic insomnia also have some perpetuating factors that reinforce the insomnia. Negative conditioning about sleep is particularly common (e.g., people might say, "I'm so tense about my sleeping problem that as soon as I go into my bedroom, I'm worried sick that I'm not going to sleep that night, and I lie awake for hours."). People with negative conditioning about sleep can lie in bed and sleep poorly. How can you relax and get to sleep when you are filled with tension and worry? Drugs, whether sleeping pills, caffeine, alcohol, or illicit drugs, can precipitate sleeping problems. Performance anxiety (e.g., "If I'm not asleep in the next ten minutes, I won't be able to do my job tomorrow.") is a common problem. A common perpetuating factor is poor sleep hygiene.

Sleep Hygiene

The best intervention for insomnia is a behavioral approach called sleep hygiene, or the development and maintenance of sleeping habits. The goal is to practice good sleeping habits so you sleep better and to avoid bad sleeping habits, which will make you sleep more poorly.

For good sleep hygiene:

- Maintain a regular schedule for going to bed and waking up, regardless of your weekend and weekday schedules.
- Avoid excessive time in bed. Spending too much time in bed can lead to frustration at not sleeping, and that will add to the insomnia problem.
- Avoid taking naps during the day. Taking a nap to catch up on sleep during the day means less sleep that night, reinforcing the bad sleeping pattern at night. Depending on your reasons for being sleep deprived, naps can be very beneficial or detrimental.
- Use the bed and bedroom for sleeping and sex only. Make the bed a pleasant place to be, not filled with anxiety. Sleeping and sex are pleasant activities that will be associated with positive conditioning.
- Do not watch the clock while in bed; this reinforces how much time has gone by and how worried you are about not sleeping.
- Do something relaxing before going to bed.
- Make the bedroom quiet and comfortable.
- Avoid taking the troubles of the day to bed with you.
- Avoid alcohol and caffeine.
- Try to get regular exercise, but not within two hours of bedtime.

Avoid using sleep medications if possible. Most people can make significant improvement by focusing on sleep hygiene.

Obstructive Sleep Apnea

Obstructive sleep apnea is estimated to affect 2–4 percent of the general population. Sleep apnea is a condition in which one stops breathing while sleeping. In adults, sleep apnea is almost always obstructive, meaning that the airway closes off and blocks breathing. The person tries to breathe and makes bigger and bigger efforts at breathing. Finally, the mind interrupts the sleeping pattern to restart the breathing again. The airway opens, and the breathing resumes, but this causes a disturbance in the brainwave sleeping pattern so that the person is not rested in the morning. Generally, there is a reduction in the blood oxygen level as a result of the absence of breathing. The body continues all its normal metabolic activities and uses up oxygen while the person is not breathing. Obstructive sleep apnea is a fairly common disorder, and it is diagnosable and treatable. The expert witness in cases of sleep apnea is often the sleep partner, and it's very important in the sleep clinic to talk to the sleep partner. The patient usually is unaware of the sleep apnea, and the sleep partner often can provide reliable information about the presence of snoring and episodes of interrupted breathing.

Treatment for Obstructive Sleep Apnea

There are a number of different treatments for obstructive sleep apnea:

- Weight loss is commonly recommended in sleep apnea because most patients with sleep apnea are overweight. Weight gain creates deposits of tissue in the neck. This accumulation makes the airways smaller and predisposes patients to sleep apnea. Patients who do lose weight generally reduce the severity of their sleep apnea.
- It is also recommended to avoid alcohol and sedatives near bedtime. Alcohol relaxes the muscles in the windpipe, making it more likely that your airways will close off and block breathing.
- Postural training involves sleeping only on your side rather than on your back. Many people with sleep apnea have more breathing problems when they sleep on their back, and patients are encouraged to sleep on their side. If sleeping on your side helps, sew one or two tennis balls in back of an old T-shirt so that if you roll over onto your back, you'll feel the tennis ball and roll back over on your side.
- Continuous positive airway pressure (CPAP) remains the most effective treatment. It is a recent treatment that involves wearing a mask that covers the nose; straps hold the mask in place, and an air hose connects the mask to a small air compressor that sits at the side of the bed. During sleep apnea, the throat muscles relax, and the airway locks shut. Blowing positive pressure into the windpipe helps keep the airway open to maintain normal breathing. Although cumbersome, CPAP treatment can eliminate 90–100 percent of the sleep apnea in affected people.
- Oral appliances are plastic bridges that fit the upper and lower teeth to hold the jaw in a more forward position. They are worn during sleep on an ongoing basis to provide some improvement.
- Surgery can be done for sleep apnea. Surgery offered a lot of promise originally, but it is not always successful, and CPAP often is used as the first treatment option. The value of surgery for sleep apnea depends on the severity of the sleep apnea and the patient's anatomy. Despite the risks and potential failure of surgery to cure apnea, it is clearly appropriate for some patients.

Circadian Rhythms

Circadian rhythms are rhythms of behavioral and physiological processing, which occur approximately every twenty-four hours. The strongest stimulus for circadian rhythms is sunlight, which makes sense from an evolutionary point of view, although social cues and exercise can also have an effect. This is how your mind and body know when to lie down and go to sleep and when it's time to wake up. Circadian rhythms are disrupted in two common situations: jet lag and shift work. In jet lag, the physical stimuli of bright sunlight and social interactions encourage realignment, and most people can adjust their circadian rhythms one to two hours per day according to sunlight and social activity.

In shift work, the physical stimuli—light and the social stimuli of family and friends—are both oriented to keeping you awake during the daytime. Most people with shift work try to sleep during the daylight hours several days per week but sleep at night on the weekends. The most effective way to perform shift work from a sleep point of view is to sleep during the daytime seven days a week. If you go back and forth, you're essentially getting jet lag from weekend to weekend, and your circadian rhythms usually stay oriented more toward being awake during the sunlight hours and sleeping at night. Most people in their twenties and thirties can handle shift work, but when they reach their fifties or sixties, it becomes too difficult.

Your need for sleep varies depending in part on your activities and habits (not all people need eight hours of sleep nightly). Prolonged lack of sleep reduces efficiency and the ability to function. How you sleep is important, too. If sleeping pills or pain medications are helpful in obtaining an adequate night's rest, they should be used. Resolving any perplexing and annoying emotional problems helps immeasurably. The use of relaxation techniques, meditation, and biofeedback is often invaluable.

Sleep Medications

If behavioral treatments (e.g., sleep hygiene) and symptom-specific medications (e.g., controlling pain with appropriate medications) are ineffective for treating insomnia, then a range of medication options are available. These include hypnotics, sedatives, and antidepressants. Hypnotics typically are shorter-acting medications with less chance of causing morning drowsiness. Sedatives typically have a longer duration of action and are more helpful if anxiety is also present. Antidepressants can be given to help reduce depression and anxiety (in order to help reduce insomnia) or as a sedating medication at bedtime. It is important to discuss with your physician which of these medications might be most helpful for you.

Understanding the multitude of physical and psychological problems that can disturb the sleep of cancer patients is the first step in finding appropriate assistance from the medical team or from family and friends. The first step to improve insomnia is to practice the good sleeping habits outlined in this chapter. Sleep disorders are diagnosable and treatable, and they should be discussed with the treating medical team. Improved sleep can help patients cope with the physical and psychological problems that occur in the setting of cancer.

25 Changes in Sexuality and Sexual Dysfunction[1]

Christine M. Derzko, M.D., David G. Bullard, Ph.D., and Ernest H. Rosenbaum, M.D., F.A.C.P.

Cancer affects all aspects of your life, so it's not surprising that it can affect your sexual feelings and the ways you express those feelings. You and your spouse or partner remain sexual beings and may have the same needs and desires as you had before the illness struck.

Sexuality can be expressed in many ways: in how we dress, move, and speak and through kissing, touching, masturbation, and intercourse. Changes in body image, tolerance for activity, and anxieties about survival, family, or finances can strain the expression of sexuality and can create concerns about sexual desirability. But if you were comfortable with and enjoyed your sexuality before your illness, the chances are excellent that you will be able to keep or regain a good sexual self-image despite any changes brought about by cancer.

Many people, particularly those dealing with an illness, find that being sexually active is not important to maintaining a loving, intimate relationship. This can be a healthy, rational choice for any individual or couple. However, the loss of interest may be transient for others, and they may be quite distressed by their loss of libido (sexual interest) or by their inability to respond or perform sexually as they had in the past. If sexual intimacy has been a joy and comfort to you, you may want to resume or continue being sexually active even after your cancer has been diagnosed and treated or while it is being treated.

Becoming sexually active again may entail some adaptation of your normal sexual patterns, and it might be difficult to change them. Support groups can give understanding and encouragement, and open, comfortable communication with your partner is essential. Make a point of sharing your concerns with your partner: He or she wants and needs to help sort out the problems. You may also need specific information and guidance from your doctor. The subject of sexual health for people with chronic illnesses, especially cancer, has been neglected for far too long. Members of your medical team may find it hard to initiate discussions about sexual problems. But don't make the mistake of trying to be a "good" patient by suffering in silence. Sexuality is a legitimate area of concern. Don't be shy: Take the initiative and ask your doctor any questions you have about your sexuality. Seek referral to a sexual counselor if needed. You can overcome many problems, reduce tensions, and get much more sexual satisfaction.

The Phases of Sexuality

Understanding the phases of sexuality and how cancer can affect one or more of them can help you increase your satisfaction with sex.

Desire

Desire varies from person to person, ranging from an uninterested, indifferent attitude that may or may not change with time to a very active desire for sex. Desire can often be increased by physical, visual, or fantasy stimulation. The initial emotional impact of a cancer diagnosis and its treatment may leave little or no energy for sexual desire. Depression or certain classes of medications can directly lower desire, as can treatment that alters hormone levels. Discussing your lack of interest with your doctor is important. It may be that alternative medications can be prescribed that do not have such a negative effect. Indeed, with some conditions, hormone replacement therapy, which may correct or at least improve the symptoms, may be appropriate. The important thing to remember is that you do have options. Explore them!

Excitement

The body reacts to stimulation with increased blood flow in the sex organs and increased heart rate and blood pressure. Sexual interest and stimulation are popularly thought to be characterized by an erection in men and increased vaginal lubrication in women. On the other hand, particularly after cancer therapy, a person may feel desire, yet those physiological responses may not follow.

Sexual problems often occur during the excitement phase. This can lead to anxiety and distress. Men may lose the ability to get or keep an erection. Women may not have enough vaginal lubrication for comfortable penetration, making intercourse difficult or painful.

Orgasm

This is a peak of pleasurable expression, followed by a gratifying relaxation. It is both a physical release and an emotional high.

Some men might ejaculate only after prolonged stimulation. Sometimes nothing happens despite prolonged effort. Or the ejaculate might be reversed into the bladder (retrograde) rather than going forward and out through the penis. In this case, orgasm still occurs, but there is no semen or liquid.

For women, the painful intercourse (dyspareunia) that sometimes follows cancer treatment can inhibit both enjoyment and orgasm. A number of treatments are available, so don't give up before you have explored the possibilities available to you.

Resolution

Many people feel relaxed and satisfied after sex regardless of whether they reach orgasm. For others who experience problems during the desire, excitement, or orgasm phases, the satisfying resolution may be replaced by sexual tension, discomfort in the pelvis, or emotional frustration.

Sexuality and Cancer

Treatment for some cancers may have little effect on sexuality beyond the effects of fatigue, pain, weakness, or other temporary side effects. However, two distinct questions and concerns may arise. First, the younger patient might wonder whether the treatment will affect his or her ability to have a family in the future and, if so, what can be done about it. The patient may also wonder whether the treatment will directly affect his or her sexual functioning and quality of life. It is important to recognize that lengthy treatments and impaired fertility may cause marital stress unless both partners are encouraged and willing to communicate their feelings. Chapter 26 deals specifically with fertility issues related to cancer therapy.

The Sexual Problems of Specific Cancers

The treatment of several kinds of cancer may directly affect sexual function.

Bladder Cancer

Surgical therapy for bladder cancer can lead to decreased desire, a reduced ability for men to get an erection, retrograde ejaculation, and orgasm problems, including a lower intensity. About half of women who undergo this therapy end up with a shorter and narrower vagina, making penetration more difficult. Communication with her partner will become especially important in such cases, as will the use of lubricants.

Breast Cancer

Psychological counseling and support groups are helpful for many women treated for breast cancer, given the symbolic sexual significance of the female breast. Thirty to 40 percent of women who have a modified radical mastectomy report sexual concerns; fewer sexual problems are reported if only a lumpectomy is performed, which results in less change to body image, but even 10 percent of women who have a benign biopsy may want to discuss sexual concerns.

Premature menopause after chemotherapy, hormone therapies, or radiation can cause a woman to feel loss of desire or even aversion for sex. When it can be done safely, treatment with low dosages of testosterone cream (not commercially available, but can be prepared by a compounding pharmacy) applied vaginally may help women regain desire and sexual enjoyment. It is hoped that women may have another option soon: the testosterone patch, which has been widely tested and shown to be effective in both naturally and surgically menopausal women distressed about their low sexual desire. Taking more time with sexual activities other than intercourse, using vaginal lubricants, reading erotic literature or watching erotic videotapes, and using sensory enhancements such as music, scented candles, and massage lotion are additional things to try. Of course, having a warm, caring, and communicative relationship with your partner is one of the best enhancers of sexual pleasure. The same applies to people without a partner, who can and should treat themselves with love and nurturing.

Colon Cancer

There is twice the amount of sexual dysfunction after surgery for colon cancer as there is after surgery for benign conditions such as an ileostomy for ulcerative colitis. Some preliminary data suggest that after endoscopic colectomy there may be less sexual dysfunction because there is less surgical disruption of pelvic innervation. People with ostomies may be embarrassed or worry about their partner's reaction, which might interfere with their sexual responsiveness. Direct communication with and reassurance from a partner can be very helpful.

Gynecological Tumors

A woman who undergoes gynecological cancer surgery with removal of the ovaries will have a sudden loss of estrogen, resulting in premature menopause. Sudden loss of ovarian function is associated with very intense symptoms of menopause: severe hot flashes, joint and muscle aches and pains, mood swings, sleeping problems, anxiety, and depression. Sexual partners often have a hard time coping with these changes. All this can reduce a couple's ability to have sex or their inclination to even think about it. With the feelings of abandonment and rejection that often follow, the relationship can suffer. But the right kind of help and counseling can help the couple talk about and cope with these problems. Seeking this help may be an important first step. Hormonal replacement therapy may also resolve some of these problems.

Hysterectomy and radiation treatment to the female genitals may lead to problems in the excitement phase. The surgery might also affect orgasm, and painful intercourse can be the result of lack of hormone (estrogen), caused by the premature failure of the ovaries, or of the radiation effects on the tissues. As a result, the frequency of intercourse might be reduced. Some women who have had hysterectomies for benign disease report similar problems: a decrease in sexual desire, especially in the first six months after the operation, with desire often returning to normal within a year.

Radical surgery to the vagina and vulva can change the physical aspects of the genitalia so that sexual activity can become very difficult both physically and psychologically because of the fear of pain or bleeding during intercourse. Plastic surgery to reconstruct the organs, along with sexual counseling, can be very helpful to some, whereas others may learn to enjoy lovemaking without intercourse.

Hodgkin's Disease

About 20 percent of men and women with this type of cancer lose energy and interest in sex. Hodgkin's disease doesn't usually affect the ability to get an erection, but in women, premature failure of the ovaries with the resulting lack of circulating estrogen may cause vaginal dryness, leading to painful intercourse. Although the ovarian failure may be permanent, return of ovarian function particularly in young women may occur, even several years later. In general, the shorter the treatment, the lower the dosage, and the younger the patient, the better the chance is that some recovery of ovarian function will occur.

Cancer of the Penis and Testicles

As challenging as it sounds, men who lose part of their penis may still be capable of getting erections, having orgasms, and ejaculating. Removal of the whole penis naturally can cause very severe sexual difficulties. But orgasm may still be possible with stimulation of the bones, pubis, perineum, and scrotum, and ejaculation through an urethrostomy is possible.

With testicular cancer, the sexual problems depend on the type of tumor. With nonseminoma, removal of a testicle and the lymph nodes in the area usually results in a decrease in fertility and sexual activity. Some men with seminoma who have had a testicle removed plus radiation therapy report low or no sexual activity, decreased desire, problems with erections and orgasms, and decreased volume of semen. Others continue to function and enjoy their sexuality. Individual responses vary widely, as in any aspect of sexuality.

Prostate

The diagnostic biopsy for prostate cancer might result in less ejaculate. Surgical removal of the prostate can cause similar problems, and with hormonal therapy the ability to get an erection and ejaculate may be lost or diminished. After treatment such as surgery, urinary incontinence might be a problem for some men, but this usually resolves within six months, although a few patients may take up to eighteen months to heal. Some men may require an absorbent pad for stress incontinence. It is important to consult with a urologist about aggressive therapy for erectile functioning after prostate surgery. This might entail injections or oral medication to help the erectile tissue heal.

Radiation produces problems, too, but only half as many as surgery. When the pelvic lymph nodes are removed and a radiation implant is used for localized tumors, 15–25 percent of men have difficulties with erections and about 30 percent have retrograde ejaculation. New nerve-sparing surgical approaches and new chemotherapy treatments help reduce erection and ejaculation problems. The phosphodiesterase 5 inhibitors, such as tadalafil (Cialis), vardenafil (Levitra), and sildenafil (Viagra), may help men regain erectile functioning after prostate cancer treatment. Radiation proctitis (rectal/anal inflammation) and cystitis (bladder inflammation) are other possible side effects of radiation to the prostate. Men who experience these conditions should consult with their physicians about symptom relief.

In one study, physical activity was positively correlated with sexual functioning for those who underwent external beam radiotherapy, but these results should be replicated and explored in a larger, longitudinal sample to ascertain whether the effects of physical activity in this at-risk population extend over time and protect men from treatment-related decrements in sexual functioning.[2]

Testosterone is important for libido and sexual performance in men. Hypogonadism (small testicles) caused by androgen deprivation therapy (ADT) causes a decrease in sexual desire, early morning erections, and potency. Other factors include age and social conditions. Only about 2 percent of androgen-deprived men can have intercourse. Unfortunately, there's no way to improve libido in these survivors. Some who do retain libido have erectile dysfunction, and recently drugs such as sildenafil (Viagra) help improve performance.

Drugs That Affect Sexual Desire and Activity

Most cancers occur in people over fifty, many of whom have already experienced some decrease in sexual activity. The diagnosis of cancer itself may result in a significant reduction in sexual desire, as can such diseases as diabetes, alcoholism, and psychological problems. Furthermore, it is important to know that a great many drugs can lower sexual desire and activity and therefore can lead to sexual dysfunction.

Use of some medications in the following categories may be associated with sexual difficulties. It is always important to take the medication your medical provider prescribes for you. But if you are experiencing sexual difficulties and you are taking any drugs from the following categories, you should be aware that the problem may be related to your medication. It is worthwhile to ask whether your problem is drug related and whether an alternative preparation or drug is available and appropriate.

- Alcohol
- Anticancer drugs and hormones
- Anticonvulsants
- Antidepressants
- Antihypertensives, including beta blockers (at high dosages)
- Carbonic anhydrase inhibitors
- Codeine or other narcotics
- Cytotoxic drugs
- Digitalis family
- Diuretics
- H_2 receptor antagonists
- Hallucinogenic drugs
- Hormone blockers
- Nonsteroidal anti-inflammatory drugs
- Opiates
- Pain medications
- Psychedelic drugs
- Recreational drugs
  - Tobacco
  - Alcohol
  - Opiates
- Sleep medications
- Tranquilizers

Treatments to the Genitals or Reproductive Organs

Even the prospect of surgery or radiation treatments for these cancers can make you intensely concerned about your body image. But it is usually impossible to predict the effects of treatment for any one person. Treatment can affect some people's ability to get erections, ejaculate, or have intercourse. The same treatment for someone else might result in little or no change in sexual functioning.

Anxiety

Sexual problems that seem to be the physical results of treatment may actually be caused by anxiety. You can reduce your worry by discussing potential problems and possible solutions before or after treatment with your doctor, other members of the healthcare team, or support group members who have gone through similar experiences. This discussion will also reassure you that if problems do come up there are ways of handling them. Because in most situations physical and emotional causes of sexual problems interact, your exploration and experimentation about what you can do are very important. Your diagnosis does not dictate what is possible for you sexually.

Painful Intercourse

You may find that intercourse is painful not only after treatment for a genital cancer but also if pelvic or total body radiation has been part of your therapy. There are four common reasons why this problem may arise:

- Infections of the bladder or vagina (this may be a recurring problem)
- Lack of lubrication
- Vaginal shortening
- Anxiety with resulting spasm of the vaginal muscles

Ask your doctor for a gynecological examination to find the cause.

Infection

Vaginal or bladder infections are common and may cause painful intercourse in any woman, including a woman recovering from cancer therapy. These conditions are readily treatable. Vaginal infections can be treated either *locally* (with vaginal cream or suppositories) or *systemically;* whereas bladder infections are treated with systemic antibiotics. A yeast infection (with or without a discharge) may result from treatment with some systemic antibiotics, and this possibility should be considered when intercourse becomes uncomfortable or painful during or after a course of antibiotics.

Lack of Lubrication

The vagina may feel dry in the presence of a yeast infection. But if this cause is ruled out, commonly there are two other reasons: inadequate estrogen effect and lack of adequate sexual arousal.

Estrogen is produced normally during reproductive life by the ovaries. Surgical removal of the ovaries permanently deprives the body of this natural source of female hormones. Chemotherapy and radiation therapy may temporarily or permanently stop the production of estrogen. This removal of estrogen may be a necessary part of the treatment of the primary cancer (e.g., breast cancer and uterine [endometrial] cancer but not cervical cancer). Your doctor will be able to tell you whether it is necessary, and you should therefore feel free to discuss the question with him or her. Unless estrogen deprivation is essential to your management, and particularly if you are in your forties or younger, hormonal therapy with an estrogen is almost certainly appropriate for you and can be prescribed by your doctor. This may be true even after breast cancer therapy, particularly if the disease is receptor negative. However, any decision to initiate hormone treatment must be made in conjunction with your oncologist or gynecologist.

Hormonal therapy (HT) may take the form of either *systemic* medication such as pills, patches, gels, injections, or implants or *local* vaginal applications of creams, an estrogen-containing vaginal ring, vaginal tablets, or suppositories. Often, despite use of adequate systemic dosages of hormones, additional vaginal estrogen therapy is needed to relieve vaginal dryness.

It may take many months for HT, local or systemic, to return the vagina to normal and improve lubrication. A change of dosage is sometimes needed to achieve more rapid relief from symptoms. More commonly, though, healing brought about by time is what is needed. Keep in mind that many couples, even those without any health problems, find that they need to use a vaginal lubricant for intercourse. Estrogen cream is not meant to be used for this purpose.

If the cause is not enough lubrication, use of saliva, a natural lubricant, or water-soluble lubricants can reduce friction. Artificial lubricants such as K-Y Jelly, Astroglide, and other creams may make coitus (intercourse) possible where the lack of circulating estrogens has caused dryness. Replens (a nonhormonal vaginal gel that is available without prescription in the United States and Canada) is a vaginal moisturizer that is applied three times a week and may improve lubrication for sexual arousal and intercourse. In some cases, small amounts (one-third to one-half an applicator) of a poorly absorbed estrogen such as Premarin may help restore lubrication and atrophy of the vagina. However, if breast cancer has been diagnosed, use of even small amounts of estrogen may be discouraged. Discuss this with your doctor.

Shortening of the Vagina

Surgery or radiation therapy can cause shortening of the vagina or make the vagina less elastic. Either situation may make intercourse difficult. Your doctor may recommend dilators to exercise and stretch the vagina. Getting back to intercourse soon after treatment can also help prevent these problems. Different positions during intercourse, especially sitting or lying on top of your partner, may let you move in pleasurable ways. Although significant improvement can be expected after the first month of treatment with local estrogen-containing products (e.g., Premarin cream, Vagifem vaginal estrogen tablets, or the Estring vaginal estradiol ring), it often takes six to twelve months, or more, to fully restore the genitourinary tract to its normal state. This time lag also occurs when systemic therapy is used.

Vaginal dilators require prolonged regular use before they achieve maximal lengthening and stretching of the vagina. If treatment is begun early, a more rapid response can be expected. The penis is an excellent dilator; therefore, repeated attempts at intercourse with adequate lubrication (natural or artificial), gentleness, and persistence are likely to succeed.

Do not be discouraged if initial attempts at penetration or complete penetration are unsuccessful or painful. Several months of treatment with hormone creams may be needed before the tissues soften adequately to allow penetration to occur.

Anxiety

Fear and anxiety may prevent the normal flow of vaginal fluids in response to sexual stimulation. Correction of this situation entails a number of combined treatments: application of a lubricating cream or gel, relaxation, and, most importantly, communication with your partner. Taking a little more time to enjoy foreplay may promote relaxation, enhance sexual response, and increase vaginal lubrication.

Sometimes anxiety can lead to a spasm of the pelvic muscles, which blocks the vaginal passage and prevents penetration. Forceful attempts at penetration may be both painful and frustrating. Consultation with a sex counselor may help you overcome the problem. This condition is readily treatable, so do not be discouraged if your initial attempts are unsuccessful.

Time, patience, sharing your feelings with your partner and support group members, and seeking help from your doctor and possibly also a sexual counselor are your best guarantees of improving your sexual and intimate experiences.

Expressing Yourself Sexually After Treatment

With all the possible effects of cancer treatment, the prospect of having a normal sex life may seem out of reach. But whatever your cancer, there are steps you can take that will help you increase your sexual enjoyment.

If You've Had an Ostomy

People with ostomies and their partners have to learn about ostomy appearance, care, and control. Women may be comfortable wearing special undergarments that cover a pouch while still permitting sexual stimulation. Specially designed and aesthetically attractive pouches are available.

If You've Had a Laryngectomy

Laryngectomy patients should learn how to deal with sounds and odors escaping from their stomas. Wearing a stoma shield or T-shirt will muffle the sound of breathing and will keep your partner from feeling the air that is pushed through the stoma.

If You've Had a Mastectomy

After a mastectomy, you may be worried about how you look. Undressing in front of your partner or sleeping in the nude may feel awkward. That's natural, especially in light of the overemphasis our culture places on the sexual significance of breasts. Grieving over what you have lost is important. But with time and patience, most women overcome their self-consciousness and feel secure and comfortable with their bodies again.

- Some women have found it helpful to explore and touch their bodies, including the area of the scar, while nude in front of a mirror. You may want to try this alone at first and then with a spouse, lover, or close friend. Share your feelings about your new body.
- Be aware that your partner may not know what to say. Your spouse or lover may not know how or when to bring up the topic of sexuality and so may wait for you to do it. Your partner may be afraid of hurting or embarrassing you and want to protect your feelings. Sometimes this "protection" may feel like rejection. Although you might feel that it's risky to break the ice and approach the topic yourself, most patients and their partners feel relieved once they've done it.
- You both may also worry about pain. If your incision or muscles are tender, minimize the pressure on your chest area. If you lie on your unaffected side, you can have more control over your movements and reduce any irritation to the incision. If your partner is on top, you may protect the affected area by putting your hand under your chin and your arm against your chest.
- If you feel any pain, stop and let your partner know why you are stopping. If he or she knows that you'll speak up when you notice any pain, you will both feel more relaxed and less inhibited in exploring and experimenting. Taking a rest or changing position may help you relax, and relaxing will usually decrease any pain. You can also apply extra lubrication. With communication and cooperation, you can work together to find positions and activities that give you the most pleasure.
- Experimentation and time seem to be the keys to finding satisfactory ways of adapting to the loss of such a symbolically important part of the body as the breast. Talking with other women who have had mastectomies—women from the American Cancer Society's or the Canadian Cancer Society's Reach to Recovery programs or other support groups, for example—can provide support, encouragement, and suggestions about clothes and prostheses.
- Some women find breast reconstruction important for their emotional well-being, whereas others find that they learn to love and appreciate their altered bodies over time.
- Treatment with testosterone cream may also be beneficial.

If You Have Trouble Reaching Orgasm

The natural interruption in the ability to experience sexual pleasure after an illness may make having orgasms more difficult for some women. If this is a problem for you, learning to reexplore pleasurable body sensations may be helpful.

It is important to do this when you can be alone and not distracted by having to please or perform for your partner. So find a comfortable place where you can be alone—your bedroom or bathroom—and a time when you won't be interrupted. Undress slowly and gently stroke your whole body. Then focus on the most sensitive areas—your neck, breasts, thighs, genitals, or any other area that feels good to you.

Use different kinds of touch, soft and light, firm and strong. Try moistening your hands with oil, lotion, or soap. Pay attention to the sensations you feel and discover which ones are most pleasurable. Learning which kinds of touch feel best will help you heighten your sensation and will give you information to share with your partner. There are many excellent books on women's sexuality that can help to make you comfortable with this kind of exploration.

If You're Having Trouble with Erections

Because some drugs can temporarily interfere with the ability to have erections, you may want to ask your physician about possible side effects of your treatment.

Physical and Emotional Causes

If you can get an erection by masturbating or you wake up with an erection in the night or morning, it is most likely that anxiety or trying too hard is the cause, and it's not a physical problem. If you are not sure of the cause, ask your doctor to refer you to a urologist or sex therapist for evaluation and treatment.

Taking the Pressure Off

The more options you have for sexual expression, the less pressure there is on having erections. This in turn makes it more likely that they will happen. Many couples report that they have learned to have very pleasurable sexual experiences without erections or intercourse. Many kinds of sexual expression and stimulation do not require an erect penis. It may be reassuring to know that to have an orgasm many women need or prefer direct stimulation by hand or mouth on or around the clitoris. This is stimulation that even an erect penis in a vagina can't provide.

If you explore other kinds of sexual touching and expression for a while, you may discover that erections will return with time or that the increased variety of sexual options satisfies both you and your partner. Patience, communication, and time are critical factors in developing pleasurable sexual experiences.

Counseling

If erections don't come back and intercourse is important to you and your partner, ask your doctor to refer you to a sex therapist for counseling. Counseling will help you with relaxation techniques, planning time for proper stimulation, and methods for using visual stimulation and fantasy. Cancer survivors who have had the same problem report that group counseling can also help.

A number of new medications for erection problems have come on the market in the last few years. Taken before a sexual encounter, these medications increase blood flow to the penis, resulting in erections. The first of these, sildenafil (Viagra), became available in late 1997, followed by vardenafil (Levitra) and tadalafil (Cialis). They differ in onset of action, duration of action, and interaction with food. Sildenafil and vardenafil should be taken on an empty stomach for optimal effect and have an onset of action of thirty to sixty minutes and a duration of action of about four hours. On the other hand, tadalafil can be taken without regard to meals and has an onset of action of about forty-five minutes and a duration of action of twenty-four to thirty-six hours. Side effects include headaches, visual disturbances, and flushing. Though considered generally safe for most men (including those using most blood pressure medications), sildenafil, vardenafil, and tadalafil should not be used by men taking nitrates. Medical clearance is essential before use of these drugs. Other medications are becoming available, so discuss the appropriateness of their use in your case.

If even with the help of these medications you are still not getting erections, the counselor may refer you to a urologist. Together with you and your counselor, the urologist can explore options such as use of a vacuum pump, injection therapy, or a penile implant.

Hormone Deprivation Therapy for Prostate Cancer

Prostate cancer is the most common form of male cancer, and the most common treatment is androgen deprivation therapy (ADT) by either surgical orchiectomy (removal of the testicles) or medical orchiectomy with gonadotropin-releasing hormone. In addition to the possible side effects of osteoporosis and metabolic syndrome, it can cause sexual dysfunction, hot flashes, and gynecomastia (enlarged breasts).

Hot Flashes

The major effect on quality of life is hot flashes. This vasomotor instability involves a sudden perception of heat, usually in the upper body, reddening of the skin, sudden sweating, and often a chill that lasts for seconds to hours. Hot flashes can be mild or severe. Occasionally anxiety, agitation, and impaired cognition occur. Estrogen deficiency may affect the brain's hypothalamic thermoregulatory zone, which then triggers a heat loss mechanism, resulting in a hot flash.[3]

Men with even mild hypogonadism (small testicles) can have hot flashes. In older adults this is often associated with decreased testosterone levels. Estradiol is produced mainly via aromatization of testosterone. Estradiol levels are also low in hypergonadal men. Hot flashes are common in patients undergoing ADT: Approximately 70 percent are symptomatic with hot flashes. Therapy includes the following:

- Estrogen as a means of castration
- Complete androgen blockade (orchiectomy or gonadotropin-releasing hormone analogs plus flutamide)
- The use of transdermal estrogen
- Low-dose estrogen (0.05–0.10 mg)
- 20 mg megestrol twice a day to reduce the frequency of hot flashes
- Antidepressants, such as venlafaxine (Effexor) 12.5 mg twice a day, to reduce the frequency of hot flashes.

Gynecomastia (Enlarged Breasts)

Gynecomastia, a benign proliferation of glandular breast tissue in the breast area, is a common side effect of ADT, which causes an increase in the ratio of estrogen to testosterone. Men receiving antiandrogens (flutamide, bicalutamide [Casodex]) have a 60–80 percent higher incidence of gynecomastia than those in the general population. This is probably because the androgen receptors on the pituitary gland result in loss of negative feedback by circulating androgens. This leads to an increase in leuteinizing hormone and testosterone levels, ultimately resulting in higher estrogen levels. The incidence is 13–32 percent.[4]

Treatments include subcutaneous mastectomy or liposuction. Prophylactic radiation before ADT therapy has had good results. Tamoxifen 10 mg per day in men on bicalutamide was comparable to radiation therapy. One study showed that tamoxifen was superior to anastrozole (aromatase inhibitor) in preventing gynecomastia.

Hormone Replacement Therapy in Women

Estrogens from Reproductive Life to Menopause

From puberty to menopause the ovaries produce estrogen (estradiol), and when ovulation occurs, progesterone is added. The ovaries also produce the male hormones testosterone and androstenedione. Estrogen and progesterone act on their target organs, so called because they contain specific receptors or receiving areas where these hormones can enter the cell and produce the necessary effect. The target organs for estrogen and progesterone are the breasts, vulva, vagina, uterus, urethra, bladder, skin, and parts of the brain that control mood, sleep (insomnia), and temperature (hot flashes).

After menopause, the ovaries secrete very little estradiol, so the total amount of estrogen in the body drops to only a fraction of that produced during reproductive life. As a result, an alternative but small source of estrogen becomes significant. Male hormones continue to be produced by the adrenal gland—and, importantly, also by the ovary—for about five years after menopause. The increased facial hair which many women report in the early postmenopausal years is the result of the male hormones that continue to be secreted. These male hormones are carried to the skin, liver, body fat, and brain, where they are converted to a weak but effective estrogen, estrone. Body fat is a particularly important site of estrone production; it has long been recognized that women with more body fat have higher circulating estrone levels.

Why Is Estrogen Important?

The degree to which estrogen affects the tissues becomes evident after menopause, when levels of estrogen drop. After menopause, the deficiency in estrogen causes obvious symptoms such as hot flashes, insomnia, vaginal dryness, increased urinary frequency, increased incidence of bladder and vaginal infections, and, in the long term, osteoporosis and a predisposition to arteriosclerosis. Hormone therapy (HT) provides symptomatic relief whenever it is begun, and it is particularly important when the production of estrogen stops prematurely (before the age of forty)[5] because the long-term consequences (bone loss and cardiovascular problems) often are even more significant.

What Are Menopause and Premature Ovarian Failure?

Menopause means that the periods *(menses)* have stopped *(pause)*. Menopause occurs naturally around age fifty. However, radiation, chemotherapy, or surgical removal of the ovaries before menopause results in ovarian hormone deficiency even earlier. In younger women who have experienced premature ovarian failure as a result of chemotherapy or radiation therapy, the ovaries may begin to function again later. Although we are unable to predict whether this will occur, factors that appear to play a role are the woman's age and the type and amount of chemotherapy or radiation. Until ovarian function resumes, these women should be on hormonal replacement therapy and, if pregnancy is not desired, on some form of contraception.

Hormone therapy prescribed after menopause often is called estrogen therapy or hormone therapy (HT), which usually means estrogen with progestin. The use of progestin is currently being reevaluated, so consult your doctor.

HT Medications

There are many possibilities for hormonal replacement therapy. Nonsmoking reproductive-aged women with premature ovarian failure often are best treated with birth control pills (oral contraceptives), which contain adequate amounts of both estrogen and progestin. The advantage of this approach is that the higher dosage of hormones in birth control pills is what is often needed to control estrogen deficiency symptoms in younger women, and it provides contraceptive protection if the ovaries begin to function again. *Because of the risk of breast and endometrial cancer, use of these hormones should be discussed with your doctor.*

When vaginal or urinary symptoms persist despite systemic HT, local HT may be added. This may be in the form of estrogen vaginal cream (Premarin), vaginal estrogen tablets (Vagifem), or a vaginal estrogen ring (Estring).

Standard HT consists of estrogen preparations, which include oral estrogens such as conjugated estrogen tablets (Premarin), estropipate (Ogen), and estradiol (Estrace); estrogen gel (EstroGel); or a transdermal estrogen patch (Estradot, Estraderm, or Climara). Women who have not had a hysterectomy need to add a progestin—either medroxyprogesterone acetate (Provera), norethindrone (Norlutate), or progesterone (Prometrium). Estrogen–progestin combinations may be used together, continuously (nonstop) or cyclically (i.e., estrogen alone for about two weeks, then estrogen with the addition of a progestin for an additional ten to fifteen days). Two products that contain a combination of estrogen and progestin are available: Estalis, a transdermal estradiol–norethindrone patch, and FemHRT, an oral pill that contains ethinyl estradiol and norethindrone. *Because of the risk of breast and endometrial cancer, use of these hormones should be discussed with your doctor.*

Another possibility is an implant under the skin (subdermal implant of 17ß estradiol), which must be replaced every six months. This preparation is not available for use in Canada. For many years a popular form of postmenopausal replacement therapy has been an injection of Climacteron, Depo-Testadiol, or Dura-Testin, which is a combination of estradiol and testosterone that is given intramuscularly every six weeks. This preparation not only treats estrogen deficiency symptoms but also may improve libido as a result of the testosterone in the mixture. Occasionally, a small dose of testosterone is prescribed alone, specifically to treat problems of decreased libido. Oral tablets of testosterone undecanoate (Andriol) may be used two to three times per week, and are available on prescription. Testosterone creams and gels in dosages appropriate for women are not commercially available but can be compounded by some pharmacies for topical transdermal applications. A testosterone patch (Intrinsa) has been widely tested in North America and found to be effective in the treatment of women distressed about their problem of low libido. The testosterone patch is under review by Health Canada, and it is hoped that they will approve the use of this product in the near future.

Treatment Regimens

Estrogen with or without a progestin may be given cyclically (resulting in menstrual periods) or in a continuous combined nonstop regimen (no menstrual periods). A common regimen using both estrogen and progestin is to give estrogen alone for fourteen to fifteen days, then add progestin (such as Provera) for seven to fourteen days. Both hormones are then stopped, and a period follows in one or two days. The cycle is repeated monthly.

Similarly, if continuous estrogen is given and progestin is added only for twelve to fourteen days, a period is expected one or two days after the progestin is stopped. This regimen is commonly used with transdermal preparations. *Because of the risk of breast and endometrial cancer, use of these hormones should be discussed with your doctor.*

For women who do not want to have a period but need HT, a combined regimen of estrogen and progestin is given continuously. After a short adjustment period (approximately six months) during which some vaginal bleeding may occur, most women enjoy all the benefits of HT, including relief of hot flashes, insomnia, and vaginal and urinary symptoms. Obvious early benefits include a reduction in hot flashes and night sweats and more restful sleep. Some women also report a sense of increased well-being.

After a few months of treatment, women may notice other beneficial effects. The vagina and cervix can be expected to become healthier and more moist with increased vaginal secretion and better lubrication during intercourse. Many women also report increased sexual awareness and enhanced sexual response after starting HT. In addition, fewer bladder and vaginal infections occur. However, there may be some normal but undesirable effects as well, including increased sensitivity and sometimes tenderness of the breasts, increased vaginal discharge, and the return of menstruation.

Patients with breast cancer should consult with their doctor about taking progesterone.

Is HT for You?

Whether systemic HT is appropriate or likely to prove beneficial for you can best be determined by your doctor. Talk to him or her about the possibility of this treatment. You may be an ideal candidate. This is particularly likely if your periods have stopped and menopause has occurred in your early forties or before.

Management of Menopausal Symptoms Without Hormonal Replacement

You may want or need to manage your symptoms without hormones. Standard estrogen therapy may not be safe or appropriate for some, so it is heartening that research has been directed to finding other nonhormonal and nonmedical approaches that can improve sexual functioning and menopausal symptoms after breast cancer. These include giving patients access to educational pamphlets discussing menopause, estrogen replacement therapy, urinary incontinence, tamoxifen, and sexuality and teaching them the use of slow abdominal breathing (for hot flashes), Kegel pelvic floor muscle exercises (for urinary incontinence and sexual response), and the use of moisturizers such as Replens and lubricants such as Astroglide (for vaginal dryness). Also, patients with particular psychosocial stressors benefit from referral to counseling or support groups.

General Guidelines for Resuming Sexual Activity

Whenever you are sick, your usual sense of control over your body may be shaken. You may feel inadequate and helpless. An illness can change the way you experience your body, or it might actually change the way you look because of surgery, amputation, scarring, or weight change. These changes can create painful anxiety. You wonder whether you'll be able to function in your usual social, sexual, and vocational roles. You wonder what people will think of you. This anxiety and the depression and fatigue that often go along with it understandably make sexuality seem less important. But once the immediate crisis passes, sexual feelings and how to express them may become important again.

Feeling anxious about resuming sexual activity is normal and natural. It is easy to get out of practice. You may have questions about whether sexual activity will hurt you in some way. You may wonder how you will be able to experience sexual pleasure, and your partner may share the same worries. He or she may be especially concerned about tiring you out or hurting you somehow. But once you resume sexual relations, your comfort and confidence should gradually increase. If not, sexual counseling may help you discover ways to deal with whatever problems you are having. For many people, a new start—by themselves or through counseling—is refreshing. It might even create opportunities for greater intimacy and sharing than ever before.

What to Do When You Are in the Hospital

Your cancer treatment might involve long stays in the hospital and long separations from those you love. Hospitals or convalescent facilities don't usually provide much privacy, so there may be little opportunity for sexual expression unless you speak up.

Although healthcare facilities are rarely designed to ensure patients' privacy, there is no reason why you and your partner can't have time for intimate physical contact in the hospital. With a little friendly intervention doctors might be able to arrange for a special room where you and a loved one can spend some time alone. Or you can always make a sign reading "Do Not Disturb Until ___ o'clock" or "Please Knock" and hang it on the door to your room. The nurses will respect your wishes.

If this sounds important to you, ask your doctor to speak to the hospital staff and help foster a caring and respectful attitude toward your need to express your sexuality with guaranteed privacy. It takes some education and maybe a change in the hospital routine but may be well worth the effort.

Developing Helpful Attitudes and Practices

Whenever you are ready to become sexually active again, there are a few things you should keep in mind:

- *You are loved for who you are, not just for your appearance.* If you were considered lovable or sexually desirable before you got cancer, chances are that you will be afterward, too. Your partner, your family, and your friends will still love you and value you, as long as you let them.
- *We are all sexual beings.* Whether we are sexually active or not, sexuality is part of who we are. It is not defined just by what we do or how often we do it.
- *Survival overshadows sexuality.* If you've lost your good health, it is normal and natural for stress, depression, worry, and fatigue to lower your interest in sex. Just coping with basic everyday decisions can seem like a burden. But take one day at a time and be patient. Sexual interest and feelings probably will come back when the immediate crisis has passed.
- *Share your feelings.* Making relationships work is a task we all face, but it can be made more difficult by worries about our worth and attractiveness. Whether you are looking for a new relationship or already have a regular partner, you may find yourself in the position of having to share your sexual feelings with someone, perhaps for the first time.

  This sharing may feel awkward at first. Learning how and when to talk about sexual issues may not come easily. You may feel shy or nervous about exploring new and different ways of finding sexual pleasure. You may wait for your partner to make the first move while your partner is waiting for you to make the advances. This familiar waiting game is often misunderstood as rejection by both people. It may be frightening to think of breaking the silence yourself. Yet it's good to make the first move. Try sharing some of the myths or expectations you grew up with about sexuality. Often this is humorous and may break the ice in starting a frank discussion about your sexual needs and concerns. Try not to make broad, generalized statements. Talk about what is important to *you* and about how *you* feel. The payoff is greater understanding of each other's needs and concerns, and that is worth the effort.
- *Expect the unexpected.* The first time you have sex after treatment, physical limitations or fears about your performance, appearance, or rejection may keep you from focusing on the sheer pleasure of physical contact. On the other hand, you may be surprised by unfamiliar pleasurable sensations. If you expect some changes as part of the natural recovery process, they will be less likely to distract you from sexual pleasure if they do happen.
- *Give yourself time.* You and your partner may be frightened of, or even repulsed by, scars, unfamiliar appliances, or other physical changes. That's natural too. But such feelings are usually temporary. Talking about them is often the first step to mutual support and acceptance. Don't pressure yourself about having to work

on sex. A satisfactory and enjoyable sex life will happen one step at a time. You may want to spend some time by yourself exploring your body, becoming familiar with changes, and rediscovering your unique body texture and sensations. Once you feel relaxed doing this, move on to mutual body exploration with a partner.

- *Take the pressure off intercourse.* Almost all of us were brought up to believe that intercourse is the only real or appropriate way of expressing ourselves sexually. Yet sexual expression can encompass many forms of touching and pleasuring that are satisfying psychologically and physically.

  When you resume sexual activity, try spending some time in pleasurable activities—touching, fondling, kissing, and being close—without having intercourse. Reexperience the pleasure of playing, of holding and of being held without having to worry about erections and orgasms. When you feel comfortable, proceed at your own pace to other ways of being sexual, including intercourse if you like.

  Experiment and explore to discover what feels best and what is acceptable. If radiation therapy has made intercourse painful, for example, try oral or manual stimulation to orgasm or intercourse between thighs or breasts. If you are exhausted by the disease or movement is painful, just cuddling or lying quietly next to your partner can be a wonderfully satisfying form of intimacy.
- *Don't let your diagnosis dictate what you can do sexually.* Your sexuality cannot be "diagnosed." You will never know what pleasures you are capable of experiencing if you don't explore. Try new positions, new touches, and, above all, new attitudes.

Remember:

- *Your brain is your best and most important sex organ.* And its ability to experience sensation is virtually limitless.
- *Plan sex around your changing energy levels.* Life with cancer can be exhausting. Fatigue, depression, and just feeling sick are almost normal for cancer patients at certain times. The amount of energy you have for all kinds of activities, including sex, can vary from day to day or week to week. So plan sexual activities to coincide with the times when you think you will feel best.
- *Ask for help if you need it.* Don't hesitate to seek counseling or information if you have problems. Help is available from a wide range of sources. If you want to discuss any problems, bring them up with your healthcare providers. Ask them to recommend competent sex counselors or therapists in your area. There may also be other resources available nearby, such as people who have had both cancer and experience in talking about sexual concerns.
- *Be patient.* The important thing is to be patient, with both yourself and your partner. You won't adjust overnight. Give yourself time to explore and share your feelings about your body changes and time to again see yourself as a desirable sexual being. When you can accept the way your body looks and recognize your potential for sexual pleasure, it will be easier to imagine someone else doing the same.

The satisfaction and good feelings—emotional and physical—that can come from a sexual relationship require patience, communication, respect, cooperation, and a willingness to remember that in some respects the relationship must be learned all over again, physically if not emotionally. Everything may not work properly at first. Everything may not be enjoyable at first. But for those for whom sexuality is still an important component of their intimacy, continuing to have the courage and confidence to keep trying should bring healing results.

26 Infertility Problems in Cancer Survivors

Mitchell Rosen, M.D., and Ernest H. Rosenbaum, M.D. F.A.C.P.

Infertility is a common problem for those who have had cancer and cancer therapy. In recent years, improvements in cancer treatments have been developed to both prolong life and reduce the risk of infertility. New treatment options are making fertility a possibility for many cancer survivors.[1]

The human reproductive system is complex and unique for both sexes. The reproductive system is affected by many cancer-related therapies, with the end result of difficulty conceiving. Cancer therapy effects on fertility depend on the patient's age, type of cancer, and method of treatment. In order to understand the causes of infertility related to cancer and cancer therapies, we will review the reproductive axis and processes of ovulation, sperm production, and fertilization.

Reproductive System

The reproductive axis is made up of the pituitary gland, the gonads (ovaries or testes), and the reproductive tract (the vagina, uterus, and fallopian tubes in women and the epididymis, vas deferens, penile urethra, and glands in men). In men, the seminal vesicles and prostate are the major glands responsible for semen production.

Women

A woman's oocytes (eggs) are completely formed during fetal development and stored in a resting pool in her two ovaries. After birth, the oocytes do not regenerate but rather decline with age; their depletion results in ovarian failure (menopause). The oocytes continually leave the resting pool, enter the growth phase, and die. When a woman reaches puberty, a complex cyclic process begins—the menstrual cycle—which rescues one of the oocytes from death and causes ovulation, which culminates in either pregnancy or a period (menses). The ovulatory cycle continues until menopause, which occurs on average at fifty-one years of age. Ovulation is controlled by follicle-stimulating hormone (FSH) and luteinizing hormone (LH), which are produced by the pituitary gland. Once expelled from the ovary, the oocyte is captured by the fallopian tube and is ready to be fertilized. If it is fertilized, the resulting embryo moves into the uterus and attaches to the uterine lining to continue development. During the ovulatory cycle the ovaries also produce estrogen and progesterone, which prepare the lining of the uterus for the embryo, thereby facilitating implantation and maintenance of a pregnancy. If the oocyte is not fertilized, the lining of the uterus is shed, resulting in a period.

Men

In contrast to the female reproductive system, in the male reproductive system sperm production is initiated at puberty and continues throughout life. The testes contain stem cells that continually replenish the sperm pool. The ability to produce sperm depends on adequate amounts of FSH, LH, and testosterone. The sperm are stored in the epididymis until ejaculation. During intercourse, the sperm are transported through ducts along with secretions from the glands and are ejaculated through the penile urethra. The process of ejaculation requires intact nerves in the pelvis. The testes also produce testosterone, which controls sex drive and the ability to achieve an erection.

Cancer Therapy and Reproduction

Cancer therapies can cause a spectrum of damage to the reproductive axis. The damage may be severe and result in sterility (ovarian or testicular failure) or partial injury resulting in early menopause and infertility (inability to conceive within twelve months). Symptoms of ovarian failure include absence of menses, hot flashes, and vaginal dryness. Testicular failure can lead to loss of sex drive and ejaculation or erection difficulties.

The treatments for cancer that can affect the reproductive system include the following:

- Surgery on the reproductive organs
- Chemotherapy
- Radiotherapy to abdomen and pelvis

Surgery

Operations for cancer that do not involve the reproductive axis do not affect a woman's ability to achieve pregnancy. However, if the operation involves removing parts of the reproductive system, it may cause sterility or infertility. For example, treatment for gynecological cancer may involve the removal of the uterus (a hysterectomy), ovaries (a bilateral oophorectomy), or some portion of the reproductive tract such as the cervix, vulva, or vagina. Some operations may involve these organs but spare reproductive function. However, the scar tissue that develops after surgery may hinder conception. The surgery that is performed will depend on the type of cancer and whether it has spread to other organs.

For a man, surgery may involve removing both testicles (a bilateral orchidectomy), which results in sterility. Operations that spare one or both testicles preserve the capacity to conceive; however, other surgeries that involve removing the prostate, bladder, or bowel or that cause damage to the nerves in the pelvic area can result in infertility or erectile dysfunction. Surgery in the pelvic area involving the lymph nodes may result in ejaculation difficulties.

Chemotherapy

Chemotherapy targets tissues with actively dividing cells, such as skin, hair, the digestive tract, and the reproductive organs. The sperm and supporting cells of the oocyte divide during development. Therefore, all chemotherapies are potentially damaging to the ovaries and testes and may reduce the number of oocytes and sperm. Whether chemotherapy results in infertility depends on the patient's age, the type of chemotherapeutic drugs used, and the dosage of drugs given.

Results of a recent study showed that chemotherapy-induced amenorrhea (lack of menses) is a probable risk in the first year after treatment.[2] The incidence of no menses after chemotherapy in women under forty years of age ranges from 5–54 percent, and for those over forty years of age, it ranges from 76–92 percent. However, menses may return several years after treatment. The chance of return after two years of follow-up is 28 percent for those younger than forty years old and 8 percent for those over forty years of age. At age forty-five, women who undergo chemotherapy have about an 85 percent chance of going into permanent menopause. The younger the patient at the time of the treatment, the more likely she is to experience temporary amenorrhea and then resume normal menstrual function, although this can take several years. For prepubertal patients, the likelihood of early menopause and infertility is lower.

Alkylating chemotherapy agents (such as Cytoxan) are most harmful to oocytes. In one study, 42 percent of women treated with this type of chemotherapy were in premature menopause by the age of thirty-one, although some returned to normal menses.[3] However, having normal periods does not mean a woman is fertile. Adriamycin and docetaxel are also gonadal (ovary and testes) toxic. Of women exposed to chemotherapy, only 5–35 percent achieve spontaneous pregnancy. Chemotherapy can result in partial ovarian injury (decreasing the number of oocytes) such that cancer survivors have normal menstrual cycles but don't realize they are infertile until they try to conceive. Cancer treatment may push patients out of the reproductive window and into the early stages of menopause with no particular signs or symptoms.

In men, alkylating agents are similarly most harmful to sperm production. However, the testosterone-producing cells (Leydig cells) are more resistant to chemotherapy than oocytes. Therefore, sterility may not be readily apparent. Damage to sperm production may result in low sperm count (oligozoospermia), however, with the end result of infertility. The damage caused by chemotherapy can be temporary or permanent. If the injury is directly to the sperm and does not destroy the stem cells, then recovery is possible, often with minimal residual effect. High dosages of chemotherapy can damage the Leydig cells, resulting in loss of sex drive and ejaculation and erection difficulties.

Radiation

The gonads (testes or ovaries) can be temporarily or permanently damaged by radiation therapy. The severity of damaging effects is related to the radiation dosage, the number of treatments, the location of the treatment field, and the patient's age. Radioactive iodine does not cause infertility. In contrast to chemotherapy, prepubertal age provides no protection against radiation effects to the reproductive system.

Radiation therapy affects the number of oocytes remaining in the resting pool and stem cells in the testes. The dosage that causes ovarian failure depends on age. In younger women, more oocytes are present. Therefore, at a given dosage of radiation young women have less chance of menopause than older women. In one study, radiation dosages less than 2,000 cGy resulted in ovarian failure more often in women thirteen to twenty years of age than in girls less than thirteen years old. At dosages greater than 2,000 cGy, the incidence of ovarian failure was more than 70 percent regardless of age. In women older than twenty years, dosages as low as 800 cGy can result in menopause. However, even low dosages can be harmful for both sperm and oocytes, rendering one infertile, and this result is highly unpredictable. If pelvic radiation is given at higher dosages, the uterus is also vulnerable to muscular or vascular injury.[4] Symptoms include intrauterine growth retardation, spontaneous miscarriages, and preterm labor. Radiation at lower dosages to the testes may affect the sperm only, sparing the Leydig cells, yet still result in infertility. With normal supporting cells, children would experience normal pubertal development, and adults may have a normal sex drive and be capable of erections and ejaculation.

The Psychological Impact of Infertility

Infertility can be an emotionally devastating experience for anyone. In the case of cancer survivors, the possibility of infertility adds an additional burden to the many challenges created by the short- and long-term side effects of therapy and the potential for recurrence or a new cancer.

One of the domains of *symbolic immortality,* as described by Robert Jay Lifton, M.D., of Harvard University in his 1979 book *The Broken Connection: On Death and the Continuity of Life,* is the hope of leaving something behind through a biological family. Infertility often leads to grieving and loss, and although the goal of cancer therapy is survival, the possibility of being unable to continue one's family line threatens one of the most basic dreams of life.

Patients suffering grief, loss, or anxiety may need professional counseling and psychosocial therapy to aid in psychological adjustment. The hope is that fertility may return, reinforcing the survivor's commitment to life.

Some survivors fear having children when they are at risk for experiencing a cancer recurrence, developing a new cancer, or dying prematurely. This can cause both negative feelings and a negative approach to becoming fertile. There is also the fear that offspring conceived after cancer therapy might be born with a congenital abnormality. Thus far, a higher risk of congenital malformation is not supported by current research, which has found abnormalities in about 3.4 percent of cancer survivors' offspring, compared with 3.1 percent of cancer-free siblings' offspring. The genetic propensity for abnormalities in the general population is about 5 percent.[5]

Those fortunate enough to conceive after cancer treatment experience a greater sense of a normal life. Fertility is a high priority despite the risks, making it possible to be a parent and watch one's progeny grow and develop, one of the most valued and coveted of life's experiences.

Even for those who have not had cancer, infertility can be a major challenge, necessitating many physician visits, treatments, and often high costs that are not always covered by insurance. The distress from failures is an additional cost that is not always balanced by the gratification of success. Recently, there have been many advances in the treatment of infertility. If success cannot be achieved, adoption often is considered, although this approach also presents costs, both financial and emotional, in the struggle to find a suitable baby. Patients often go overseas, where more children are available for adoption, accepting the additional costs and risks of dealing with unfamiliar legal and medical systems. For many, however, adoption does not satisfy their desire to sustain the family and genetic life history.

Although a majority of infertile cancer survivors have considered adoption, another option is the third-party approach, in which a surrogate carries the baby. Alternatively, a cancer survivor may consider using a donated embryo, egg, or sperm. Some religions, such as Roman Catholicism and Islam, are against third-party reproduction. Having one's own biological child through use of current advanced technology is becoming a potentially more accessible approach.

Preserving Fertility

The improved long-term survival and cure rates for many cancers have made future fertility a question to be considered in reproductive-age patients, preferably before the cancer treatment begins. The importance of this question has been recognized, and although the existing options are limited, particularly in women, this is an area of active research, and it is likely that in the near future other options will become available.

Clearly, cancer treatment that entails surgical removal of the testes or the ovary renders the patient sterile. To preserve fertility, the most important step for those diagnosed with cancer is to discuss their concerns with their doctor. If possible, alternative treatments, such as different chemotherapeutic agents or radiation exposure, may help decrease the incidence of infertility. Before beginning treatment, discuss alternative options for fertility preservation with your doctor so that he or she can refer you to a fertility clinic. Some of the available options can be performed after treatment, but the most effective methods are used before cancer treatment.

Men

Men have the option of freezing (cryopreserving) sperm for later use. This process is available in most major medical centers and is a simple and affordable method. Semen cryopreservation has been used successfully for more than fifty years. Sperm banking should be completed before the initiation of radiation therapy or chemotherapy in case the sperm count and quality do not return to normal after treatment. The sperm can be stored indefinitely without significant damage. When ready for use, the sperm are thawed and available for intrauterine insemination (IUI) or assisted reproductive techniques (ARTs). Unfortunately, men often are not advised of this option before therapy. It has been estimated that only 10–30 percent of patients use the option of stored semen.[6]

Men with cancer often have abnormal sperm counts before treatment. In the past, low sperm counts were a reason not to bank sperm because poor samples yield a low pregnancy rate with IUI. However, with ARTs, such as in vitro fertilization and intracytoplasmic (into egg) sperm injection, there is a high success rate for successful fertilizations and pregnancy.[7]

Boys and young adolescents who have not experienced puberty do not make sperm and therefore are unable to use sperm banking. For these patients, encouraging approaches in the experimental phase include the following:

- *Gonadotropin-releasing hormone (GnRH) agonists:* This hormonal therapy is administered by injection every month or every three months. It temporarily shuts down the reproductive system, thereby decreasing the number of dividing cells in the testes. Thus far, there are no proven studies of a GnRH agonist successfully protecting males from high-dose chemotherapy damage. Although older studies have shown no protection against chemotherapy, recent studies have suggested a possible benefit.
- *Cryopreserved testicular tissue for future transplantation:* Testicular tissue is obtained surgically and cryopreserved. When ready for use, the tissue is transplanted back into the testes, making spontaneous conception possible. This is an option for prepubertal patients. Research on this option is in progress, and to date there have been no live births from this method.
- *Testicular sperm extraction (TESE):* In men with no sperm in their ejaculate, TESE is an option. It is a well-established procedure to overcome severe male infertility and has a high pregnancy success rate. The chance of obtaining sperm is 30–70 percent. TESE may also be an option for prepubertal patients but is still in the experimental phase, with no pregnancies to date.

Options after cancer treatment depend on the severity of damage to the testes. If sperm are present, IUI and ART are available options. If there are no sperm in the ejaculate, TESE may be attempted. Hormonal therapies such as FSH and LH to increase sperm production are being investigated.

Women

In women, the damage done to ovaries by cancer treatment depends on a number of factors, including the patient's age at the time of treatment, the dosage and particular chemotherapeutic drug used, and the dosage and fractionation schedule of radiation.

For women, there are a number of strategies for preserving fertility:

- *Embryo cryopreservation:* The most well-established option is embryo cryopreservation. It is a common technique used with couples to overcome infertility. It is available only for women who have experienced puberty and have a partner or are willing to use donor sperm. The success rate depends on the woman's age and the number of oocytes recovered from the ovary. The process entails a two- to six-week time commitment and should be performed before the initiation of cancer treatment. It begins with ovarian stimulation, which allows multiple oocytes to be produced. The ovarian stimulation requires FSH and LH and results in increases in estrogen production. In cases of hormone-sensitive cancer (i.e., breast cancer), techniques to reduce estrogen production are available. The oocytes are collected by a surgical procedure, using an ultrasound-guided needle that is passed through the vagina into the ovaries to collect oocytes. Once the oocytes are recovered, they are fertilized and stored for later use. When the patient is ready for pregnancy, the embryos are thawed and transferred into the uterus. In some cases, it may not be possible to delay cancer treatments long enough to do ovarian stimulation. If this procedure is desired, the patient should discuss it with her doctor as soon as possible so that the possible delay in cancer treatment is minimized.

The other options available to women are in the experimental phase and include the following:

- *Egg (oocyte) cryopreservation:* A question that often arises is, "Can I bank my eggs just like men can bank their sperm?" The process is similar to embryo cryopreservation. However, the oocyte is not fertilized. Therefore, the need for a partner or donor sperm is avoided. Unfortunately, at present this is not routinely possible. However, in a few centers it is being performed on an experimental basis under the strict supervision of institutional research committees. The success depends on the woman's age and the number of oocytes recovered. The reported success is 2–4 percent live births per oocyte recovered. The lower survival rate of frozen eggs after thawing and the less than optimal pregnancy yield makes freezing of ova obtained before cancer treatment not yet widely available as a clinical option. This area is of great research interest, and advancements are continually developing, with corresponding improvements in pregnancy rates, so it is likely that egg banking will be feasible in the near future.
- *Ovarian transposition (oophoropexy):* Oophoropexy can protect the ovaries from radiation. The operation places the ovaries out of the radiation field. This technique has been used for years to shield the ovaries from radiation during pelvic irradiation, but the results are variable for fertility protection, ranging between 0–90 percent.[8] The variability in success is attributed to the difficulty of keeping the ovary out of the radiation field and the concurrent use of chemotherapy in addition to radiation. In the past this procedure entailed a long recovery time, thereby delaying radiation treatment. Newer oophoropexy techniques under investigation show promising results.

- *Ovarian cryopreservation (tissue freezing):* Another approach being studied is that of freezing ovarian tissue in the hope that later, after successful treatment of the cancer, it can be transplanted back into the patient and still function. This procedure is not widely available at this time. This process has no time requirement and therefore avoids any delay in cancer treatment. It does not require ovarian stimulation or a partner and is an option for prepubertal patients. The tissue is obtained surgically and cryopreserved. When the patient is ready, the tissue is transplanted (autotransplantation) by either of two methods:
  - *Orthotopic transplant:* The ovarian tissue is transplanted back into the native ovaries. This process would potentially produce sex steroids, resume menstrual cycles, and allow spontaneous conception. To date, two reported live births have occurred after orthotopic transplant.
  - *Heterotropic transplant:* The ovarian tissue is transplanted under the skin (e.g., in the arm). This process would potentially produce sex steroids and resume menstrual cycles but would not allow spontaneous conception. In order to conceive, ART would be needed. No live births to date have been recorded after heterotropic transplantation.

  A major concern for ovarian transplantation is the possibility of reintroducing malignant cells from the ovarian tissue to a cancer survivor. The ovarian tissue removed before treatment could contain latent malignant cells, and cryopreservation does not kill cancer cells. Investigations are being performed to reliably screen for cancer cells in the ovarian tissue.
- *GnRH analogs:* This hormonal therapy is administered by injection every month or every three months. It temporarily shuts down the reproductive system, decreasing the number of dividing cells in the ovaries. Evidence suggests that GnRH agonists may be a beneficial option for postpubertal females receiving chemotherapy. The treatment should be administered before chemotherapy begins but may be beneficial even during treatment. Studies have shown that use of GnRH analogs does not protect against radiation.
- *Gynecological cancer treatments that spare reproductive function:* The options available depend on the type of cancer and whether it has spread to other places.
  - *Cervical cancer:* Trachelectomy, removal of the cervix from early stage cervical cancer, takes special surgical expertise and appears to be a safe way to preserve the uterus for pregnancy.
  - *Uterine cancer:* Hormonal treatments may treat early stages of uterine cancer.
  - *Ovarian cancer:* Early stages may necessitate removal of only one ovary and tube.

Options after treatment include use of ARTs and surrogacy if a hysterectomy has been performed.

Pregnancy After Cancer Treatment

Follow-up studies indicate that the toxic effects of chemotherapy given to women before pregnancy do not appear to be a risk to children conceived naturally. However, animal studies suggest that natural conception within six months after treatment in females increases the chance of fetal abnormalities. In males, the only risks of fetal abnormality were found in those conceived during or immediately after chemotherapy.

There is new evidence to suggest that pregnancy after cancer treatment does not increase a breast cancer survivor's risk of recurrence or shorten her life. However, it is wise for breast cancer patients to wait two years after completing their cancer treatment before trying to conceive a child, as that is the highest risk period for breast cancer recurrence.[9] If the proper steps are taken before treatment to preserve fertility, surgery and radiation therapy have not been shown to affect a breast cancer patient's ability to conceive a child or to have a normal child. Chemotherapy, however, may cause amenorrhea and an increased possibility of infertility. Breast cancer patients should consult with their physicians about their future pregnancy plans before starting cancer treatments.

Although cancer survival has continued to increase in recent years, infertility remains a major challenge for cancer survivors. Cancer patients interested in future fertility should receive appropriate psychological support and early referral to specialized fertility clinics and perinatal care services. It is important to note that there are no guarantees of preserving fertility with any of the aforementioned options. Cancer survivors unable to use their own eggs or sperm may still achieve pregnancy using donated eggs or sperm. The process of donating eggs or sperm is well established and has high pregnancy rates. The recipient has many options for donors, including various individual characteristics and genetic backgrounds.

A nonprofit organization, Fertile Hope, provides fertility resources for cancer patients and can be contacted at www.fertilehope.org, 888-994-HOPE, or by mail at 65 Broadway, Suite 603, New York, NY 10006.

27 Body Image, Wigs, and Makeup

Gerd Mairandres,
Alexandra Andrews,
Chris Wilhite, and
Ernest H. Rosenbaum,
M.D., F.A.C.P.

A cancer diagnosis and treatment can severely compromise self-esteem. Sources of self-esteem that can be threatened by cancer and the effects of medical treatments include appearance, physical abilities, activity levels, health, and independence. Quality of life diminishes very quickly when one is fearful, fatigued, in pain, enduring side effects of therapy, or contemplating the possibility of treatment failure and death. Therefore, your first task in dealing with cancer is to regain your equilibrium by addressing these very real issues and creating a support system tailored to your needs.

One of the most devastating side effects of therapy is loss of hair, and many cancer patients who lose their hair choose to get a wig. Anything that can enhance the way a person feels about himself or herself and promote well-being is significant. It is not about the face you present to the world but the face you see in the mirror. Think of a wig and simple makeup as an opportunity to reinvent yourself.

Wigs

Choosing a Wig

Wig Material

- Natural hair wigs need labor-intensive maintenance. They are more expensive.
- Synthetic hair wigs are easy to maintain. They cost less, making it possible to purchase several wigs, which minimizes maintenance and allows you to change your look.

Types of Wigs

- *Wefted wigs:* Hair is woven onto threads, producing rows of hair that are attached to stretch foundations. These are the least expensive.
- *Knotted wigs:* Hair is individually knotted onto a mesh foundation. These are the most expensive and most realistic looking.
- *Machined wigs:* These approximate knotted wigs. Sometimes half the wig is knotted onto a monofilament base and the rest is wefted. These wigs are a good alternative to knotted wigs.

- *Wigs with microfilament foundation on top:* These wigs imitate the look of scalp and therefore stand up to closer scrutiny.

Wig Choices

- Elastic in the foundation of the wig makes for a better fit.
- Shorter wigs are easier to maintain.
- Before hair loss, cutting your hair in a style similar to the wig you have chosen may create an easier transition.
- A stylist can trim your wig using thinning shears.
- Find a wig that has more than one color. Many wigs have color blends for a more natural look.
- Choose a wig color that is a shade or two lighter than your own hair color. Lighter wigs can appear less dense and give a better appearance in daylight and artificial light.

Wig Care

- Use dishwashing soap or mild detergent to wash your wig. There is no need to purchase a special shampoo.
- Use cold water to wash and rinse the synthetic wig. Hot water will affect the texture and consequently the style of your wig.
- Shake out any extra water and allow the wig to air-dry.

Wearing the Wig

- *Mesh caps:* Mesh caps are lighter and cooler than a nylon stocking cap. If the elastic is too tight on your forehead, then turn the cap around, placing the elastic at the back of your head. Caps worn under wigs are necessary only when you need to contain hair under the wig. There is no need for a cap if you have little or no hair.
- *Putting on the wig:*
  - Shake out the wig before putting it on to get some air into the style.
  - Make sure you place the wig on your head evenly. Use the tabs at the ear area and check to see that the wig is straight.
  - Don't place the wig hairline lower on your forehead than your natural hairline.
  - Don't be afraid to show your ears.
  - Use your fingers to fluff the wig. Fingers are a terrific tool and can produce a natural appearance.
  - Avoid flat spots. Remember to check the back of your head.
  - Your wig may need a tune-up. Revisit your stylist.
- *Dos and Don'ts:*
  - Your wig is easily damaged. In particular, wigs containing synthetic fibers react to heat and may melt. Don't open your oven to check a roast or turkey while wearing your wig. Be careful around open flames and extreme heat such as an oven, broiler, or stovetop. Similarly, don't use a curling iron on your wig, and be careful using hot rollers.
  - Don't panic if you get caught in the rain. Your wig will not be damaged by a sudden downpour. Unlike hair, the fiber will not absorb the rain easily. Your hairstyle will remain intact.
  - Don't be surprised if your hair regrowth after the end of therapy is different. Your hair may have a different texture (chemo curl) and color than your prior hair type.

Simple Makeup Ideas

- *Eyebrows:* Many times with cancer therapies one loses facial hair. Eyebrows are the punctuation marks of your expression, so having no eyebrows can give a blank look. To maintain thinning eyebrows or create the look of eyebrows with makeup:
  - Use eye shadow to sketch in eyebrows. Choose a color that is a few shades lighter than your wig.

- To define, add a few lines with an eyebrow pencil. Concentrate the color on the outer portion of the eyebrow.
- Use a soft toothbrush or eyebrow brush to brush your eyebrows.
- First do the eyebrow opposite the dominant hand. For instance, if you are right handed, your normal tendency would be to first do your right eyebrow. Instead, do the left eyebrow and then do the right eyebrow. This will help you match both eyebrows.

- *Lips:* Dry lip liner helps prevent lipstick from bleeding or flowing into lip lines.
- *Cheeks:* You can use a tiny amount of lipstick for your cheek color.
  - Don't use dark lipstick.
  - Make sure you apply the color to the apple of your cheek. Remember, a little goes a long way. If you do not wear foundation, lipstick rouge is a dandy trick for quick color.
- *Other tips:*
  - Art supply stores can be good sources for makeup brushes. Chisel-point brushes are useful for eyebrows.
  - If you find your eyebrow, lip, or eyeliner pencil too hard, hold it near a light to soften it.

The Look Good . . . Feel Better Cosmetic Program by the Cosmetic, Toiletry, and Fragrance Association Foundation[1]

Just about everyone's quality of life is seriously diminished during cancer treatment. Fatigue and changes in daily routine and physical appearance, personal emotions, and reactions from family, friends, and colleagues can all weigh heavily on cancer patients.

If you are a woman getting cancer treatment, you may find that physical changes are especially hard to bear. Your personal appearance directly affects your self-image and psychological well-being. And if you are experiencing some of the common side effects of radiation or chemotherapy, you may start to believe that you're in worse medical shape than you really are. The face you see in the mirror each morning is a harsh reminder of your disease. Every day, you can't escape your loss of hair, eyelashes, and eyebrows or the changes in your skin tone and texture.

Looking in that mirror, you may start thinking that you can't possibly lead a normal life. But in today's world, leading a normal life—with all the family relationships, work, and social demands normal life involves—is essential while you are getting cancer treatments. What you need to get back to a good quality of life is help overcoming the changes in appearance that cancer treatments bring.

Fortunately, to help you do that, Look Good . . . Feel Better (LGFB) is a free national public service program designed to teach women with cancer, through practical hands-on experience, beauty techniques that help restore their appearance during chemotherapy and radiation treatments.

So while your medical treatment helps heal the inside of your body, the LGFB program helps you renew your self-esteem by enhancing your appearance. It encourages you to pay attention to yourself during a time of dramatic physical changes.

How the LGFB Program Works

LGFB began in 1989, when three national organizations pooled their resources to develop the service and make it available to women across the country. The program was founded and developed by the Cosmetic, Toiletry, and Fragrance Association (CTFA) Foundation, a charitable organization supported by the members of the cosmetic industry's trade association, in collaboration with the American

Cancer Society (ACS) and the National Cosmetology Association (NCA). The NCA is a national organization that represents hairstylists, wig experts, aestheticians, makeup artists, and nail technicians, among others.

LGFB provides the following:

- Free beauty tips and techniques to cancer patients—through group workshops or individual sessions—by volunteer cosmetologists and beauty advisors.
- Complimentary makeup kits for everyone participating in a group program.
- Free self-help program materials.

The LGFB program is administered nationwide by the ACS and is designed to meet the needs of local communities. The NCA organizes volunteer cosmetologists who can evaluate your skin and hair needs and who will teach you the appropriate techniques to deal with the appearance-related side effects of cancer treatments. The CTFA Foundation provides the makeup, materials, and financial support for the program. LGFB is product neutral and does not promote any specific cosmetic product line or manufacturer. All volunteers for LGFB are trained and certified for participation by the ACS at local, state, or regional workshops. The purpose of this training is not only to discuss important hygienic guidelines and helpful cosmetic tips but also to promote sensitivity and understanding about what a cancer patient goes through during treatment. This is a necessary step for each volunteer.

Group Sessions

Each group session usually consists of six to ten women led through a two-hour program by beauty professionals. Through hands-on experience, the women learn a twelve-step makeup program and are shown beauty tips about hair, wigs, turbans, and scarves. To ensure that every participant gets the same working tools, each woman in a group program receives a complimentary bag of makeup containing twelve items, which match the twelve-step makeup program: cleanser, moisturizer, concealer, foundation, powder, blush, eyeshadow, eyeliner, eyebrow pencil, mascara, lipliner, and lipstick.

LGFB group programs are located in comprehensive cancer centers, hospitals, ACS offices, and community centers.

Personal Consultation

A free one-time consultation in a salon by a participating volunteer may also be available, depending on where you live. The makeup kit is not provided at one-on-one consultations. A list of volunteers willing to provide this service is compiled and distributed to all ACS divisions and is available through the LGFB toll-free number (1-800-395-LOOK).

LGFB for Teens

LGFB for Teens was launched in 1996. This program is designed to address the needs and concerns of teenage cancer patients, both girls and boys, about the appearance side effects of treatment and the possible effects on self-esteem. Like LGFB for adults, the teen program includes instruction on skin care and makeup and alternatives for coping with hair loss, all geared to teens. In addition, the teen program addresses some of the important social, fitness, and nutrition issues unique to teenagers battling cancer.

LGFB for Teens is offered as a group program in eighteen designated children's hospitals. Information about the teen program can be obtained through the national LGFB toll-free number (1-800-395-LOOK). LGFB for Teens information is also available online through www.2bMe.org or through www.lookgoodfeelbetter.org (click on "Teens").

How and Where to Find Programs in Your Community

Many doctors, nurses, social workers, and other medical professionals recognize how important outward appearance is to their patients. And with their help, LGFB is reaching out to tens of thousands of women across the United States.

The growth of the program has been remarkably rapid and widespread. Two pilot programs were successfully operated at the Memorial Sloan-Kettering Cancer Center in New York City and the Vincent T. Lombardi Cancer Research Center at Georgetown University Hospital in Washington, DC, in the fall of 1988. By March 1989, the program was up and running. Since then, LGFB has been implemented in all fifty states and the District of Columbia and most of the National Cancer Institute–designated comprehensive cancer centers. Group programs served 50,000 women with cancer in 2005. LGFB materials are also available in Spanish, and bilingual programs are available in some cities.

For more information, or to find out about programs in your area, call your local ACS office or the LGFB toll-free number (1-800-395-LOOK), or visit the LGFB Web site at www.lookgoodfeelbetter.org.

28 Falls: A Major Cause of Disability[1]

Ernest H. Rosenbaum, M.D., F.A.C.P.

Falls are the leading cause of injury and associated deaths in older adults and one of the most common causes of nonfatal injuries and hospital admissions. With age, there is a decline in the activities of daily living and an increase in the chance of being institutionalized. Impaired coordination and balance, lower limb weakness, impaired gait, poor vision, and the use of psychotropic medicines are factors promoting falls.

Older adults are more susceptible to dizzy episodes, confusion, or sleepiness, which can also lead to falls. Other factors include unsteadiness caused by changes in blood pressure, vision, and hearing and poor nutrition and hydration status.

Insomnia may be a significant risk factor for falls. A study of 34,000 nursing home residents with a mean age of eighty-four years (76 percent were women) found that 43 percent of participants had a fall within a six-month period, with 2.5 percent sustaining a hip fracture. The study noted that there was a 47 percent elevated risk of falls in patients with moderate insomnia and an 80 percent risk for those with severe insomnia. Evidence from recent studies shows that those who used hypnotic drugs (sleeping pills) had less insomnia and a lower risk of falls.[2]

The ancient practice of tai chi (a low-impact movement exercise) has been found to improve coordination and balance. Tai chi reduces the fear of falling and the rate of falling by almost 50 percent. It appears that there is value in tai chi for preventing falls in older adults, and more research is ongoing. Tai chi is not recommended for those with severe osteoporosis, acute knee and back problems, sprains, or fractures.[3]

It has been shown that balance training studies with computerized balance testing equipment can be even more effective than tai chi in promoting balance.

The Relationship of Noise, Colors, and Falls in Older Adults[4]

An ounce of prevention is worth a pound of cure, particularly in efforts to reduce the risk of falls in older adults.

Colors, contrasts, and distractions often make people feel dizzy, with resultant falls. Homes and buildings often are not designed in a manner to help prevent falls. For example, color-coordinated walls blend in with similarly colored stairs, which may be a precipitating factor for falls. In addition, sounds can distract people, leading to poor balance and falls.

When designing a home or room for older adults, it is best to use contrasting colors between the floors or carpets, stairs, and walls to improve depth perception. Using different colors that are calm but distinct can help by delineating passageways. Pastel colors appear to have a calming effect, whereas bright oranges and reds can promote agitation. Bold and contrasting furniture and carpet patterns are more protective than smaller patterns and result in less dizziness. Avoid loose rugs or electric cords.

Adequate lighting and rails for stairs are essential to prevent falls. A nightlight should be kept on in the bathrooms, with adequate rails near toilets and in baths and showers to prevent falls. Noise control is also important because noise can be very distracting and lead to confusion and dizziness. Both vision and hearing tests must be performed periodically because these two senses decline with age. Correcting these senses as much as possible will improve depth perception and sound orientation and thereby reduce the risk of falls.

Improperly fitted shoes and the resulting calluses, bunions, corns, and ingrown toenails are common problems promoting falls. The use of a cane or walker will improve balance and thus help reduce the risk of falls.

Frequent blood pressure checks and appropriate medication changes are needed to control hypertension (high blood pressure) without episodes of low pressure, which can cause dizziness and fainting. Likewise, good control of diabetic medication is mandatory to avoid episodes of hypoglycemia (low blood sugar), which causes confusion and fainting.

A periodic review of medications with the treating physician is important because the need for medication changes with age and various conditions. Many medications have a dual usage, such as the antidepressant amitriptyline (Elavil), which is also used for relief of neuritic and general pain caused by diabetic neuropathy. Care must be taken to avoid adverse drug effects because many medications have a wide variety of side effects that can affect balance and cause dizziness, which can lead to falls and injury.

Patients should also learn how to fall properly, sitting down rather than falling forward, sideways, or backward, causing injuries to the head or hips. Wearing protective hip pads, which are available at orthopedic appliance stores, can help prevent hip fractures.

29 Lymphedema

John P. Cooke, M.D., Ph.D.,
Andrzej Szuba, M.D., and
Ernest H. Rosenbaum,
M.D., F.A.C.P.

Modified from *Everyone's Guide to Cancer Supportive Care.*

What Is Lymphedema?

Lymphedema is a swelling caused by a buildup of fluid (lymph) in the soft tissues of the limbs. It rarely occurs in other parts of the body, such as the head and trunk. This buildup often occurs after surgical removal of lymph nodes or radiotherapy to lymph nodes (because of blockage of the lymphatic system) and sometimes after chemotherapy.

Lymphedema happens when the lymphatic vessels become incompetent and no longer drain lymph fluid from the extremities, resulting in a swollen limb. It occurs after a tight constriction of an affected limb, such as use of a blood pressure cuff, tight clothing, or jewelry, and can trigger a buildup of tissue lymph fluid from damaged lymphatic vessels. Lymphedema usually is a chronic problem, but it may be permanent, causing distress, pain, loss of function, and anxiety. One indication of lymphedema is a circumference of the limb on the affected side more than 2 centimeters greater or 10 percent larger than the unaffected side.

A major cause of lymphedema can be an infection in the limb, caused by even a minor cut or bruise. Other causes include strenuous exercise or heavy lifting, excessive limb heat, or vigorous massage, resulting in excessive limb fluid buildup. Lymphedema sometimes may occur without an identified cause. In rare cases, lymphedema may be caused by a genetic abnormality (mutation), and family members may be affected. Gaps in our understanding of lymphedema have limited treatment options, but recent advances in genetic studies and imaging (x-rays, dye scans, and ultrasound) and insights gained from physiological studies hold promise of a more definitive therapy.

Lymphedema can be a daily reminder of a persistent cancer problem. It may develop soon after surgery or radiotherapy or months or years after therapy. There are fewer cases today because newer treatments such as sentinel node biopsies are used rather than axillary lymph node dissection. Radiotherapy treatment planning has improved, minimizing the extent of the radiotherapy field and thus minimizing collateral damage.

Where cancer is involved, lymphedema is most common after breast surgery or radiotherapy; 15–30 percent of women develop lymphedema after breast cancer treatment.[1] In a recent study of women who underwent sentinel node biopsy instead of axillary dissection, 6.9–22 percent experienced lymphedema.[2] However, it may occur in upper or lower extremities (arms or legs) in connection with almost any other malignancy (e.g., malignant melanoma or ovarian, cervical, testicular, or prostate cancer). In lymphedema related to cancer treatment, it is surgical lymph node dissection and radiotherapy that cause damage to the lymphatic system.

Chronic lymphedema may result in minor swelling and discomfort. Occasionally it leads to grave disability and disfigurement. Unfortunately, one cannot predict which patients will develop lymphedema. Therefore, all patients should be advised that this is a possible treatment complication.

A limb affected with lymphedema is more prone to infections (cellulitis). Infection may begin suddenly and progress rapidly. Oral antibiotics usually can cure such infections, but in severe cases, hospitalization for intravenous antibiotics might be necessary. In some cancer survivors, lymphedema does not occur until after a skin infection involving the affected arm occurs.

Precautions for People with Lymphedema

The following precautions will help survivors avoid infections and control lymphedema.[3]

- Avoid limb injuries, especially cuts, bruises, and animal scratches.
- Keep extremities dry and clean.
- Keep skin lubricated with moisturizing creams or oils to prevent chafing.
- Protect skin from excessive sunlight by covering up or using sunscreen.
- Protect skin from bug bites by using insect repellants.
- Protect your fingers. For example, wear gloves to avoid injury, especially when gardening or doing manual work.
- Avoid cutting your cuticles and use extra care when cutting your nails.
- Use an electric razor rather than a blade for shaving the affected limb to avoid nicks and skin irritation.
- Avoid blood draws and injections in the affected limb if possible.
- See your physician if the limb is red or if rash, swelling, pain, or fever occurs.
- Avoid the use of blood pressure cuffs on the affected limb.
- Take care of cuts or injuries to the limbs; clean small wounds with warm, soapy water and apply antibiotic ointment under bandages. Change dressings often. See your doctor if you have any questions.
- Avoid wearing jewelry on the affected arm or leg.
- Avoid heavy lifting.
- When traveling in airplanes, support the limb with a compression garment. Decreased air pressure in airplane cabins can increase tissue fluids, causing the onset of lymphedema. Prophylactically wearing a compression garment can be helpful.
- Avoid prolonged heat exposure (more than fifteen minutes) in hot tubs, steam rooms, and saunas. Baths should be less than 102 degrees.
- When washing dishes, avoid putting the affected arm in hot water because excessive heat might increase swelling. Try to wash dishes with the unaffected arm. Let the dirty dishes soak in hot water, then scrub and rinse them with tepid water.

Lymphedema and Quality of Life

Emotional problems associated with lymphedema are not uncommon and often are neglected by physicians. The need to address the psychological aspects of long-term disfigurement, especially with adolescent patients, cannot be overemphasized. Patients should be realistic about the possibility of progression but should remember that they can modify the course of lymphedema through careful attention to the details of the medical program.

Some people become sedentary in response to uncomfortable or heavy sensations in the affected limb. Reduced physical activity at work and at home leads to apathy and malaise; these can be avoided by performing physical activity with proper support hose. Regular exercise appears to reduce lymphedema as long as elastic support (or hydrostatic pressure) is applied. Swimming is a particularly good activity because the surrounding hydrostatic pressure of the water means compressive support isn't needed.

A study of breast cancer survivors with lymphedema at baseline engaging in twice-a-week weight training supported the hypothesis that resistant exercise did not increase the risk or exacerbate symptoms of lymphedema.[4] Use of exercise programs (including isometrics and gentle stretching exercises) carefully monitored by a specialized lymphedema physical therapist did not aggravate lymphedema. Discontinue repetitive range-of-motion exercises if lymphedema worsens. Exercise can help stimulate lymphatic drainage.

Management of Lymphedema

Special physiotherapy is an effective way to treat extremity lymphedema. Several variants of this treatment have been developed in different centers. Vodder, Foldi, and Casley-Smith are among the pioneers of physiotherapy treatments for lymphedema; their schools provide training for physiotherapists around the world. Principles of physiotherapy for lymphedema were outlined in the Consensus Document of the International Society of Lymphology. Physiotherapy treatment of lymphedema has several key elements:

- Manual lymphatic drainage, a special type of light massage that stimulates function of the lymphatic system and increases lymphatic flow.
- Compressive bandaging, or multilayered wrapping with low-stretch bandages that provide gradient compression of the arm or leg (no elastic or ACE bandages).
- Decongestive exercises, special exercises designed to alleviate edema.
- Meticulous skin care to avoid skin infections. Treat skin infections immediately.

Decongestive Lymphatic Therapy

Decongestive lymphatic therapy (decongestive physiotherapy, complex decongestive therapy, or manual lymphatic therapy) is the gold standard treatment for lymphedema. It usually takes several days to achieve significant volume reduction. After edema is sufficiently reduced, the arm or leg is fitted for a compressive garment that should be used daily. Daily manual lymphatic drainage treatments for two or three weeks may be needed to initially control lymphedema by gently stimulating the lymphatic system and redirecting lymphatic fluid for decongestion. A reported edema reduction of 40–90 percent is possible after intensive treatment.

Typical treatment starts with establishing a daily routine:

- A skin protection program is implemented, using moisturizing oils or creams. Meticulous skin care is necessary to prevent skin breaks and subsequent infections.
- Manual lymphatic massage (usually twenty to sixty minutes daily) is performed. Massage is first applied to the contralateral quadrant of the trunk, then to the distal (fingers or toes) part of the affected extremity, and finally to the proximal (upper) part of the limb. Massage sessions are performed once or twice daily for a period sufficient to reduce edema of the limb. This may vary from one to six or more weeks. At the time of therapy, patients and their families are taught techniques of massage self-care, which

include self-applied lymphatic massage, bandaging, and exercises. Follow-up visits are recommended to ensure that control is adequate.

- Multilayer compressive bandaging follows the massage. Low-stretch bandages are applied to the whole extremity, including fingers or toes. Proper wrapping of bandages provides gradual compression, with the highest pressure applied distally and a lower pressure applied at the proximal part of the limb. The pressure from bandages should not be too high because there is a small risk of arterial or nerve compression.

Patients may also be fitted with a compression garment. The garment is measured after initial lymphedema control is attained. This is important because the stocking does not reduce the size of the leg but only maintains the circumference to which it is fitted. If the limb is fitted for a stocking while in a swollen state, the stocking will maintain it in a swollen state. An improperly fitted sleeve garment can provoke lymphedema rather than support the lymphatic system. The garment should be worn daily (with hand gauntlet as needed) for as long as necessary. It should be put on first thing in the morning, before the patient gets out of bed. It is particularly important to wear the compression garment during airplane flights and exercises. Some patients benefit from devices such as the Reid sleeve.

Pneumatic compression pumps might be used in conjunction or separately to reduce or maintain arm or leg volume if needed. Consult with your doctor.

- Decongestive exercises are specially designed to help evacuate lymphatic fluid. Exercises are performed daily, with bandages or a compression garment worn. Bandages are worn overnight until the next massage session. It is important to use proper low-stretch bandages for wrapping. *High-stretch bandages (such as ACE wraps) are inappropriate for treatment of lymphedema and pose a significant risk (e.g., worsening edema or compromising circulation in the limb).*

30 Urinary Incontinence[1]

Ernest H. Rosenbaum, M.D., F.A.C.P.

As people age, urinary incontinence may become more prevalent. Women accept it better than men, who are often more embarrassed. It is a problem that patients often delay reporting to physicians, and therefore it is underdiagnosed and undertreated. In one study, it was seen to affect 35 percent of women and 22 percent of men over age sixty-five, costing approximately $16.3 billion for incontinence care per year. Incontinence often becomes so severe that patients reduce drinking water, confine themselves to home, and stop socializing. Fortunately, many things can be done to help alleviate or reduce this problem.

The first step is to talk it over with your physician. Often, physicians notice the condition in those wearing pads and having a urine smell. Urinary infections and neurological problems are ruled out because these may be more easily treated. The physical examination includes a pelvic and rectal examination, urinalysis, and postvoid procedural tests (less than 100 cc of urine in the bladder is considered normal).

Causes

- *Urge incontinence:* Involuntary contractions of the detrusor bladder muscles cause a precipitous urge to void, often followed by small amounts of urine volume.
- *Stress incontinence:* Failure of the bladder sphincter to remain closed during periods of increased abdominal pressure, such as sneezing or coughing, may be the cause.
- *Mixed incontinence:* This is a combination of stress and urge incontinence.
- *Overflow incontinence:* This is more common in men, who often dribble, have a weak urinary stream, and get up at night to go to the bathroom (nocturia) because of detrusor muscle underactivity or bladder outlet obstruction. Benign prostatic hypertrophy or neurological conditions, such as diabetic neuropathy or spinal injury, can be the cause.
- *Functional incontinence:* Patients have physical impairment and decreased mobility, making toileting difficult, or they may have a cognitive status problem.

Behavioral Treatments

Behavioral treatments are the first options to try:

- Setting up a voiding schedule, such as voiding upon awakening, before and after meals, and at bedtime, may be helpful. Results should be seen within three or four days.
- Changing drinking patterns may also help. Eliminating coffee and other caffeinated beverages may improve incontinence problems.
- A bladder diary can be used to record voidings and incontinence problems to see whether there is a pattern. This makes people more aware of when they need to empty their bladders.
- Kegel exercises tighten the muscles that control the rectum and bladder. They are nonrhythmic exercises in which the bladder and rectal sphincters are tightened as though resisting urges for diarrhea or urination. Contract the muscles for several seconds, then rest and repeat. These very easy and effective exercises have been practiced for years. During pelvic examinations or during a man's rectal examination, physicians can observe how, on command, muscles properly contract.

  Five minutes of Kegels three times a day may help reduce stress incontinence by training the patient to tense bladder muscles, especially when sneezing or coughing, resulting in fewer leaks. These exercises can also be helpful for problems of anal stool incontinence. For urge incontinence, rather than racing to the bathroom, stand still for thirty to sixty seconds, trying to control the bladder urge, and then walk when the urge subsides. This works in many cases. Some suggest doing Kegels earlier in life, before incontinence becomes a problem.

Use of Drugs and Side Effects

Medication can decrease incontinence by up to 70 percent in many patients. Anticholinergic drugs inhibit the parasympathetic nerves and reduce smooth muscle bladder spasms. These include oral oxybutynin (Ditropan and Ditropan XL) or a transdermal patch (Oxytrol), tolterodine (Detrol and Detrol LA), darifenacin (Enablex), trospium (Sanctura), and solifenacin (VESIcare).

In frail older adults anticholinergic drugs should be used carefully to avoid side effects. It has been noted that there may be fewer side effects with longer-acting formulations.

Some of the side effects of drugs used to treat incontinence include dry mouth, blurred vision, and constipation. It is recommended to start at a lower dosage and build up as directed by your physician.

Alpha-adrenergic agonists such as pseudoephedrine (Sudafed) can increase pressure in the muscles of the bladder neck and urethra (the tube exiting the bladder) and can cause urinary retention.

Postmenopausal women can often benefit by applying a small amount of estrogen cream (Premarin) once or twice a day to the vaginal urethra (where urine is excreted) because often urethral tissues lacking estrogen are atrophic, causing incontinence. Estrogen decreases urethral blood vessels and thickens the muscles and can help improve control of urethral pressure. However, one recent study found that estrogens could make the condition worse in some cases.[2]

Surgical Options

There are many surgical options, such as bladder suspension; sling procedures, using supportive hammocklike approaches to partially close the urethra; collagen injections, adding bulk to the urethral lining to help it close properly; and InterStim therapy, in which a surgical device is placed so electrical impulses to the sacral nerves can be activated to help control bladder spasms.

What to Do If Problems Persist

Patients should undergo a more complete evaluation and may need to see a urologist or someone specializing in incontinence therapy. The use of sanitary napkins or urinary incontinence pads can be helpful for frequent incontinence. The goal is to help gain control.

Extra care must be taken for older adults, who are more susceptible to delirium and confusion, especially on medications. Try to control infections, if present. In women, the use of local vaginal estrogens may help relieve symptoms. Also, the use of drug therapy and reduction of caffeine, diuretics, anti-Parkinson's medications, hypnotics, and antispasmodics should be evaluated. In addition, depression, anxiety, and stress can contribute to incontinence, and physician counseling may help relieve these problems. A bathroom and house check should be done and necessary modification made so that patients with limited mobility can have better access to a toilet. When driving, know potential bathroom rest stops or gas stations. Check with restaurants or performance spaces so you know where a bathroom is available. Also, check for stool impactions because they can exacerbate incontinence.

31 Infections

Lawrence Mintz,
M.D., F.I.D.S.A.

Infections pose a serious and ongoing risk for cancer survivors, particularly those whose treatment or underlying disease compromises their immune systems. Once an infection is established, medical treatment should be obtained promptly. However, the purpose of this chapter is to describe ways to prevent infection from occurring in the first place. We all live in a sea of bacteria, viruses, and fungi, and it is impossible to completely avoid the possibility of infection. Still, some simple and routine procedures can greatly reduce the risk of acquiring one. The two major approaches described here are hand washing and immunization. As we shall see, some immunizations provide the benefit not only of preventing infections but also, in certain instances, of preventing the development of cancer itself.

Hand Washing

Of the preventive techniques, the simplest yet most important is proper hand washing. This must be practiced by those caring for patients (medical staff, other caregivers, family, and friends) and by the patients themselves. Although hand washing was proved effective 160 years ago, it is grossly underused. Even today, numerous hospital studies have confirmed that only a quarter to a half of all caregivers regularly and appropriately wash their hands.

History[1]

In 1846, Ignaz Semmelweis, a Viennese-trained Hungarian physician, was serving as the senior house officer in the First Obstetrical Clinic of the Vienna General Hospital. At that time, a disease called puerperal fever, or childbed fever, was rampant among women giving birth in hospitals. This fact was so well known by the general public that most wealthy and educated women chose to give birth at home, and many poor women chose to give birth in the streets rather than in hospitals. Semmelweis observed that 13–20 percent of the women in his First Obstetrical Clinic died of childbed fever. On the other hand, the maternal death rate in the Second Obstetrical Clinic was only 2 percent. Both wards had the same equipment and used the same delivery techniques. Semmelweis noted that the First Clinic was staffed by medical students, whereas the Second Clinic was used to train midwives.

In 1847 a friend and colleague of Semmelweis died from an infection after cutting his finger with a knife while performing an autopsy on a childbed fever victim. His colleague's autopsy revealed features similar to those of women dying from puerperal fever. The twenty-eight-year-old Semmelweis put these observations together and realized that the medical students performed autopsies on their expired patients, whereas the student midwives did not. He further noted that after autopsies, medical students often went directly to the clinic without washing their bloody, contaminated hands. Although the germ theory of infection was not developed for several more decades, Semmelweis concluded that the physicians and medical students must be carrying some unknown infecting particles on their hands from the cadavers to the patients they examined in the First Clinic, thereby causing childbed fever.

To test his hypothesis, Semmelweis mandated that on his ward, hands be scrubbed with a brush in a solution of chlorinated lime between autopsy work and the examination of patients. Maintaining meticulous records, he showed that the death rate from puerperal fever dropped precipitously, from more than 12 percent to about 2 percent. The next year he extended his washing protocol to include all instruments used on patients in labor, and childbed fever was virtually eliminated from his hospital ward.

Despite the seemingly incontrovertible proof that his theory was correct, doctors' practices did not change. Some colleagues were even offended by his claims: It was impossible that doctors could be killing their patients. Far from being hailed, Semmelweis was dismissed from his job. He returned to Budapest in 1850, where he built a successful obstetrical practice. Using his hand- and instrument-washing techniques, he reduced the mortality of childbed fever to less than 1 percent. He did not publish his discoveries until 1861, but they were generally scorned and ignored by the European medical community. Thereafter, he suffered several years of mental deterioration. In 1865 he was committed to a mental institution. Considered to be violent, he was beaten by the asylum personnel and, within two weeks, was dead from his injuries at the age of forty-seven.

In the 1870s and 1880s the germ theory of infection was conclusively proven by Louis Pasteur in France, Joseph Lister in England, and Robert Koch in Germany. Even so, their findings were only slowly accepted by the general medical community. The pioneering theories of Ignaz Semmelweis were ultimately vindicated several decades after his death. Today, hand washing is considered the cornerstone of infection prevention, yet it is grossly underused by many healthcare professionals in both inpatient and outpatient settings.

The Mechanism of Skin Contamination

Human skin is not sterile. A number of benign or nonpathogenic bacteria normally colonize the skin surface, where they reside in minute skin creases and crevices. The hands, as well as the armpits and groin, generally harbor 10–20 percent more bacteria than other skin areas. The highest accumulation is generally under the fingernails. These normal skin bacteria adhere quite tightly to the surface of skin cells and are not easily removed. More problematic, however, are the pathogenic, or disease-causing, bacteria that may contaminate the hands after contact with infected wounds, feces, and other contaminated substances. Fortunately, these bacteria (such as *Staphylococcus aureus, Salmonella,* and *Pseudomonas*) do not adhere as avidly to skin cells and are more easily removed. Bacteria do not penetrate intact skin. However, once on the hands, pathogenic bacteria can enter the body by touching open wounds or even normal but sensitive areas such as the mucous membranes of the eyes, lips, mouth, and nose. Even the benign skin bacteria can cause infections if they gain access to normally sterile areas of the body. This occurs most often when one is inserting or manipulating medical devices that enter sterile sites, such as intravenous lines and urinary catheters.

Viruses, particularly those that cause respiratory diseases such as flu or the common cold, can also be carried on the hands. They are acquired by touching surfaces that have been contaminated by infected people. Examples include shaking hands with an infected person or touching doorknobs or other objects recently handled by such people. Like bacteria, respiratory viruses do not penetrate intact skin but are introduced into the body when contaminated hands or fingers touch mucous membranes. Unlike some bacteria, viruses do not adhere firmly to skin cells. Therefore, even the simplest hand washing will readily remove these viruses.

Hand-Washing Techniques

Most routine hand washing consists of sanitizing or decontaminating the hands. For this purpose, a good fifteen- to thirty-second wash of the hands and wrists with plain soap and warm water, using friction, does a perfectly adequate job. The detergents in soap remove loose dirt, grime, viruses, poorly adherent pathogenic bacteria, and dead skin cells with their adherent normal skin bacteria. For the general population, including most cancer survivors, hands should be washed in this manner after any activity that causes hand contamination. Typical examples include urinating and defecating, touching potentially contaminated surfaces, touching plants or soil, or handling uncooked meats and poultry, which may be contaminated with strains of *Escherichia coli* and *Salmonella,* bacteria that can cause severe gastrointestinal illness and diarrhea. Cutting boards and other surfaces in contact with raw meats and poultry should also be washed with soap and warm water before other foodstuffs are placed on them.

For caregivers and patients who will be manipulating open wounds or inserting catheters or other invasive medical devices, more thorough hand washing is necessary. In these situations, high-level disinfection or sterile technique is called for. On your doctor's recommendation you may need to use soaps containing such antibacterial products as chlorhexidine or iodine-containing substances such as povidone–iodine. These products usually are available only by prescription. Before using these products, remove rings, watches, and other jewelry. After wetting the hands, lather the medicated soap with friction on all surfaces, including the wrists and lower third of the forearms, for a full thirty seconds, followed by a thirty-second rinse with warm running water. Dry hands with a clean, disposable towel, which is then used to turn off the faucets. Blotting rather than wiping the hands is preferable in order to avoid irritation and chapping. Again, on your doctor's advice, you should put on clean or sterile vinyl or latex gloves after hand washing and before certain procedures (e.g., changing a dressing or flushing and intravenous catheter). After the procedure, remove gloves by peeling them off inside out and discarding them in a suitable receptacle where they will not be touched again by you or others. Except during these sterile procedures, antibacterial hand washing is generally necessary only for patients whose immune systems are depressed by chemotherapy or by persistent or recurrent cancer. Once again, the type of hand washing needed should be guided by the advice of your health-care provider.

Another type of hand-washing product is rinses, foams, or gels containing 50–90 percent alcohol. These are most commonly used in hospitals, where they are found in wall-mounted dispensers in patient rooms or just outside their doors. Because they can be applied in about fifteen seconds and dry automatically by evaporation, they offer speed and convenience to hospital personnel, who must wash their hands many times each day. Alcohol-based rinses also contain moisturizers or emollients, so they produce less skin chapping and irritation than would occur if soap and water hand washing were done fifty or more times a day. They do have drawbacks, however. They do not kill spores (thick-walled, dormant forms of certain bacteria), and they do not remove debris and dead skin cells as well as does washing with soap and running water. Because the alcohol evaporates quickly, it does not leave any residual antibacterial activity on the hands, as do most medicated antibacterial soaps. Therefore, they are a temporary measure for convenience only. Hospital personnel who use these alcohol rubs must also frequently wash their hands in the typical manner, especially before and after performing any procedure necessitating high-level skin disinfection or sterile technique.

Many over-the-counter soaps for home use are labeled "antibacterial." They usually contain a chemical called triclosan, which is listed on the bottle label. Earlier studies suggested that exposure of bacteria to triclosan might lead to the emergence of triclosan-resistant organisms, which could then colonize household areas such as sinks, faucet handles, drains, and countertops. More disturbing still, there was evidence that exposure to triclosan could induce bacteria to become resistant to many important antibiotics. The results of more recent studies are less clear-cut on this issue, although it is still possible that resistant bacteria may emerge "after longer-term or higher-dose exposure of bacteria to triclosan in the community setting."[2] Therefore, it is advisable for patients and their household members to avoid routine use of triclosan-containing hand washing soaps (unless directed to do so by their physicians) until more definitive evidence of these products' efficacy is available.

Immunization

Influenza

Influenza ("the flu") is a viral respiratory illness that recurs every winter. Outbreaks vary in severity from year to year. In a mild flu season, 15,000 to 20,000 Americans may die from flu or its complications, and in severe epidemic years, 50,000 to 70,000 or more deaths may occur. Every twenty to fifty years, on average, a severe worldwide flu pandemic may occur. The worst of these in modern times occurred in 1918–1919, when half a million Americans and anywhere from 10 to 20 million people worldwide died. Those most at risk of dying from influenza or its complications are the very young, those over sixty-five years of age, and those with chronic medical conditions, including depressed immune systems.

Influenza viruses genetically mutate each year. The greater the degree of genetic mutation, the more likely it is that immunity from prior infections or vaccinations will be ineffective in providing protection against the current mutated strain. Therefore, vaccine manufacturers change the vaccine composition each year, based on the genetic changes noted in the virus during the previous year. For optimal protection, people should receive the latest vaccine preparation each year.

Because it takes about two weeks to develop protective antibodies after vaccination, influenza vaccine should be taken between mid-October and early November, several weeks before flu is expected to arrive in the community. In general, flu vaccine is up to 85 percent effective in preventing or decreasing the severity of influenza. Because of a general weakening of the body's immune response with increasing age, the vaccine tends to be less effective in older adults, although one is never too old to obtain some benefit from vaccination.

Because the vaccine is produced in chicken eggs, people with severe egg allergy, or those who have had a well-documented allergic reaction to a previous flu shot, should not be vaccinated. Aside from some mild discomfort at the injection site and a possible low-grade fever during the twenty-four hours after the shot, the vaccine is extremely safe. These mild side effects should not be interpreted as an allergic reaction and should definitely not discourage people from receiving future annual influenza vaccinations. Because the vaccine contains a killed rather than a live virus, it can safely be given to all cancer and other patients, even those with depressed immunity.

A common misconception holds that the flu vaccine can actually cause influenza. Again, because it is a killed virus vaccine, it does not multiply in the body and is completely incapable of causing influenza. Shortly after vaccination, some people might coincidentally come down with a different viral illness, or even the flu itself, if it was already incubating at the time the vaccine was received. Similarly, because the vaccine is not 100 percent effective (especially in years when the virus undergoes a major mutation, rendering the current vaccine less effective), a person may still come down with the flu after being vaccinated. However, in neither case is the vaccine the cause of the subsequent illness, and this should never be a reason for refusing an annual influenza vaccination.

Tetanus and Diphtheria

Everyone should receive a tetanus and diphtheria booster immunization every ten years. Tetanus toxoid (T) is combined with low-dose diphtheria vaccine (d) in a preparation known as Td vaccine. Like the influenza vaccine, Td contains no live organisms and can safely be given to immune-compromised patients.

Recently, a highly contagious and serious childhood infection called pertussis (whooping cough) has been found to infect adults to a much greater degree than previously suspected. Accordingly, the U.S. Centers for Disease Control and Prevention (CDC) now recommends that all adults under sixty-five years of age receive a single dose of a special combined tetanus–diphtheria–pertussis vaccine (Tdap), marketed as Adacel, at the time of their next routine tetanus booster dose. Thereafter, adults can return to their regular schedule of routine Td booster vaccinations every ten years.

Shingles

Shingles, or herpes zoster, is a viral disease that manifests itself as a painful, blistering rash in a bandlike distribution a few inches wide on one side of the body, usually on the trunk. The rash generally extends from the back, near the spine, and around the body, stopping at the midline in front. It lasts several days and then slowly heals as the blisters scab over and fall off over the course of about ten to fourteen days or longer. The pain can be intense and, in a significant proportion of patients, can last weeks, months, or even years, a condition called postherpetic neuralgia.

Shingles is caused by *Varicella zoster* virus, the cause of chickenpox. Eighty-five percent of people develop chickenpox during childhood. Although almost all children easily recover from the infection, the virus never completely leaves the body. Some virus survives in the nerve roots emerging from the spinal cord, but the body's immune system keeps the virus suppressed and dormant. As immunity wanes with age, particularly after age sixty or so, the virus in a single nerve root may reactivate and travel down the nerve, where it emerges on the skin supplied by that nerve in the form of the characteristic rash. By age eighty-five, approximately half of all adults will have experienced an attack of shingles. About a million new cases of shingles occur each year in the United States.

Shingles is particularly common in cancer patients whose disease or chemotherapy suppresses their immunity. Treatment with antiviral drugs, if given within seventy-two hours of the onset of rash, may reduce the severity and duration of the pain by half or more.

In October 2006 the U.S. Food and Drug Administration (FDA) approved a new shingles vaccine (Zostavax) for people sixty years of age and older. When given to those in their sixties, the vaccine was 50 percent effective in preventing attacks of shingles and more than 67 percent effective in preventing postherpetic neuralgia. When administered to those eighty years of age or older, the vaccine was 18 percent and 39 percent effective in preventing shingles and postherpetic neuralgia, respectively. A single vaccination is effective for at least four years, but longer-term studies are needed to determine the full duration of its protective effects.

Although the vaccine is now licensed and available, it is quite expensive (about $150 per dose); it remains to be seen whether insurance companies will cover its cost. In addition, it is a live virus vaccine and therefore should not be given to those with impaired immunity, such as people with AIDS, immunosuppressive cancers such as lymphoma and certain leukemias, and those receiving immunosuppressive chemotherapy. However, it can be given to currently immune-competent people who are expected to become immunosuppressed, such as patients with early, asymptomatic HIV infection and those with cancers and other conditions who plan to receive chemotherapy and other immune-suppressive therapies in the future.

Hepatitis B

Hepatitis B is a viral infection transmitted by sexual contact with, or exposure to blood from, infected people. Those at greatest risk of acquiring hepatitis B in the United States are people with multiple sexual partners, monogamous sex partners of hepatitis B carriers, injection drug users, and household contacts of a hepatitis B carrier. The infection can also be transmitted from an infected woman to her newborn at the time of delivery. A single milliliter of blood from an infected person (about a fifth of a teaspoon of blood) can contain up to a billion infectious viral particles. Because even the smallest amount of infected blood is capable of transmitting the infection, sharing toothbrushes or razors with an infected household member poses a risk of infection. Blood transfusions were once a great risk for infection, but with the current screening and blood testing practices used by blood banks this risk has been reduced to less than 1 in 5,000 transfusions.

The symptoms of infection (jaundice, fatigue, loss of appetite, and right upper abdominal discomfort, pain, or tenderness) occur in 30–80 percent of acutely infected adults, whereas infected infants and young children rarely develop any symptoms at all. Most symptomatic people recover clinically in about one to three months and completely clear the virus from their liver and blood within six months, thus developing lifelong immunity to reinfection. However, about 5 percent of infected older children and adults fail to clear the virus and become chronic carriers of the virus in their blood. The rate of chronic infection rises to about 30 percent for children infected between one and five years of age. For infants infected at birth, an astounding 90 percent or more become lifelong chronic viral carriers.

Patients with chronic hepatitis B may initially be asymptomatic or may exhibit only mild, nonspecific symptoms such as fatigue. However, the virus causes ongoing and slowly progressive liver damage. After five years, up to 20 percent of adult patients have developed cirrhosis of the liver, and this percentage increases with time. Cirrhosis usually results in progressive decompensation of liver function (i.e., liver failure), at a rate of 20–25 percent of patients per year. Once liver decompensation occurs, only about a third of patients will survive for five years.

Approximately 6–15 percent of hepatitis B patients with cirrhosis will develop hepatocellular carcinoma, a liver cancer that is highly fatal. Chronic hepatitis B patients who drink alcohol have a four times greater risk of liver cancer than those who do not drink. Overall, 15–25 percent of patients with chronic hepatitis B will die of chronic liver disease (cirrhosis, liver failure, or liver cancer).

Fortunately, vaccination against hepatitis B prevents acute infection and the chronic complications of cirrhosis, liver failure, and liver cancer. Thus, hepatitis B vaccine, introduced more than a quarter century ago, was the first vaccine shown to prevent cancer (specifically hepatocellular carcinoma). In the United States, routine hepatitis B vaccination is recommended for all people. Ideally, the first dose should be given at birth, the second one to two months later, and the third six months after the first dose.

For those in whom vaccination was not begun at birth and who do not belong to high-risk groups for acquiring hepatitis B, a three-dose vaccination series can be begun at any age, using a similar dosage timing of zero, one to two, and six months. Of course, the later the vaccine series is begun, the more likely the person is to be already infected. Once a person has acquired hepatitis B infection, vaccination provides no benefit.

For people at high risk of acquiring hepatitis B (those with multiple sexual partners, sexual contacts of hepatitis B carriers, injection drug users, and household contacts of a hepatitis B carrier), it is more cost-effective to screen them first with a blood test for the presence of hepatitis B infection. If the screening test is negative, the vaccination series should be begun without delay.

One other group deserving special mention is those who have just been exposed to infectious hepatitis B. This group includes people with very recent exposure to an infected or high-risk person, such as through sexual contact, needle-stick exposure, blood splash to a mucous membrane (eye or mouth), or birth to an infected mother. In these people the hepatitis B virus has already entered their bodies but has not yet become established. Treatment of these people is called postexposure prophylaxis. In addition to beginning the vaccine series, these people must also receive an intramuscular dose of hepatitis B immune globulin (HBIG), a serum with extremely high levels of antibody against hepatitis B. These antibodies will begin to neutralize the hepatitis B virus already introduced into the body during the time it takes for the vaccine to stimulate the immune system to produce its own antihepatitis B antibodies. To be effective, HBIG should be given within twenty-four hours (and preferably within twelve hours) of exposure. The first dose of hepatitis B vaccine should be given at the same time but at a separate site on the body from the HBIG injection. The second and third doses of hepatitis B vaccine should be given at the time intervals described earlier.

Cervical Cancer

Cervical cancer is the second most common cancer in women worldwide. Each year nearly 10,000 women in the United States are newly diagnosed with cervical cancer and nearly 4,000 women die from it. Infection with the human papillomavirus (HPV) is now known to be the primary cause of cervical cancer.[3]

Of the more than 100 types of HPV, about 40 are known to be spread by sexual contact. Approximately 6 million genital HPV infections occur annually, making it the most common viral sexually transmitted disease in the United States. More than half of all sexually active men and women become infected with one or more types of HPV at some point during their lives.[4] The most common conditions caused by sexually transmitted HPV are genital warts, which are acquired by up to half a million Americans annually. Ninety percent of these warts are caused by HPV types 6 and 11.

Of greater concern is the association of genital HPV infection with cervical cancer. Although several HPV types can cause cervical cancer, types 16 and 18 account for 70 percent of all cases. In about 90 percent of people infected with genital HPV, the virus is eliminated from the body within two years, leaving them immune to reinfection with that specific HPV type. The 10 percent of women who develop persistent HPV infection constitute the risk group for subsequent cervical cancer. Persistent infection with high-risk types of HPV in women and men is also associated with the development of at least some cases of cancer of the vagina, vulva, penis, and anus. Fortunately, these cancers are far less common than cervical cancer.

In June 2006 the FDA licensed Gardasil, a vaccine that protects against the four major types of HPV (types 6, 11, 16, and 18). The vaccine was tested in more than 11,000 girls and women nine to twenty-six years of age. During five years of follow-up, the vaccine proved to be nearly 100 percent effective in preventing cervical, vaginal, and vulvar precancerous lesions and genital warts caused by the four HPV types included in the vaccine. It is not known, at present, how long vaccine immunity will last. Longer-term follow-up studies will determine whether and when vaccine booster doses might be needed.

The vaccine is remarkably safe. The predominant side effect is mild pain at the injection site. Because the vaccine contains no live virus, it can safely be given to immune-suppressed people; however, immune compromise might decrease the vaccine's efficacy. The vaccine contains no thimerosal or mercury.

Like the shingles vaccine, Gardasil is quite expensive ($120 per dose, $360 for the full three-dose series). The details of insurance coverage for this vaccine remain to be determined.

Ideally, the vaccine should be given before sexual activity begins. The American College of Immunization Practices recommends the vaccine be given to girls and women nine to twenty-six years of age, preferably at ages eleven to twelve years. It can also be given to older adolescents and adults. It will provide no benefit against any of the four HPV types with which a woman might already have become infected, but it will protect against the remaining types. It offers no protection against any of the HPV types not included in the vaccine.

Limited studies reveal no ill effects when the vaccine was given to pregnant women. Until more extensive studies are conducted, however, it is currently recommended that pregnant women delay vaccination until after delivery.

A second HPV vaccine, Cervarix, has been developed to prevent cervical cancer in women over twenty-five years of age. It provides protection only against HPV types 16 and 18, the strains responsible for 70 percent of cervical cancer. It is expected to be approved by the FDA in 2007. There is no reason to believe that Gardasil would not be effective in this age group as well. The only reason Gardasil is not licensed for women older than twenty-six years is that it was not studied in them.

Despite the availability of the HPV vaccine, women should still receive routine cervical cancer screening with a standard Pap smear or the newer liquid-based Pap test. A new test that detects the presence of HPV DNA in cervical cells is also available. The reason for continuing routine screening is that 30 percent of cervical cancers are caused by HPV types not included in the current vaccines. By the same token, women whose Pap smears show precancerous changes or whose DNA tests are positive for the presence of HPV virus are still eligible to receive the HPV vaccine because their current infection might be caused by an HPV strain other than the ones present in the vaccine.

More information on the HPV vaccine can be obtained from the Centers for Disease Control and Prevention Web site, which is listed in Appendix C.[5]

Other Preventive Measures

Other routine measures can help protect against infection. Most viral respiratory infections, including influenza, are spread when droplets expelled by coughing or sneezing contact the mucous membranes of the mouth, nose, or eyes. Covering the mouth and nose with a tissue or handkerchief when coughing or sneezing effectively blocks transmission of most of these droplets. Patients should ask family members, friends, and associates to cover their coughs and sneezes, and they should do so themselves when they have a respiratory illness in order to avoid spreading infection to others. Because expelled droplets travel a distance of only 4 feet at most, maintaining a safe distance from a coughing or sneezing person is also a reasonable precaution. During the cold and flu season it is wise to avoid crowded areas (e.g., buses, theaters) when practical to do so. Wearing a paper or cloth surgical mask does not effectively shield the wearer from exposure to airborne infectious droplets, and their use is not recommended as a protective measure.

Diseases such as gingivitis and periodontitis damage the mucous membranes of the gums, allowing bacteria from the mouth to enter the tissues and even the bloodstream itself. Proper oral hygiene and routine dental prophylaxis and care therefore are essential in preventing infection in cancer survivors.

Breaks in the skin are another possible portal of entry for infection-producing bacteria. Small cuts and abrasions should be dealt with promptly by carefully washing and drying the area, covering it with a clean dressing, and keeping it dry until a scab has formed. Wet dressings should be removed, the wound should be gently dried, and a fresh clean dressing reapplied as soon as possible.

Care should be taken when trimming fingernails and toenails to avoid skin cuts. Skin conditions such as athlete's foot should be treated promptly to prevent entry of bacteria through damaged, broken skin. This is particularly important during periods of chemotherapy-induced immune suppression and for all patients with diabetes.

Malnutrition increases the risk of infection by suppressing the immune system[6] and generally impairing the body's healing mechanisms. In the United States, undernutrition affects 15 percent of all outpatients[7] and up to 65 percent of long-term care and hospitalized patients. The importance of maintaining a nourishing, balanced diet cannot be overemphasized.

PART VI

Improved Survival with Creative Expression

32 The Importance of Creative Expression[1]

Ernest H. Rosenbaum, M.D., F.A.C.P., Isadora R. Rosenbaum, M.A., and Cynthia D. Perlis, B.S.

Attitude

Attitude has a major influence on your life and has become one of the important ingredients in living well and longer. It is shaped in part by our experiences, education, failures, and successes. A positive attitude can help increase our ability to cope with life's problems or with a disease. We have a chance each day when we get up to make this a great day and achieve what we wish or to merely accept events that occur and not try to improve our lot or set new goals. Some things in life are more difficult to change than others. Therefore, how we live is controlled in part by our attitude toward life, which becomes the pivot on which the future hinges.

The Will to Live

The will to live is nurtured by a positive attitude. A negative attitude can diminish or undermine the mind through fear, anger, or loss of self-esteem. When unresolved, these emotions can lead to hopelessness, futility, resignation, and the loss of the will to live. Here are a few examples:

- The phrase "frightened to death" is more than a figure of speech. An early reference to stress and fear is recorded in the Bible, in Acts 5, when Ananias and his wife, Sapphira, suddenly die after being castigated by Peter for withholding from the disciples some of the money paid for the sale of land. Their deaths have been attributed to sudden coronary death from stress.
- In primitive societies people have been literally frightened to death by the imposition of a curse or spell, known as bone pointing. When a person who believed in the phenomenon was "boned," he or she withdrew from the world, stopped eating, and waited to die. Death could take place in a few weeks. Such deaths have not been explained medically, even with an autopsy, but it seems apparent that the paralyzing effect of fear played an important role. The victim's fear stems from ignorance and superstition. He or she has been encouraged to believe in the power of the curse. Thus, ignorance and superstition play a role in how the mind functions to help or hinder a person in living.

People with a positive attitude are able to be open, to talk about their problems with their family, friends, and physicians. They feel good about themselves and generally have been that way all their lives.

It is often very hard to change lifelong patterns such as your psychological reaction to daily living. The will to live therefore is a spiritual, emotional, and ethical commodity. It needs nurturing and development and, if controlled, can strengthen a person's resolve to survive. We soon discover that the mind plays an important role in trying to control life, that there is a direct correlation between a person's mental and emotional states.

We measure successes and failures in life by our standards and ideals as we strive for goals in work, relationships, and health. Mere survival makes for a shallow life. Victory is for those who have the courage and stamina to fight and endure each of life's many struggles and who always have goals and the satisfaction of aspiring to reach them, whether they succeed or fail. This is the challenge of life.

The Role of Creating Art in Health

A hundred years ago, it was commonly believed that people could not be creative past middle age. Now, reports Lydia Bronte in *The Longevity Factor,* most Americans can expect a "second middle age"—a stage of adulthood between fifty and seventy-five that has not existed before. Today, people in middle age and beyond sometimes feel that life is just beginning. A new sense of identity is discovered and defined along with an enhanced sense of self. During these years, art can be a healing force.

Artistic expression is an important psychosocial activity. We can create art by ourselves, alone in a studio, or we can attend classes ranging from beginning drawing to advanced printmaking. Sometimes we can express ourselves visually when we are unable to express ourselves verbally. Art can help us express what we are feeling in the present, yet it can also help us to express a memory, a moment that has happened that we do not want to forget. Music, drawing, painting, and creating sculpture provide a means of communication and self-expression and a way to alleviate stress.

Art also helps us to change our moods, come out of depression, or simply relax.

Art can be richly therapeutic for people, including older adults, with a serious illness such as cancer. Suzanne, a woman approaching eighty who is living a full and energetic life despite her advanced cancer, has continued to teach art classes, take printmaking classes, and work in her home studio. Her recent works have included drawings and watercolors that express what it feels like to cope with life-threatening illness. She has created drawings that tell the story of her disease. One watercolor, *The Cell of Positive Thinking,* was created when she began a course of chemotherapy.

Suzanne says that creating art improves her self-worth and leaves a permanent gift to be enjoyed by all. She has received constant encouragement and support from her friends and family. They drive her to art classes and create along with her. Together they are participating in a shared experience, a shared community of meaning—the essence of what it means to be human.

You do not have to have artistic ability to be creative. Sometimes just doodling or experimenting with art materials can open up a wide range of ideas. People often become too critical of their work or are afraid others will judge their ability. It is important to express yourself for yourself and not for anyone's approval. There really is no right or wrong in expressing who you are. For instance, if you feel you cannot draw, try making collages from pictures cut from magazines.

Creating art at any age gives people an opportunity to express what they are feeling. Creating art provides the ability to make decisions for oneself. With the opportunity to make decisions, to exercise control over choice, people enhance their quality of life, improve self-esteem, and create ways to relate to others in a meaningful way. A whole life or one experience can be shared in a work of art. One artist writes, "No, I will never say my work is finished. I must live forever—on and on. The reason we artists enjoy such longevity is that we are always looking ahead to the 'masterpiece' to come."

Here are some recommended creative art activities:

- Draw a self-portrait. Include words to describe who you are.
- Create a family tree. Ask everyone to draw his or her own portrait on the tree.
- Take painting, drawing, or sculpture classes at your local community college. If you feel you're not good enough, take a beginners' class; everyone will be in the same boat.
- Draw your dreams.
- Make a collage with pictures cut out of magazines. Decide on a theme before you start or let the theme evolve.
- Do a drawing with a friend, child, grandchild, or spouse.
- Take photographs.
- Learn needlepoint or knitting.
- Buy fabric paint and paint on T-shirts.
- Don't be judgmental—there is no right or wrong, no rules, no grades.
- Smile as you create.

Breast Cancer Quilts

Inspired by the AIDS quilt, in the summer of 1996, Dr. Rosenbaum suggested to the Susan G. Komen Breast Cancer Foundation a project designed to give women with breast cancer a creative voice. The tradition of quiltmaking has been nurturing and creative for countless women throughout history and, as it had for people with AIDS, could alert women about breast cancer in a moving and beautiful way.

Cynthia Perlis, director of Art for Recovery at the University of California at San Francisco Mount Zion Comprehensive Cancer Center, remembered the touching stories and drawings that women with breast cancer had shared with her. It was time to give these women a voice in the larger community, to let them speak through their creative spirits and to share their pain, their hopes, and their dreams with their families and friends. Women recovering from and coping with breast cancer would be able to express visually their feelings about this illness. The Breast Cancer Quilts Project became a project of Art for Recovery through quilt workshops and meetings with women at the bedside quiltblocks.

These squares began to represent the entire scope of this devastating illness. One square read, "I WON THE LOTTERY NO ONE CARED TO ENTER." On another piece of fabric, written in ballpoint pen, was the entire story of one woman's breast cancer experience. Another woman embroidered "THE GIFT OF A LIFETIME" and dedicated the square to her doctor. The quiltmaker then sewed the fabric squares into a beautiful quilt.

One year later, there are five quilts, each measuring 8 feet by 8 feet and each including images by or in memory of twenty-five women with breast cancer. In 2006, more than fifty quilts were made, and the number is growing by five quilts a year. The quilts have been on display across the country. One of the most poignant parts of this project is the stories women have written about their own squares that tell the painful reality of breast cancer. Here is one example:

> I wanted to make this square as a thank you to my three daughters who have been so loving and supportive these past ten months. The design idea came from a beautiful Christmas tree ornament given to me by my second daughter. I was extremely touched by this gift and displayed it prominently on our tree.
>
> I didn't really understand why it made such an impact on me and I'm not sure I

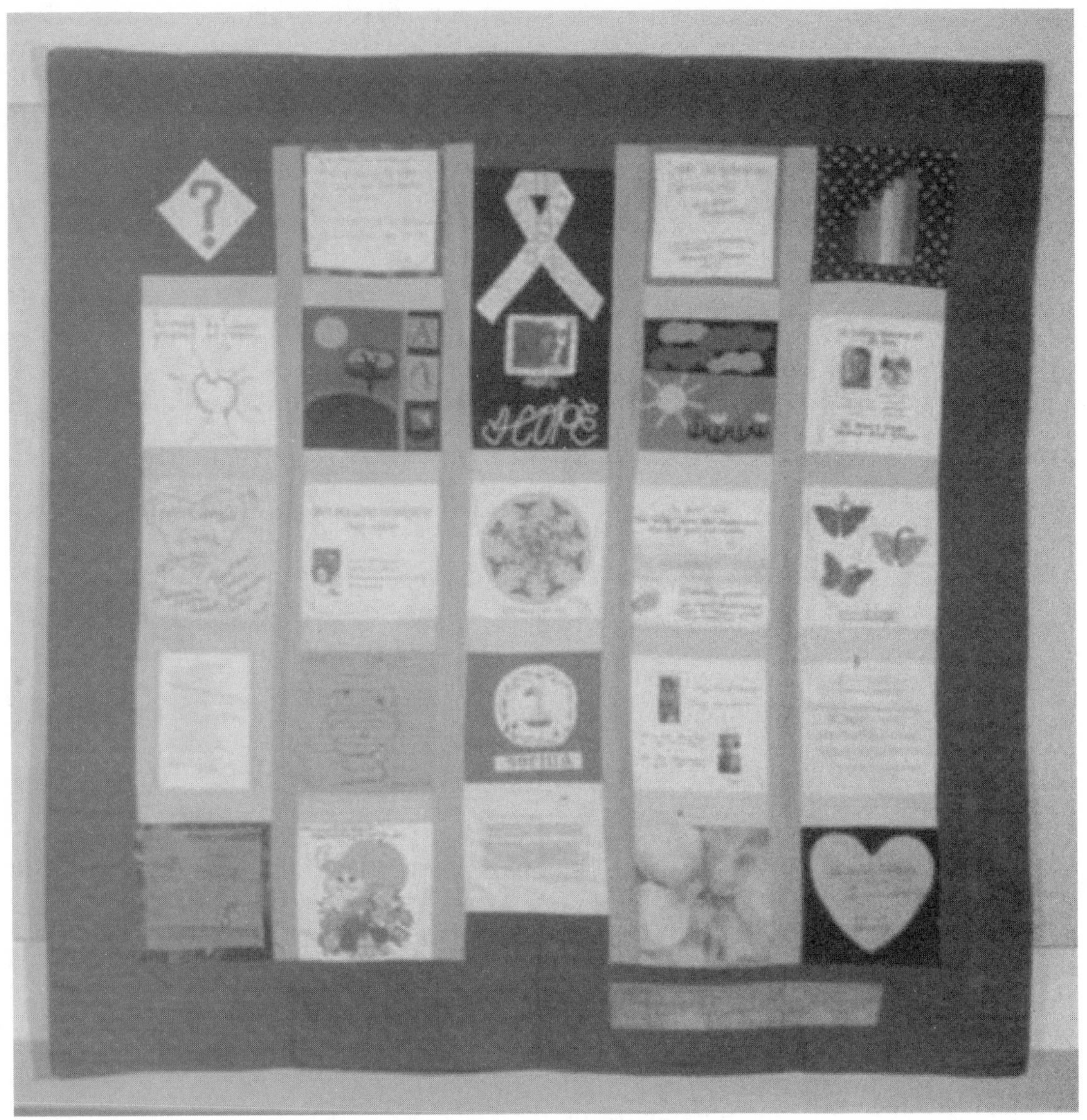

Art for Recovery Breast Cancer Quilt

know the answer yet. However, I suspect one of the reasons was that it was possible to have something beautiful represent a difficult and challenging time in my life. It also served as a daily reminder to be ever-vigilant and to never forget. I wear a pink ribbon of some kind every day now to continue to remind myself, my thirtyish daughters, and the world that the ENEMY is still out there ready to strike 180,000 more women this year alone.

—Elisa Bambi Schwartz

The Breast Cancer Quilts Project continues to invite women from around the country to create images for the quilts. In May 1998, eleven quilts were exhibited at the National Institutes of Health as part of the National Cancer Institute's Breast Cancer Think Tank to support other women battling cancer and increase public awareness of the disease. As a result of this prestigious exhibition, calls continue coming to Art for Recovery from all over the United States wanting information about participating in this significant project. Learn more about this project at cancer.ucsf.edu/afr/quilts.html.

33 The Role of Poetry and Prose in Health

Ernest H. Rosenbaum, M.D., F.A.C.P., and Isadora R. Rosenbaum, M.A.

"The Veil of Illusion"

The night time is brutal,
there is no "snuggling in."
All of the aches and pains and horrors
come to haunt me.
In the deep dark stillness of the night
I am left with myself,
A loneliness I can't describe
Nothing seems real.
Even the light of a beautiful day
can't diminish the darkness.
The hustle, bustle of Saturday morning sounds
can't break the silence, the stillness.
But once in a while
in a blissful moment of distraction
I can almost remember the other side
when I still wore the veil.
—Elisa Bambi Schwartz

Since the development of written language, people have tried to capture their lives and history through writing. The ancients used pictures and signs to record their lives and thoughts. Over the centuries this has evolved into written history and literature. Like art and music, literature, whether prose or poetry, is another way to support and enhance patient care and well-being. Like art and music, literature can be the best medicine and, through the benefits of self-expression, can have healing powers.

Reading or writing poetry or prose can reduce boredom and help relieve depression. It can divert your mind from your medical situation, providing creative stimulation and helping you to communicate your feelings with your family, friends, and medical team. Enjoying the use of your creative spirit and intelligence can provide a vital force to improve your state of wellness, daily living, and quality of life.

You may feel unsure about your ability to create literature, but do not be too critical of your early efforts because it takes time to learn techniques and to discover your unique voice. Your talent will develop if you give yourself a chance. Many people find that taking a creative writing class or joining a poetry or fiction writers' group provides guidance and reduces their initial frustrations.

When people are seriously ill or depressed, they often feel hopeless. Such feelings can be heightened by bad news about their disease or treatment. Even during recovery, people may feel sadness and a heaviness of heart. Reading great literature, whether prose or poetry, and attempting to express your own feelings of sorrow and loss through writing can raise your spirits, provide relaxation, and give creative satisfaction. Working with others in a class or group can also help to prevent isolation.

A patient who is a poet described the deep effect that reading Pushkin, Lermontov, and Pasternak has on her heart and spirit. She also said, "Sometimes when I have had a sad or hard day, I create poetry myself. Poetry makes my heart 'burn bright' through its magical strength. It also pleases me with an unusual inner feeling when people read my poetry, which for me is a 'lyric confession.' They appreciate my lyric confession when they understand my point of view and this creates an impulse to create more and more poetry."

This poet is also a journalist and writes articles and reviews on art, dance, and music. She says, "I have also enjoyed the recognition I have received. It has led to important moments in my life during the past two and a half years, such as when a small four-page Russian newspaper *Odessky Listok* told stories [I had written] of people from other cities and countries. Readers appreciated the stories about people's adventures and life which is not only a personal declaration of their importance on earth but for mankind as well."

"I want to live—to think and suffer"
The poet said, and I agree.
I want to live to sing in poems
The taste of life, its smell, its joy, its dreams.
I want to share my deepest feelings
How free and happy—I am blessed to live
In Golden State—unique and gorgeous
In the mysterious Bay waves.
I want to suffer, but not from pain
Not from the evil—my inevitable fate
I want to cry from love, to love again,
Be loved, forget my age, be able to create.

—Tamara Belorusets,
translation by Yelena Nechay

Alexander Morrison, also a poet, said, "I also have written poetry for many years. I find it interesting to observe how, in different ways, I expressed the same philosophy at 18 as I do now. I was amazed then as I am now at how the human being, screwed by circumstances beyond all belief, can manage to stand up despite the unmitigating bullshit that presses down on him. I'm talking about mankind and people like myself—the survivors and the contributors, the people I think have become successful human beings."

Trace the affinity
Of the will to be
with the ability
To be no longer.
Ah . . . such a narrow way divides.
And yet, in the precarious clime
Of this most eccentric inch
A world of men lived
Triumphant!

—Alexander Morrison

According to Morrison, "I'm looking for the same answers I looked for at 18. I haven't changed, but I do know that even with the odds tremendously against you, most of us manage somehow to make it."

The vulgar splendor of a noise
Contents the appetite of ears
Insensitive to subtleties
The really loud occurrence falls
without the benefit of sound
How silently are these:
The awakening to love,
The audacity to dream,
The will to live.

—Alexander Morrison

"The Recovery"

No longer can I bear
To dwell in this misbegotten state
Of involuntary confinement
The sorrow is too deep
The truth of it too great
For human comprehension
And so, with anxious hands I break away
The larval crust and shake myself free!
Outside carillon bells
Sing of my resurrection and celebrate
My reawakening with soft murmurs
Bird songs and forgotten lullabies
They call to me, beckon me
Into the blazing light of day
And direct me toward the path
Of undisturbed freedom!
With grateful tears
I squint into the blinding sun
And with an innocence of childhood born
I join the living once again
All is forgotten
—Diane Behar

My breast, my womanhood, my life.
These things I took for granted.
But that all changed just
as the New Year began.
No, it couldn't be happening—not to me.
It just doesn't happen so fast.
I was just checked.
It doesn't run in my family.
It's just my imagination.
It's probably nothing.
Or is it?
It's a Saturday night.
How long should I wait?
Then Monday came.
My doctor's on vacation.
Find someone else, I can't wait.
"Just a cyst," they said,
"This doesn't look good."
"What does that mean?" I said.
"Don't worry, it's probably nothing,
but get it checked IMMEDIATELY."
"Don't panic," they said, as if I could stop.
It's all so unreal,
like I'm in a padded tunnel.
More tests, more worried looks, no answers.
"See a surgeon," they said, "ASAP."
I felt so alone, so small, so scared.
Why me? Will I die? Will I be mutilated?
Will Chris still want me?
"We'll call you tomorrow, just relax."
As if I could!
Who are they kidding?
Somehow I slept that night.
I can't remember what I dreamed.
It's probably better that way.
We met the surgeon the next morning;
I vaguely remember.
"I'll have to operate," he said,
"Go home, wait for the results."
The hours seemed endless.
Then the call came.
Oh, God! It can't be true!!
Not cancer! Not me!
I nearly collapsed.
Chris looked so helpless.
My life flashed before me.
Not so much the past,
but the future I was so scared of losing.
I'm too young to die.
I'm not finished living.
So back to the surgeon we went.
"It's a nasty one," he said.
"We'll operate tomorrow,
no time to wait."
What will I look like?
How much will they take?
Has it spread?
Will it come back?
Will my life ever be the same?
—Holly Kurzman 1999

"Poster Girl"

I want to be the poster girl
For this cancer that has invaded me
I want the doctors (after treatments)
To say, "There's no cancer I can see."
How did this cancer get inside of me?
I did not invite it here

And since it is not welcome
Why should I fear it?
It's true that it is awesome
But my God is awesomer
So, cancer, you got to go
As I'm sure you must know
Do you think that I saved this body
For a poison such as you?
Do you think that I will lay down
And accept you as my due?
Not 'til I've declared war
And fought my very best
I won't let up until I've destroyed you
You most unwelcome pest
—Josie Teal, 7/21/2000

Poetic Medicine: Using Poetry to Deepen Your Connection to Self and Others

John Fox, C.P.T.

We human beings are at our best when we enjoy poetry. Sometimes all you need is to reflect in your mind one poem that says, "I can make it through."
—Maya Angelou

Support is a major issue in coping with cancer or any illness that requires intense medical intervention and time. The sheer logistical requirements of doctor visits and hospital treatments can be exhausting. Indeed, it can be difficult when you are ill to make it through a day without the help of a friend or family member acting as advocate and companion, the support of a medical professional offering treatment, or the help of a counselor or minister.

Support may come in the form of stress-relieving practical information, advocacy, friendship, and counsel, but there is a particular kind of support that offers nourishment to your creative spark. This creative spark is accessible to us even when we are ill. We may experience a pull toward imaginative expression as a form of healing, but when you are dealing with the necessities of illness, your creative voice may be given short shrift.

The encouragement to write down your feelings will nourish your creativity. How can you get even more out of your creative expression and the healing art of poem making? Giving attention to this creative spark may support your desire to live life as fully as possible. People find that the expression of feelings, images, and metaphor meets some of their deepest needs in being human while coping with cancer and, at the same time, taps into their spiritual strength, playfulness, and search for meaning. Creative expression helps you hold on to your core self while facing the demands of a disease such as cancer. Poetry reminds you that you are more.

How can you get started? You can start by putting your pen to the page. You don't have to share your writing with anyone; however, you might find it a surprising source of inspiration and support when you do so.

Ask a receptive friend (perhaps a few friends) or a family member with whom you are comfortable to share in the writing and reading of poems. Ask someone to share their favorite poem with you. Robert Pinsky, poet laureate of the United States, appears regularly on *The NewsHour* to share Americans' favorite poems.

You could ask a nurse, caregiver, or doctor whether he or she is open to listening to your poems and perhaps to share his or her own. There is a growing interest among nurses and doctors in poetry. Medical humanities courses are increasingly popular at medical schools. Poems regularly appear in the *Journal of the American Medical Association*. You can encourage this healthy trend.

The opportunity to share poems, to speak poems you've written, and to listen to others speak their poems can deepen your connection with what matters to you. There is a spiritual dimension to this creative bond that allows a deep and vulnerable place in a person to be received and honored. This is sharing at a level that fosters honesty and compassion.

Your poetry can explore joy and grief, insight and confusion, pain and pleasure, fear and love, what you do and do not know, your enjoyment of the natural world, and your intuitive awareness of spirit poems that speak to these things and feed the bonds of relationship and the soul of each person.

Laura is a close friend of Kathy, a woman with ovarian cancer. Laura accompanied Kathy through many aspects of her illness and treatment. They formed a special bond by sharing poems together. When Kathy had to leave a writing group she joined with Laura because of her illness, she continued to meet with Laura to share the writing and reading of poems. Laura says of their experience, "Having the chance to work on poetry together brings Kathy back from getting lost in the medical reality. I know it is a return to wholeness for her and it helps me to see her wholeness too." She adds, "To be with someone coping with serious illness can at times be heavy and stressful but because we are sharing with one another in this creative way there is a deepening of our friendship that is nourished by poetry. Poetry keeps us receptive to moments of joy, connection, and compassion." Laura also notes, "Writing makes us aware of a place that holds a deeper meaning than the medical reality. It carves out a time and a space where the illness is not totally in control. Listening to the voice of poetry is liberating. It's a chance for both of us to be ourselves."

Keeping your writing in a special and meaningful journal may also inspire your writing. As Kathy notes, "Laura just bought me a new blank journal and I love it. The cover is wine-color, magenta and a couple of shades of blue. It is very personal, especially when you can also include drawing. I love the colors, I want to hug it. It's perfect for me."

It is important to establish a safe environment when exploring healing issues through writing. Trust and empathy, acceptance and honesty, playfulness and respect—these are threads that weave the fabric of relationships. These qualities become more crucial in relationships when we are ill. Nurturing these qualities will be helpful in drawing out creative expression when, under the pressure of illness, our safety is threatened.

Illness forces us to enter the unknown—a loss of identity, for instance—and that can be frightening. Poetry can be a companion for this difficult journey and offer a way to navigate in the darkness. Kathy comments about writing and sharing poems, "Writing poems helps me to remember who I am. What I love. The writing brings me to life again. It brings back my love of creating things I enjoyed before I got sick. I feel so much more of my value and worth—both in writing and sharing. There is something about writing that sometimes has nothing to do with illness. The following poem came to me after waking from a dream":

"The Spring of Inner Joy"

Around the spring of inner joy
We gathered, just we three
Father, Son & Holy Ghost
and their invisible me.

Out amongst the pines at night
We heard the owl call
"Strengthen, Deepen, Darken, Flyers.
I will fly for all."

And but for their abundant joy,
A gift beyond us all
We fed together in the night
All those who heard the call.

According to Kathy, "This is a mysterious poem for me. It is a celebration. I think the 'invisible me' is a part of myself that came back to me in writing the poem. This poem is very promising. Like an underground seed, this poem is a truth I am not quite aware of." She adds, "My sister begged me for a copy of this poem as did my friend Jan who said it spoke to her about her own spirituality. I was so pleased that my poem was deeply meaningful to them! That meant a lot to me."

The benefit of people supporting one another's creative voice is profound when there is respect for safety and for the unknown that we all face.

Art for Recovery/Firefly Project

Cynthia D. Perlis, B.S.

In 1992 I developed the Art for Recovery/Brandeis Pen Pal Project/Firefly Project, in which patients enjoy the art of writing letters to teenage pen pals. The idea developed from my hospital visits at the bedsides of patients for the Art for Recovery program, where I noted that although in many cases these people were quite frail, weak, and in pain, their spirits were very much alive. I felt that they had much to offer in the way of personal experiences, insight, and wisdom.

Seriously ill patients could become, in effect, teachers. I matched twelve patients, half with cancer and half with AIDS, with twenty-four seventh- and eighth-grade students (aged twelve, thirteen, and fourteen). The teens would write letters to the patients, including drawings if they chose. They could ask absolutely any question, such as, "Are you afraid to die?" "How did you ever tell your parents that you had cancer?" One twelve-year-old girl wrote to a thirty-two-year-old woman with leukemia, "How did you ever tell your parents you had cancer? I could never tell that to my parents." The patients would write about their jobs, their families, and their illnesses in response. They would answer the teens' questions about their conditions and difficulties and tell about their experiences.

The letters are exchanged for nine months. More than 100 students and as many patients have built bridges and created their own community. Thirty patients have died, some during the school year. At the end of each school year, there is a healing service where the students and the patients meet for the first time. The students read aloud blessings that they have written, and the patients bring the students symbols of healing. This experience defines the true meaning of the word *mitzvah* (a Jewish word for a good deed). This project still continues, with a book being writing and a performance piece planned.

The following letters are excerpted from the correspondence between a woman with breast cancer and her twelve-year-old pen pal:

Dear Katherine,

How did you know you had cancer? My sister has a muscular disease, so I know about muscular problems, but I don't really know anyone with a serious disease. Was it really scary when you found out you were ill? How long have you had cancer?

I'm really looking forward to writing you.

Love,

Lily

P.S. Please send a picture.

Dear Lily,

It was really nice to get your letter.

I have breast cancer and I found a lump in my breast that felt big and hard. I could also feel swollen lymph nodes under my arm. It was very scary when I first found out.

I had to go through a lot of treatment and make decisions about the treatment. That was hard. I seem to be doing well so far and hope it continues this way.

Because I am a physician I see a lot of children with serious diseases and also a lot of children who are healthy. I'm sorry to hear that your sister has a muscular disease. How has it been for you to deal with this and help her?

Thank you for your very nice picture—Write soon.

Katherine

The following letters are excerpted from the correspondence between a woman with leukemia and her twelve-year-old pen pal:

Dear Emily:

I got some bad news recently. My leukemia is back. The doctors are very surprised. It is unusual for someone who has done well for two years to get their cancer back now. I always knew there would be a chance for it to come back, but I was hoping it would be longer (or not at all).

I had thought there was nothing more the doctors could do. But they want to try a procedure on me where they get some cells from the man who donated some of his bone marrow to me before. These cells are white blood cells and they fight off infections. The doctors hope by giving me these cells, it will help boost my immune system to fight off and maybe destroy the leukemia.

It is a hard decision for me to make. It might be hard to understand why I might just decide to just let the leukemia kill me. The procedure will make me pretty sick again. And the doctors are not too sure it will work anyway. I was not very happy last time I was in the hospital and I am not looking forward to being sick again. But my friends and family seem to really want me to try this procedure because it is my only chance to live.

It is hard to realize that I have to make these kinds of decisions. I am just a regular, normal person. These kinds of things happen in the movies or TV.

Whatever happens, I would like to keep writing you. We can write about all sorts of things still. And you can ask me questions about what is happening to me if you want. The leukemia is part of my life, but not all of it.

My knees are better, I almost walk normal. But I am still pretty weak. Only my left leg can go up the stairs. It is like someone is holding me back if I try with my right leg.

Jana

Dear Jana,

I am very sad right now because you have got leukemia again. I had no idea this could happen again and I am very sorry. But I have a lot of hope that you will get better and I know you will too.

When did the leukemia come back? Is it as bad as it was before? How does your family feel about this? Are you afraid? How do you feel about coming back to the hospital after you've been out of it for so long? I have so many questions about this.

I heard from Cindy that you feel okay right now and I'm really glad about that. I hope that the new procedure the doctors are going to try will work.

It really is going to be a hard decision for you to make, but I think that if I were in this same situation, I would just try whatever the doctors think might work. I don't know why, but I hope whatever they do works and I hope you'll feel better soon.

I would like to keep writing to you too. Thanks for saying I can ask questions about what is happening. . . . I'm glad your knees are better.

Bye,

Emily

34 The Role of Humor in Health

Ernest H. Rosenbaum, M.D., F.A.C.P., Malin Dollinger, M.D., and Stu Silverstein, M.D.

Humor and laughter have been found to have a positive effect on the body's physiology and to induce relaxation. They help people cope and improve relationships between family members and friends. A lighthearted attitude can reduce the chance of illness, reduce depression, and thereby promote longevity.

Humor reduces stress almost immediately. It also helps alleviate pain. Laughter has even been used as an aid in treating disease. As Norman Cousins stated, "I made the joyous discovery that 10 minutes of genuine belly laughter had an anesthetic effect and would give me at least two hours of pain-free sleep." He discovered that watching funny movies with the Marx Brothers or the Three Stooges was therapeutic. Cousins wrote in *Anatomy of an Illness as Perceived by the Patient* that he deliberately tried to increase his laughter to improve his health.

There is an old joke that a man was wondering what the meaning of life was, and he became morbidly depressed over this question. He even tried to shoot himself in the head but missed. Finally, in desperation, he wandered randomly into a movie theater, where a Marx Brothers movie was showing. There he realized that as long as there is laughter, there is meaning to life.

Humor can do wonders to help lift the spirits. Some studies have shown that if you just smile, the body's response is a positive one. Try it and see what happens.

The Physiology of Humor and Laughter

Humor usually results in laughter, which arouses the emotions, resulting in physical changes. These include short-term increases in blood pressure, heart rate, and respiratory rate and reduction of stress.

Laughter stimulates the brain to produce endorphins (morphinelike relaxants that have a euphoric or analgesic effect). The result is muscle relaxation, with a resolution of stress and anxiety, an improvement in mental and spiritual well-being, and often a decrease in hostility and anger. Laughter also confers several long-lasting benefits on your body; in the long run it lowers blood pressure, and it also serves as a mini–aerobic workout without the expense of joining a health club. Scientific studies are looking at exactly how laughter, mirth, and a humorous perspective can have a positive effect on health and improve quality of life.

Laughter from jokes, speeches, comedies, plays, movies, operas, or other humorous events is a socially accepted way of getting a message across. It is sometimes a means of getting through personal tragedy or crisis (for those creating the humor and those responding to it). Some people find that telling jokes about themselves removes some of the heaviness they feel about their lives.

Humor can be spontaneous or specifically created, but no matter how it evolves, it can make a difference in your life. It is a healing power for both body and soul and a help in sustaining oneself through some of the depressing episodes of life.

Benefits of Humor

There are many benefits of humor. Here are some of them:

- Humor can help us expand our perspective on life and enhance creativity.
- The more we laugh, the better our chance of decreasing depression and promoting healing. Promoting laughter injects more happiness into daily life.
- Humor can improve family relationships and smooth communications.
- Humor provides physical and mental energy and rejuvenation through emotional relaxation.
- Humor helps people cooperate and communicate and decreases anger and fear.
- Humor can promote a will to live, promote energy, improve self-esteem, and increase self-worth.
- Humor is considered one of the great medicines of all time.
- Humor can reduce anxiety and thereby improve the enjoyment of social experiences such as dining.

There is an old Dutch saying that humor often comes from telling a tragic story after enough time has passed. In this way you can laugh at many hard times in your life. It wasn't funny at the time, but after you triumph over the tribulations of life the stories can later be uproariously funny.

How to Make Humor Work for You

- Collect or write down humorous anecdotes, mementos, cartoons, and jokes. Refer to them often to improve your emotional energy and revive sagging spirits.
- Create humorous cards and cartoons to make you laugh every day. Often telling personal or family stories about life is a way of sharing humor and funny events.
- Take a class on writing or telling jokes.
- Keep humorous books, articles, or cartoons nearby. Refer to them frequently to make yourself smile and laugh.
- Try to avoid frequent contact with depressing people who drain your emotional energy. Associate with positive people who use humor.
- Promote parties and fun social events, such as birthdays. You need to make them happen.
- Arrange a get-together with friends or relatives to tell jokes, recall happy and funny events, or share a funny video or movie.
- Regularly visit a local comedy club.
- Maintain a compendium of humor and philosophy to help you reduce isolation, anger, despair, or loneliness.

By using vignettes, jokes, or philosophical or practical sayings or words, you can improve your coping skills and reduce despair. A bit of humor, when appropriate, can make a sad event a little lighter and more positive. For grave or serious situations, a little humor can decrease your level of unhappiness. Apply the techniques of Norman Cousins.

Don't leave it to chance. Actively seek humor in your life. Those who laugh last laugh best!

35 The Role of Music in Health

Ernest H. Rosenbaum, M.D., F.A.C.P., Jim Murdoch, Isadora R. Rosenbaum, M.A., Malin Dollinger, M.D., and Cynthia D. Perlis, B.S.

Music has healing powers. It has been said that music hath charms to soothe the savage breast. It is said that Plato believed that health in body and mind is obtained through music. Florence Nightingale used the healing powers of music as part of nursing the ill. Music affects the physiological and psychological aspects of an illness or disability. In the Bible, David the shepherd boy played his harp to help the psychologically anxious, insomniac King Saul relax and sleep. And music was used to calm shell-shocked soldiers in World War II.

Music has a personal meaning to each of us, often recalling or eliciting a positive emotional response. It has a universal appeal, it is inexpensive, and it crosses cultural barriers. It is available by radio, TV, tape player, CD player, vinyl records, and live. It can be listened to quietly, through earphones, or out loud for all to enjoy.

There is always a place for music in our daily life. It gives us a special pleasure and enjoyment and improves our mood. It affords us a way of expressing ourselves in a nonverbal way that can give us joy, calm us down, or lead to great excitement. It can provide us an escape or reach down into our deeper soul and elicit pent-up emotions. For some people and their relatives and friends, music offers a special way to pass time that may sometimes seem endless.

It can provide a way to decrease stress, promote emotional recovery, and provide relaxation. It can also afford a means of communication without the need for a common spoken language.

Physiological and Psychological Effects

Music can increase or decrease heart rate and blood pressure, depending on the tempo and type of music. It can relax and reduce anxiety or stimulate and heighten awareness. The intense emotions evoked by music can affect the nervous system and induce endorphin production. Music can help relax muscles to decrease nervous tension. It can also reduce alienation and feelings of isolation and improve self-control and confidence.

Age, illness, and treatment can affect a person's psychological equilibrium, causing depression and negatively affecting spiritual and emotional feelings and social interactions. Music offers a bridge in helping to support a person through many of the crises in life. It reduces stress and thus reduces stress-related illnesses.

Emotional Enhancement

There is a type of music to fit any emotion or mood. John Philip Sousa's "Stars and Stripes Forever" brings cheers and elicits patriotism. Verdi's *Requiem* or Rossini's *William Tell* may elevate the mood and give waves of relaxation to reduce stress or help alleviate grief. Listening to Mendelssohn's *A Midsummer Night's Dream* or a Count Basie or Turk Murphy jazz program can provide an emotional lift. Listening to the soft sentimental music of Nat King Cole, Glenn Miller, or Tommy Dorsey is relaxing; it can also provide fun and exercise if you get up and dance.

Music offers immediate gratification. You can sit and tap your feet to the rhythm, play simple instruments, or stand up and march. You can hum a tune to yourself or sing it out, but you can also sing songs, clap your hands, or even sing in the shower. Pretend for a moment that no one else is around. Think of your favorite song, the one that brings back pleasant memories, especially of someone close to you. How do you feel now? Do you understand how powerful music can be in helping us gain emotional peace and happiness? Music is a form of communication that can be enjoyed with others. It requires no active participation unless you want it to.

A music program:

- Reduces boredom and disillusionment
- Creates and enhances a happy mood
- Recalls pleasant experiences, bringing pleasure
- Offers immediate gratification
- Creates distraction from problems of daily living
- May improve bonding between family and friends
- Opens up communication as people reminisce after enjoying music together

In the hospital or treatment setting, music:

- Helps improve coordination when it is used with physical therapy rehabilitation
- Gives psychological, social, physical, emotional, and supportive benefits
- Enhances the effectiveness of speech training in people with brain damage
- Helps reduce anxiety commonly seen during medical therapy, thereby making therapy more acceptable

We can see the benefits live music can have for hospital patients, their friends, and their families in their reactions to a musician playing for them in their rooms:

The music you played made my day. Just that one piece gave me such happiness. Thank you more than I can say.

—F.F.G., age 94

I met the hospital musician yesterday playing music for my dear friend "R" in room 832. I cannot tell you what it meant for me to see him well and enjoying music. We had a very rough week and yesterday you brightened up our day so much.

—R.B.

I was disappointed because I couldn't go home today, and then the musician came and made the day—I love music.

—E.D.

Thank you so much for providing a much needed and stimulating distraction for my mother's condition. It is so important for her to enjoy her time here as much as possible and you have helped greatly in that department. I hope you will continue this invaluable service. Thanks.

—D.S.

Music is truly a vital part of our lives—when we are well and especially when we are ill.

Getting Your Affairs in Order

Ernest H. Rosenbaum, M.D., F.A.C.P., and Isadora R. Rosenbaum, M.A.

Adapted from *Everyone's Guide to Cancer Supportive Care* by Ernest and Isadora Rosenbaum

A cheerful heart is good medicine.

Proverbs 17:22

Whether you are healthy, just growing old, or nearing the end of your life, it is a wise move and a gift of love to your family and friends to make arrangements for end-of-life care and get your affairs in order before you are either gravely ill or dying.

Your Legacy of Love for your family and friends can, with careful thought and compassion, be one of clear decisions and planned arrangements—a house swept clean of personal, financial, and business cobwebs. By sorting out your affairs now, you can spare your survivors an inheritance of scattered papers and countless details to be waded through. Instead, you can bequeath to them the gifts of clear direction, rich memories, and unique insights.

Life is full of unplanned events. Perhaps the most challenging of these events to cope with is the death of a loved one. It's been estimated that 85–90 percent of families are not prepared when a relative dies. Important documents need to be located, funeral arrangements need to be made, and vital matters need to be attended to. The following suggestions can be helpful.

It's important to realize that death is actually a shared experience. Although each of us must face our own death, our survivors are also affected and suffer. They are left to cope with both the emotional adjustment of losing a loved one and the responsibility of dealing with someone else's affairs.

How You Can Help Your Survivors

Many decisions that must be carried out by your survivors typically occur at a time of great stress. They often have to come up with answers to troubling questions—such as what last-minute medical treatments to accept or reject on your behalf, whom to notify if you die, what burial arrangements to make, how to pay tribute to your life, how to settle liabilities and disperse assets, and what memories to embrace in order to best remember you.

By taking time and care now to attend to each of these areas of importance, you'll be providing benefits to yourself and those you love. In the short term, you'll reap the benefit of peace of mind, which comes from organization and control of your affairs, and in the long term, you'll know that what will be done is what you would have wanted.

Before considering the areas listed below, first plan where you are going to store this information file so that those who will need it will know where to find it easily. Then be sure to tell those who need to know the location of your records and safety deposit box and key.

Advance Directives

By completing a Durable Power of Attorney for Health Care form or a Natural Death Act Declaration, you are providing both your family and your health care team with guidance about your medical decisions. Forms are available at any hospital.

Here are some of the treatments you might choose (or reject) in a Durable Power of Attorney for Health Care or a Natural Death Act Declaration:

1. CPR: Chest compressions, electric shock to keep your heart beating, artificial breathing, using drugs
2. Mechanical breathing (respirator, ventilator)
3. Feeding and hydration through a tube in your veins, nose, or stomach
4. Kidney dialysis, chemotherapy or radiotherapy, pain medications, or the use of antibiotics
5. Potentially painful diagnostic tests

Be sure to include the names, addresses, and phone numbers of your primary care doctor, any specialists, family members, and the executor or trustee of your estate to have this medical information in their files.

There is often confusion associated with advance directives—they can be difficult to access, are sometimes lost, and are sometimes confusing or difficult to interpret and implement in an emergency when seconds count. At the Oregon Health and Science University Hospital and in fifteen states, a new directive form, Physician Orders for Life-Sustaining Treatment (POLST), is being used. It is designed for the chronically ill, signed by the doctor at time of discharge or transfer, and carried by the patient. It is a medical order specifying the care requested by the patient for end-of-life care, and it can help patients avoid unwanted resuscitation and treatment. More information can be found at www.polst.org.

Legal Will

Preparing a will is one of the most important responsibilities you have. Make this a priority. Get in touch with your attorney.

Be sure to review your will periodically in order to keep your information up to date. If you divorce, separate, or remarry, or if the status of your named heirs changes, be sure to revise your will appropriately.

Be prepared to include information about an executor (the person you name to carry out the terms of your will), your family and children, anyone you wish to "disinherit," your assets, tax implications, gifts, trusts, revocable living trust, life insurance, and charitable contributions.

Persons to Notify

Include the names, addresses, and phone numbers of doctors, attorneys, employers, relatives, friends, business associates, the executor or trustee of your estate, and religious and social organizations.

Arrangements for Your Body

It is important to make decisions regarding organ donations and burial arrangements.

Obituary

You can help your family by providing information about your place of birth, career background, education, special achievements, military service, involvement with organizations, hobbies, and memorial contribution preferences.

Memorial Service

Your clergy can help provide guidelines regarding mourning and burial rituals. Notify family members or friends about this information.

Benefit Information

List benefits from life insurance, pensions, and profit-sharing plans, including Keogh plans, IRAs, Social Security, Medicare, supplemental medical insurance, veterans' benefits, or workers' compensation benefits.

Assets and Liabilities

Include information about banks and savings assets, loans, and first or second notes.

Insurance Information

Provide the documentation for each insurance policy as well as contact names, addresses, and phone numbers of your insurance agents.

Home and Personal Property Inventory

A household inventory is a practical way of listing your belongings, identifying each item, specifying its location, estimating its value, and naming the heir to whom you're giving it.

Your Personal or "Ethical" Will

This is a rare opportunity for you to take the time to express your innermost thoughts, wishes, and personal philosophy. You might also want to write a personal note or a rich family history for your loved ones, or specific personal messages to each of them. You might want to record your thoughts on audiotape, videotape, or DVD. Include any diaries, pictures, or journals you'd like to pass on.

To live and die with dignity and minimal suffering is the goal, leaving a feeling of deserved honor, respect, and esteem.

Summary and Review

Ernest H. Rosenbaum, M.D., F.A.C.P.

When you are diagnosed with cancer, your life has been forever changed. Even if you have gone through successful treatments and obtained a remission, and perhaps a cure, you still live with the doubts and fears of a potential recurrence, a new cancer, and the possibility of functional disability, emotional changes, and even death. Cancer survivors begin a new lifelong battle, which is best fought through a team approach. The goal is wellness through health promotion and disease prevention. Continued support is vital to help promote quality of life and a healthful future.

How you manage your healthcare needs and your attitude and philosophy of life can make a big difference in how you cope with the diagnosis and treatment of cancer. Those who are fortunate enough to have a supportive family, financial security, and a satisfying life will have an easier time coping than those who are in distress or depressed, lack family or friend support, or face physical impairment, financial instability, or the prospect of not continuing life as it was before the diagnosis of cancer.

The number of people who survive cancer has increased dramatically in the past three decades (from 3.5 million to more than 10 million people) and will continue to do so, largely because of new and improved treatments and earlier diagnosis through prevention and screening. Careful evaluation and regular checkups are needed over the next fifteen or more years to help promote better health, longevity, and quality of life. The goal of this proactive surveillance and intervention approach is to help prevent complications and early or late side effects from cancer and its therapy, to ensure early diagnosis of a recurrence or a new cancer so that it can be treated early, and to provide avenues for survivors to reduce the risk of a second primary cancer and/or comorbid diseases.

At present, the risk of lifelong side effects is being only partially controlled. Most follow-up care can be routine, not extending beyond the surveillance needed to detect recurrence or a new cancer or to detect and treat side effects. Much follow-up care is shared care with the primary physician, oncologist, and nurse specialist in a survivorship clinic. It has been found that seeing more than one physician for follow-up care is more efficient and results in better care. In addition to physical care, psychological and psychosocial problems must be addressed because they are common, affecting probably a third of cancer survivors.

The important fact to realize is that there is a definite relationship between our lifestyles and our survival after cancer therapy. Through exercise, a prudent diet, and treating comorbidities one may decrease the risk of cancer recurrence and hopefully increase survival and longevity, and reduce the risk of toxic cancer treatment–related side effects. By increasing physical activity, improving diet, and reducing tobacco exposure, one can also reduce the risk of developing cardiovascular disease, strokes, kidney disease, and type 2 diabetes. Unfortunately, not everyone wants to change his or her lifestyle. Different strategies must be created to promote better behavioral patterns. Social attitudes, values, and peer pressure play a role in lifestyle choices; family, friends, and community social support can help people choose healthful habits.

Quality of Life and Survivorship

Betty Ferrell, associate research scientist at the City of Hope, has proposed a definition of quality of life through a model for cancer survivors.[1] It involves four domains:

- The first is physical well-being, maintenance of function, independence, and symptom relief. This includes functional activities, fatigue control, strength, sleep, overall physical health, and fertility.
- The second is psychological well-being, or attempts to maintain a sense of control in the face of a life-threatening illness, with great emotional distress, changes in life priorities, and fear of an unknown future, with anxiety, depression, and distress.
- The third domain is social well-being, with efforts being made to deal with the impact of the diagnosis of cancer and its effect on relationships and the survivor's role in life. These effects include family distress, sexual dysfunction, general appearance concerns, reduced enjoyment of life, isolation, financial insecurity, and work insecurity.
- The fourth domain, spiritual well-being, is the ability to maintain hope and derive meaning from the cancer experience, which is clouded by uncertainty. This includes the meaning of the illness, religiosity, spirituality, hope of certainty, faith, inner strength, and the will to live.

These topics are reviewed in several sections in this book, including the prudent diet, exercise, smoking cessation, limiting alcohol consumption, and supportive care plans for osteoporosis, pain, lymphedema, infertility, sun exposure, sexual dysfunction, fatigue, depression, and other problems.

The Survivorship Care Plan

The possibility of late side effects from therapy (e.g., damage to heart, lung, kidneys, bone marrow, and reproductive organs), recurrent cancer, or a new cancer makes medical surveillance necessary for fifteen or more years. To ensure that guidance is given to promote better health and longevity, the healthcare team needs to implement an organized preventive medicine program that includes screening and advice on ways to improve diet, increase exercise, and obtain psychosocial support.

Parts I and II, "A Physician Guidance Program" and "A Survivor's Road Map to Health and Longevity," provided background on the essential elements of a survivorship care program and recommended screening guidelines, prevention measures, and a compendium of known cancer treatment toxicities. A survivorship care plan from the oncologist or medical team will help inform the primary care provider, the nurses, and the patient regarding diagnosis, treatment, and future care. This plan will include future screening and preventive medical tests and examinations as well as lifestyle recommendations and psychosocial support references.

A survivorship care plan summary includes the medical history, a brief review of therapy, a list of potential side effects, and future recommendations for monitoring and care. It is provided by the treating oncologist for use by all doctors and nurse specialists involved in the clinical care of the survivor and is updated periodically to reflect treatments, screening results, and other aspects of patient care. The care plan could be initiated on the first visit, making information easier to enter as it develops, while it is current and can be well summarized. The survivorship care summary plan might be located in the patient's chart in a colored folder for easy recognition, or in a computerized Internet program. It takes commitment by the patient and healthcare providers to continue the survivorship care plan summary program because it currently is not covered by Medicare or insurance in most instances, and it is a time-consuming project.

Beyond the guidance provided by the survivorship care plan summary, survivors need supportive care programs to help them promote healthful lifestyles. In 1981, Doll and Peto found that 75–80 percent of cancers in the United States could be avoided and were the result of environmental factors, such as tobacco use, alcohol consumption, an unhealthy diet, level of physical activity, and biologic factors. Exactly how the many confounding factors, such as body weight, diet, and physical activity, relate to cancer risk is not fully known, but randomized trials have shown that these and other environmental conditions do influence the risk of cancer. Of the half million cancer deaths in the United States annually, it is believed that approximately one-third are caused by tobacco exposure, about a third from diet (eating the wrong foods and excessive amounts of food), and a small percentage caused by alcohol. Genetic inheritance with cell mutations accounts for a 5–8 percent risk of cancer.

The Emotional Impact of Cancer

When you hear the frightening words, "Your diagnosis is cancer," a sequence of events occurs, sometimes overwhelming both patient and family. Feelings of hopelessness and helplessness and an inability to cope are not uncommon after a patient hears the shocking news. Often, patients are so overwhelmed and distressed that they become nonfunctional and often do not hear much of the explanations given to them, explanations that could often put their disease in perspective and help them cope with the diagnosis.

Much of the life trajectory through cancer diagnosis and treatment depends on the patient's coping abilities in handling various problems, both for life and death, and on the patient's personal and family history. With time, some of the confusion subsides, and patients move onward with their life. Working with their medical team—doctors, nurses, social workers, and supporters—patients learn to deal with the cancer, but this ability depends on a cooperative relationship between patients, families, and the medical team. Each person has an inner strength, which he or she must call on to help them deal with their cancer diagnosis and treatments and to live and cope with the disease and all its associated problems. Support programs have been very successful in helping survivors develop the coping skills they need to live with and through their cancer.

Even after treatment, patients and families strive to promote well-being and quality of life by addressing current and ongoing problems related to cancer and its treatments. This struggle varies from patient to patient, but these problems are partially solvable, and their solutions contribute to improved quality of life. Despite all this, survivors continue to have concerns and worries about whether a recurrence, a new cancer, or what new side effects will develop at a later stage of life. Psychological and physical support are becoming more available and are very helpful in relieving the physical and psychological consequences that may develop. These include infertility, sexual dysfunction, osteoporosis, pain, fatigue, and other associated problems. It is important to keep an optimistic and positive attitude, such as will to live, that will promote self-esteem and improve mental health.

Unfortunately, the financial cost of cancer treatments, recovery support, and living and working expenses often are difficult to deal with. The prospect of unemployment, insurance problems, and other difficulties of daily living are significant and affect the person's ability to maintain the will to live and find purpose and enjoyment in life.

Cancer alters the lives not only of the patients but of their families and friends. The medical team and family and friends make up the network supporting the patient through the trials and tribulations of having cancer and its treatments and the long period of recovery.

The Road Map

Because it can affect every aspect of your life, from your faith and the quality of your relationships to your physical well-being and your career, cancer is an assault on your life. Survivors have to face the reality and consequences of a cancer diagnosis:

- Physical problems such as pain, functional limitations, and changes in appearance (hair loss, amputation, or an ostomy)
- Psychosocial problems such as fear of not being in control of one's life, anxieties, depression, cognitive changes, distress from the diagnosis and treatment, and worry about a recurrence or a new cancer

Part II, "A Survivor's Road Map to Health and Longevity," presents strategies and solutions for survivors, a basic outline of what survivors need to know about how to follow their anticancer therapy, and tools and resources for dealing with workplace, insurance, and disability issues.

Healthful Lifestyles

Behavioral interventions, such as maintaining a healthy weight, eating less saturated fat, eliminating trans fats, eating more fruits and vegetables, whole grains, and legumes (beans), and increasing physical activity can make a difference in a survivor's quality of life, both psychologically and emotionally, by reducing fatigue, improving mood, and reducing many of the toxic side effects of cancer treatment. Many cancer survivors adopt more healthful lifestyles in the hopes of improving their overall health. The goal is to increase survival, reduce the risk of side effects, and reduce the risk of cancer recurrence or new cancers.

Part III, "Ways to Improve Lifestyle and Quality of Life," presents diet and exercise guidelines and information from current research on the benefits of lifestyle improvements for survivors of specific cancers. The guidelines of the American Cancer Society (ACS), the American Society of Clinical Oncology (ASCO), and the Oncology Nursing Society provide a healthy direction and information vital to those who want to reduce cancer risk and improve quality of life.

Recommended Guidelines

- Avoid weight gain, especially after menopause. Try to maintain a healthy weight by balancing the number of calories consumed with the calories expended through daily life activity and physical exercise.

  For those already overweight or obese, an active weight control program is essential.

  To maintain your weight:
  Calories consumed = Calories expended
  To lose weight:
  Calories consumed < Calories expended
- Increase intake of fruits, vegetables, and whole grain foods. Reduce dietary fats, saturated fats, and trans fats.
- Exercise at least thirty minutes to one hour a day five days a week (e.g., brisk walking).

- Limit alcohol use (no more than one drink per day for women, two per day for men).
- Don't use tobacco in any form.
- Avoid excess sun exposure and use sunscreen (skin cancer is the most common of all cancers and is preventable).
- Adopt an osteoporosis prevention program.
- Use available information on cancer prevention and ways to improve your survivorship by adopting a healthier lifestyle.

There is no guarantee that adopting healthful lifestyle activities will prevent cancer, and following these guidelines is difficult for most people. In general, Americans are eating more and engaging in less physical activity; many work at sedentary jobs, and many households need two full-time workers to make ends meet, reducing the time available to prepare nutritious meals and exercise regularly. Often, the facilities for physical activity are less accessible for those living in cities. Living a healthful lifestyle takes time and the willingness to make an extra effort.

Two-thirds of Americans are overweight or obese, and this rate is increasing. Many cancers are associated with overweight and obesity. It is also well known that weight loss may reduce the risk of breast cancer.[2] One of the mechanisms associated with these risks is the metabolism of fats and sugars, which affect hormones, including insulin, insulin-like growth factors, and estrogen (estradiol), which affect the regulation of cancer and normal cell proliferation. Excess dietary fats create free radicals, which can damage the cell membrane and cause the cell to become cancerous. Fruits and vegetables in the diet contain phytochemicals and other compounds that help neutralize excess free radicals, reducing their toxic effects. It has been estimated that 30–60 percent of cancer survivors eat in a healthier manner, with decreased meat intake and increased fruits and vegetables, and try to maintain a healthy weight.[3] Unfortunately, 25–42 percent of survivors still consume inadequate amounts of fruits and vegetables.[3] An increased consumption of fruits and vegetables is associated with a decreased risk of lung, esophageal, stomach, and colorectal cancers.[4] There is also evidence that those who eat more fruits and vegetables are less likely to be overweight or obese.[5]

Nutrition (the prudent diet) can play a vital role in preventing cancer and reducing the risk of cancer recurrence. Unfortunately, the American diet is high in fats, sugars, and refined carbohydrates. The predominance of calorie-dense foods in the American diet must be replaced with a predominance of plant foods (fruits, vegetables, and whole grains).

To reduce caloric intake:

- Limit sugar, saturated and trans fats, and alcohol consumption.
- Reduce serving sizes.
- Limit high-calorie foods and beverages, fats, and refined sugars (cookies, cakes, candy, ice cream, fried foods, and soft drinks).
- Increase use of fruits, vegetables, and whole grains to replace calorie-dense foods.[6]

Most importantly, parents should initiate a healthy lifestyle program early in their children's lives. Seventy percent of those who are overweight by adolescence will remain overweight as adults. Childhood may be the most significant time to reduce cancer risk and future risks of cardiovascular disease, hypertension, osteoporosis, stroke, and type 2 diabetes.[7]

Exercise plays a key role in reducing cancer risk and can be very beneficial in promoting better health, survival, and longevity. It is now well established that exercise promotes longevity and potentially disease control for breast cancer, prostate cancer, and colon cancer (which affect more than half of the survivors in the United States) and cardiovascular disease. The risk reduction has been confirmed in many studies, which also provide an understanding of the physiological mechanisms by which exercise reduces breast, prostate, and colorectal cancer risk and fatigue and improves quality of life while promoting survival.

Exercise has also been found to reduce the side effects of cancer treatment. Those who exercise have less fatigue, shortness of breath, depression, pain, sleep disturbance, and memory problems during treatment and had a better quality of life. Side effects of treatment were also reduced, and the conclusion was that patients who exercised had less severe side effects.[8,9,10] Adults should engage in thirty minutes or more of moderate to vigorous physical activity on five or more days a week. Children and adolescents should engage in sixty minutes per day of moderate to vigorous physical activity.[7]

The benefits of physical activity include the following:

- There is scientific evidence that physical activity may reduce the risk of many cancers, including breast, colon, prostate, and endometrial cancer. Thus, it plays a vital role in cancer prevention. It is also important for reducing the risk of heart disease, type 2 diabetes, osteoporosis, and hypertension.
- For those who are inactive, a gradual progressive exercise program is recommended and has many benefits, including prevention of weight gain and obesity.
- There are lifetime benefits of participating in an exercise program.

Tobacco use has also been shown to be important in the development of cancer. Unfortunately, the tobacco industry has invested a lot of time and money in making its products more desirable, including increasing the percentage of nicotine in cigarettes by about 10 percent in the last few years, which makes them more addictive and even more difficult to quit. However, effective smoking cessation treatments are available. It takes a lot of family and social support and personal perseverance to succeed in any endeavor to change a bad habit. Tobacco use and the corresponding lung cancer incidence and mortality rates are starting to decline and are leveling off for women after many decades of increase. Thus, behavior changes are not only possible but are also effective.

It is imperative to involve the public in efforts to change cultural modes and lifestyle patterns that do not promote health. A good example of large-scale cultural change can be seen in the decline of tobacco use since the mid-1980s, a trend that became the norm through public awareness, increased restrictions on sites where people can smoke, persistent taxation efforts, and limitations on tobacco advertising. Similar programs of public education about the risks of obesity and sedentary lifestyles are needed to reverse the increasing rates of obesity-related disease.

The Lance Armstrong Foundation in Austin, Texas, has served as an information center and catalyst for program production and support for cancer survivors. This is an evolutionary process in which many organizations, including the ASCO, the Oncology Nursing Society, the ACS, the National Coalition for Cancer Survivors (NCCS), and the Office of Cancer Survivorship, are all playing a role in providing optimal care through centers around the country. Since its beginning in 1986, the NCCS, in conjunction with the Oncology Nursing Society, the ASCO, the ACS, and the National Cancer Institute Office of Cancer Survivorship, has promoted the importance of supportive care for cancer survivors. These organizations have addressed the problems and are looking for solutions, developing guidelines based on effective practices in order to promote a better quality of life.

Survivors of cancer graduate to a new life but may face many consequences related to their cancer and their therapy, both psychological and physical. The challenges they face can best be overcome with a team approach, including their medical team, family, friends, community resources, and, most importantly, themselves.

Long-Term Consequences and Side Effects

More than 64 percent of cancer patients are now surviving for more than five years. They need guidance and programs to help improve survival and reduce the risk of recurrence by focusing on controlling the long-term consequences of cancer and its side effects and possibly helping prevent a new cancer. Parts IV and V, "Survival with Disease Prevention and Control" and "Survival with Side Effect Control," provide descriptions and prevention measures for controlling potential comorbid conditions and for coping with and controlling the side effects of cancer and its therapies.

With today's diagnostic and treatment technologies, most cancer survivors die of other diseases, such as cardiovascular disease, diabetes, and stroke. Special care is needed for cancer patients receiving anthracycline drugs (e.g., doxorubicin [Adriamycin]), Herceptin, or radiation to the left chest above the heart because they may be subject to new cancers, cancer recurrences, and/or pulmonary and cardiovascular disease posttreatment problems. For example, peripheral neuropathy, with pain, numbness, tingling, loss of sensation, or heat and cold sensitivity, is a common side effect in patients receiving paclitaxel [Taxol], docetaxel [Taxotere], platinum, vincristine [Oncovin], vinblastine [Velban], vinorelbine [Navelbine], and oxaliplatin [Eloxatin] chemotherapy.

Long-term follow up is recommended for possible congestive heart failure for twenty years or more after treatment. For those who already have cardiac problems, radiation to the heart and treatment with these drugs may cause progressive cardiac problems. Protective drugs are being developed to delay or prevent heart damage (e.g., dexrazoxane [Zinecard]).

In addition to the screening guidelines outlined in the survivor summary care plan, lifestyle behavioral changes for a better diet, scheduled routine exercise, and psychological support are important for promoting better health, reducing cancer risk, and preventing disease.

Comorbid Problems

Those who have cardiac, pulmonary, or cardiovascular disorders, kidney disease, or diabetes are more susceptible to comorbidities, and diet, exercise, and psychological support are particularly important for these patients. The ACS guidelines are consistent with the American Heart Association and the American Diabetic Association guidelines for prevention of heart disease and type 2 diabetes and for better general health.[11]

Older adults may have preexisting heart, lung, kidney, gastrointestinal, neurological, or liver problems, which can be aggravated by anticancer therapy because these organs may be more susceptible to treatment side effects.

Osteoporosis is a common problem among survivors, especially postmenopausal women and prostate cancer patients on androgen deprivation therapy. Premenopausal women are at greater risk for osteopenia and osteoporosis because of ovarian failure and the resulting loss of estrogen (estradiol) after cancer therapy. Men with prostate cancer who are treated with androgen deprivation therapy (ADT) often have problems with osteoporosis and osteopenia due to lack of testosterone. Another problem is loss of physical function, with various levels of impairment that are common in cancer survivors, which can also cause social and economic problems.

Reducing sun exposure and using sunscreen help prevent the most common cancer: skin cancer.

Creative Expression

Part VI, "Improved Survival with Creative Expression," describes the roles of art, music, health, humor, and poetry in healthy survivorship. How a person lives has a major effect on his or her health and life. A positive attitude and enjoyable activities can promote better health. Enriching one's quality of life heightens emotional experiences and reduces depression.

In Summary

Each person has an inner strength that they must call on to help them deal with their cancer diagnosis and treatments, and to live and cope with the disease and all its associated problems. Support programs have been successful in helping survivors develop the coping skills they need to live with and through their cancer. Both psychological and physical support are becoming more available and are helpful in relieving the physical and emotional consequences cancer survivors may face. It is important to maintain a positive fighting spirit, optimism, faith, and hope, which can make a major difference in your will to live, your quality of life, and your survival.

Many people with cancer are willing to make lifestyle changes to promote better health habits, increase longevity, reduce physical dysfunction and deconditioning from side effects of the cancer or the therapy, and possibly reduce the risk of a cancer recurrence or a new cancer.

The goal of this book is to provide knowledge and tools to help patients and their caregivers chart a course to a healthier survivorship. Throughout, we have provided advice on ways to improve your health, reduce side effects, and decrease the risk of cancer recurrence or new cancers. We hope that the knowledge and recommendations made here will help survivors improve their lifestyle practices for better health outcomes and quality of life and survival after cancer. These guidelines can help you maintain your health and live longer with better quality of life.

We wish you better survival through better health!

Appendix A: References

Introduction

1. Haylock PJ. The shifting paradigm of cancer care. The many needs of cancer survivors are starting to attract attention. *Am J Nurs* 2006;106(3 Suppl):16–19.

2. Brown BW, Brauner C, Minnotte MC. Noncancer deaths in white adult cancer patients. *J Natl Cancer Inst* 1993;85(12): 979–87.

Chapter 1

1. Hewitt M, Greenfield S, Stovall E, eds. *From Cancer Patient to Cancer Survivor, Lost in Transition.* Washington, DC: The National Academies Press, 2005.

2. Ganz PA, Desmond KA, Leedham B, Rowland JH, Meyerowitz BE, Belin TR. Quality of life in long-term, disease-free survivors of breast cancer: a follow-up study. *J Natl Cancer Inst* 2002;94(1):39–49.

Chapter 2

1. Sweeney C, Schmitz KH, Lazovich D, Virnig BA, Wallace RB, Folsom AR. Functional limitations in elderly female cancer survivors. *J Natl Cancer Inst* 2006;98(8):521–9.

2. Donaldson SS, Hancock SL, Hoppe RT. The Janeway Lecture. Hodgkin's disease: finding the balance between cure and late effects. *Cancer J Sci Am* 1999;5(6):325–33.

3. Hoppe RT. Hodgkin's disease: complications of therapy and excess mortality. *Ann Oncol* 1997;8(Suppl 1):115–18.

4. Mudie NY, Swerdlow AJ, Higgins CD, et al. Risk of second malignancy after non-Hodgkin's lymphoma: a British cohort study. *J Clin Oncol* 2006;24(10):1568–74.

5. Aziz NM. Cancer survivorship research: challenge and opportunity. *J Nutr* 2002;132(11 Suppl):3494S–3503S.

6. Aziz NM, Rowland JH. Trends and advances in cancer survivorship research: challenge and opportunity. *Semin Radiat Oncol* 2003;13(3):248–66. Gritz ER, Fingeret MC, Vidrine DJ, Lazev AB, Mehta NV, Reece GP. Successes and failures of the teachable moment: smoking cessation in cancer patients. *Cancer* 2006;106(1):17–27.

7. Patterson RE, Neuhouser ML, Hedderson MM, Schwartz SM, Standish LJ, Bowen DJ. Changes in diet, physical activity,

and supplement use among adults diagnosed with cancer. *J Am Diet Assoc* 2003;103(3):323–8.

8. Chlebowski RT, Blackburn GL, Elashoff RE, et al. Dietary fat reduction in postmenopausal women with primary breast cancer: phase III Women's Intervention Nutrition Study (WINS). *J Clin Oncol,* 2005 ASCO Annual Meeting Proceedings, Part I of II, 23(16S) (June 1 Supplement), 2005:10.

9. Pierce JP, Faerber S, Wright FA, et al. Feasibility of a randomized trial of a high-vegetable diet to prevent breast cancer recurrence. *Nutr Cancer* 1997;28(3):282–8.

10. Gotay CC. Behavior and cancer prevention. *J Clin Oncol* 2005;23(2):301–10.

11. Lau DC, Dhillon B, Yan H, Szmitko, PE, Verma S. Adipokines: molecular links between obesity and atheroslcerosis. *Am J Physiol Heart Circ Physiol* 2005;288:h2031–h2041.

12. Pischon T, Girman CJ, Hotamisligil GS, Rifai N, Hu FB, Rimm EB. Plasma adiponectin levels and risk of myocardial infarction in men. *JAMA* 2004;291:1730–37.

13. Oh SW, Yoon YS, Shin SA. Effects of excess weight on cancer incidence depending on cancer site and histologic findings among men: Korean National Health Insurance Corporation study. *J Clin Oncol* 2005;23(21):4742–54.

14. National Heart, Lung, and Blood Institute. *Clinical Guidelines on the Identification, Evaluation, and Treatment of Overweight and Obesity in Adults*. Bethesda, MD: Author, 1996.

15. Meyerhardt JA, Giovannucci EL, Holmes MD, et al. Physical activity and survival after colorectal cancer diagnosis. *J Clin Oncol* 2006; 24(22):3527-34. Meyerhardt JA, Heseltine D, Niedzwiecki D, et al. Impact of physical activity on cancer recurrence and survival in patients with stage III colon cancer: findings from CALGB 89803. *J Clin Oncol* 2006;24(22): 3535-41.

16. Jones LW, Courneya KS, Peddle C, Mackey JR. Oncologists' opinions toward recommending exercise to patients with cancer: a Canadian National Survey. *Support Care Cancer* 2005;13:929–37.

17. Stanton AL. Psychosocial concerns and interventions for cancer survivors. *J Clin Oncol* 2006;24(32):5132–7.

18. Michael YL, Kawachi I, Berkman LF, Holmes MD, Colditz GA. The persistent impact of breast carcinoma on functional health status: prospective evidence from the Nurses' Health Study. *Cancer* 2000;89(11):2176–86.

19. Sandgren AK, McCaul KD. Short-term effects of telephone therapy for breast cancer patients. *Health Psychol* 2003;22(3):310–15.

20. Doll R, Peto R. The causes of cancer: quantitative estimates of avoidable risks of cancer in the United States today. *J Natl Cancer Inst* 1981;66(6):1191–308.

21. Gotay CC. Behavior and cancer prevention. *J Clin Oncol* 2005;23(2):301–10.

22. Wing RR, Tate DF, Gorin AA, Raynor HA, Fava JL. A self-regulation program for maintenance of weight loss. *N Engl J Med* 2006; 355(15):1563–71.

23. Demark-Wahnefried W, Clipp E, Lipkus I, et al. Results of Fresh Start: a randomized controlled trial to improve diet and exercise behaviors in breast and prostate cancer survivors. *J Clin Oncol,* 2006 ASCO Annual Meeting Proceedings, Part I, 24(18S) (June 20 Supplement), 2006:8503.

24. Demark-Wahnefried W, Peterson B, McBride C, Lipkus I, Clipp E. Current health behaviors and readiness to pursue life-style changes among men and women diagnosed with early stage prostate and breast carcinomas. *Cancer* 2000;88(3):674–84.

25. U.S. Department of Health and Human Services. *Physical Activity and Health: A Report of the Surgeon General*. Rockville, MD: U.S. Department of Health and Human Services, Public Health Service, Center for Disease Control and Prevention, National Center for Chronic Disease Prevention and Health Promotion, 1996.

26. Steinbrook R. Imposing personal responsibility for health. *N Engl J Med* 2006; 355(8):753–6.

27. Rosoff PM. The two-edged sword of curing childhood cancer. *N Engl J Med* 2006;355 (15):1522–3.

28. Childhood cancer survivors research. *NCI Cancer Bulletin* 2006;3(40), NIH Publication No. 05-5498.

29. Oeffinger KC, Mertens AC, Sklar CA, et al. Childhood Cancer Survivor Study. Chronic health conditions in adult survivors of childhood cancer. *N Engl J Med* 2006;355(15): 1572–82.

30. Oeffinger KC, McCabe MS. Models for delivering survivorship care. *J Clin Oncol* 2006; 24(32):5117–24.

Chapter 3

1. Eliminating the suffering and death due to cancer. Special Issue, *JNCI Bulletin* 2006; 3(40).

2. Sunga AY, Eberl MM, Oeffinger KC, Hudson MM, Mahoney MC. Care of cancer survivors. *Am Fam Physician* 2005;71(4):699–706.

3. Ziegler RG, Hoover RN, Nomura AM, et al. Relative weight, weight change, height, and breast cancer risk in Asian-American women. *J Natl Cancer Inst* 1996;88(10):650–60.

4. Fenton JJ, Taplin SH, Carney PA, et al. Influence of computer-aided detection on performance of screening mammography. *N Engl J Med* 2007;356(14):1399-409.

5. Plevritis SK, Kurian AW, Sigal BM, et al. Cost-effectiveness of screening BRCA1/2 mutation carriers with breast magnetic resonance imaging. *JAMA* 2006;295(20):2374–84.

6. Guarneri V, Lenihan DJ, Valero V, et al. Long-term cardiac tolerability of trastuzumab in metastatic breast cancer. *J Clin Oncol* 2006; 1524:4107–15.

7. Courneya KS, Mackey JR, Bell GJ, Jones LW, Field CJ, Fairey AS. Randomized controlled trial of exercise training in postmenopausal breast cancer survivors: cardiopulmonary and quality of life outcomes. *J Clin Oncol* 2003;21 (9):1660–8.

8. Goodwin PJ, Chlebowski RT, Ligibel JA. *Lifestyle Modification in Women with Breast Cancer: Basic Mechanisms, Clinical Studies, and Practical Advice*. ASCO, June 2006.

9. Koutsky LA, Ault KA, Wheeler CM, et al.; Proof of Principle Study Investigators. A controlled trial of a human papillomavirus type 16 vaccine. *N Engl J Med* 2002;347(21):1645–51.

10. Pavelka JC, Brown RS, Karlan BY, et al. Effect of obesity on survival in epithelial ovarian cancer. *Cancer* 2006;107(7):1520-4.

11. Gross CP, McAvay GJ, Krumholz HM, Paltiel AD, Bhasin D, Tinetti ME. The effect of age and chronic illness on life expectancy after a diagnosis of colorectal cancer: implications for screening. *Ann Intern Med* 2006; 145(9):646–53.

12. National Institutes of Health. *Osteoporosis and Related Bone Disease,* National Resource Center, May 2006.

13. Neuner JM, Binkley N, Sparapani RA, Laud PW, Nattinger AB. Bone density testing in older women and its association with patient age. *J Am Geriatr Soc* 2006;54(3):485–9.

14. Keating NL, O'Malley AJ, Smith MR. Diabetes and cardiovascular disease during androgen deprivation therapy for prostate cancer. *J Clin Oncol* 2006;24(27):4448–56.

Chapter 5

1. Booth CM, Vardy J, Crawley A, et al. Cognitive impairment associated with chemotherapy for breast cancer: an exploratory case-control study. *J Clin Oncol,* 2006 ASCO Annual Meeting Proceedings, Part I, 24(18S) (June 20 Supplement), 2006:8501.

2. Bradbury J. Chemobrain: imaging shows changes in metabolism. *Lancet Oncol* 2006; 7(11):890. Silverman DH, Dy CJ, Castellon SA, et al. Altered frontocortical, cerebellar, and basal ganglia activity in adjuvant-treated breast cancer survivors 5–10 years after chemotherapy. *Breast Cancer Res Treat* 2006, Sept. 29.

3. Fobair P, Hoppe RT, Bloom J, Cox R, Varghese A, Spiegel D. Psychosocial problems

among survivors of Hodgkin's disease. *J Clin Oncol* 1986;4(5):805–14.

4. Bloom JR, Fobair P, Gritz E, et al. Psychosocial outcomes of cancer: a comparative analysis of Hodgkin's disease and testicular cancer. *J Clin Oncol* 1993;11(5):979–88.

5. Curt GA, Breitbart W, Cella D, et al. Impact of cancer-related fatigue on the lives of patients: new findings from the Fatigue Coalition. *Oncologist* 2000;5(5):353–60.

6. Bodurka-Bevers D, Basen-Engquist K, Carmack CL, et al. Depression, anxiety, and quality of life in patients with epithelial ovarian cancer. *Gynecol Oncol* 2000;78(3 Pt 1):302–8. Trask PC, Paterson A, Riba M, et al. Assessment of psychological distress in prospective bone marrow transplant patients. *Bone Marrow Transplant* 2002;29(11):917–25. Carlson LE, Angen M, Cullum J, et al. High levels of untreated distress and fatigue in cancer patients. *Br J Cancer* 2004;90(12):2297–304.

7. Zabora J, Brintzenhofeszoc K, Curbow B, Hooker C, Piantadosi S. The prevalence of psychological distress by cancer site. *Psychooncology* 2001;10(1):19–28.

8. Ganz PA, Desmond KA, Leedham B, Rowland JH, Meyerowitz BE, Belin TR. Quality of life in long-term, disease-free survivors of breast cancer: a follow-up study. *J Natl Cancer Inst* 2002;94(1):39–49.

9. Bodurka-Bevers D, Basen-Engquist K, Carmack CL, et al. Depression, anxiety, and quality of life in patients with epithelial ovarian cancer. *Gynecol Oncol* 2000;78(3 Pt 1): 302–8. Fobair P, Hoppe RT, Bloom J, Cox R, Varghese A, Spiegel D. Psychosocial problems among survivors of Hodgkin's disease. *J Clin Oncol* 1986;4(5):805–14.

10. Brown KW, Levy AR, Rosberger Z, Edgar L. Psychological distress and cancer survival: a follow-up 10 years after diagnosis. *Psychosom Med* 2003;65(4):636–43.

11. Taken in part from Temel JS, Jackson A, Billings A, et al. The effect of depression on survival in patients with newly diagnosed advanced non–small cell lung cancer (NSCLC). *J Clin Oncol,* ASCO Annual Meeting Proceedings, Part 1, 24(18S) (June 20 Supplement), 2006:8511.

12. Chang C, Knight SJ, Bennett CL. *J Clin Oncol,* 2006 ASCO Annual Meeting Proceedings, Part I, 24(18S) (June 20 Supplement), 2006:8510.

13. Spiegel D, Giese-Davis J. Depression and cancer: mechanisms and disease progression. *Biol Psychiatry* 2003;54(3):269–82.

14. Raison CL, Miller AH. Depression in cancer: new developments regarding diagnosis and treatment. *Biol Psychiatry* 2003;54(3): 283–94.

15. Bower JE, Ganz PA, Dickerson SS, Petersen L, Aziz N, Fahey JL. Diurnal cortisol rhythm and fatigue in breast cancer survivors. *Psychoneuroendocrinology* 2005;30(1):92–100.

16. Bower JE, Ganz PA, Aziz N, Fahey JL. Fatigue and proinflammatory cytokine activity in breast cancer survivors. *Psychosom Med* 2002; 64(4):604–11.

17. Anderson KO, Getto CJ, Mendoza TR, et al. Fatigue and sleep disturbance in patients with cancer, patients with clinical depression, and community-dwelling adults. *J Pain Symptom Manage* 2003;25(4):307–18. Koopman C, Nouriani B, Erickson V, et al. Sleep disturbances in women with metastatic breast cancer. *Breast J* 2002;8(6):362–70. Mormont MC, Waterhouse J, Bleuzen P. Marked 24-h rest/activity rhythms are associated with better quality of life, better response, and longer survival in patients with metastatic colorectal cancer and good performance status. *Clin Cancer Res* 2000;6(8):3038–45.

18. Caspi A, Sugden K, Moffitt TE, et al. Influence of life stress on depression: moderation by a polymorphism in the 5-HTT gene. *Science* 2003;301(5631):386–9. Gillespie NA, Whitfield JB, Williams B, Heath AC, Martin NG. The relationship between stressful life events, the serotonin transporter (5-HTTLPR) genotype and major depression. *Psychol Med* 2005;35(1):101–11.

19. Bultz BD, Holland JC. Emotional distress in patients with cancer. *Community Oncol* 2006;3(5):311–14.

20. Koopman C, Butler LD, Classen C, et al. Traumatic stress symptoms among women with recently diagnosed primary breast cancer. *J Trauma Stress* 2002;15(4):277–87.

21. Han WT, Collie K, Koopman C, et al. Breast cancer and problems with medical interactions: relationships with traumatic stress, emotional self-efficacy, and social support. *Psychooncology* 2005;14(4):318–30.

22. Evans DL, Charney DS, Lewis L, et al. Mood disorders in the medically ill: scientific review and recommendations. *Biol Psychiatry* 2005;58(3):175–89.

23. Classen C, Butler LD, Koopman C, et al. Supportive–expressive group therapy and distress in patients with metastatic breast cancer: a randomized clinical intervention trial. *Arch Gen Psychiatry* 2001;58(5):494–501.

24. Spiegel D, Bloom JR, Yalom I. Group support for patients with metastatic cancer. A randomized outcome study. *Arch Gen Psychiatry* 1981;38(5):527–33.

25. Spiegel D. *Living Beyond Limits.* New York: Ballantine/Fawcett, 1994. Spiegel D. A 43-year-old woman coping with cancer. *JAMA* 1999;282(4):371–8.

26. Spiegel D, Classen C. *Group Therapy for Cancer Patients: A Research-Based Handbook of Psychosocial Care.* New York: Basic Books, 2000.

27. Classen C, Butler LD, Koopman C, et al. Supportive–expressive group therapy and distress in patients with metastatic breast cancer: a randomized clinical intervention trial. *Arch Gen Psychiatry* 2001;58(5):494–501.

28. Compas BE, Haaga DA, Keefe FJ, Leitenberg H, Williams DA. Sampling of empirically supported psychological treatments from health psychology: smoking, chronic pain, cancer, and bulimia nervosa. *J Consult Clin Psychol* 1998;66(1):89–112. Andersen BL. Psychological interventions for cancer patients to enhance the quality of life. *J Consult Clin Psychol* 1992;60(4):552–68. Fawzy FI, Fawzy NW, Arndt LA, Pasnau RO. Critical review of psychosocial interventions in cancer care. *Arch Gen Psychiatry* 1995;52(2):100–13.

29. Pennebaker JW, ed. *Emotional Disclosure and Health.* Washington, DC: American Psychological Association, 1995. Lepore SJ, Helgeson VS. Social constraints, intrusive thoughts, and mental health after prostate cancer. *J Soc Clin Psychol* 1998;17:89–106.

30. Nieman DC, Cook VD, Henson DA, et al. Moderate exercise training and natural killer cell cytotoxic activity in breast cancer patients. *Int J Sports Med* 1995;16(5):334–7.

31. Benson H, Dusek JA, Sherwood JB, et al. Study of the Therapeutic Effects of Intercessory Prayer (STEP) in cardiac bypass patients: a multicenter randomized trial of uncertainty and certainty of receiving intercessory prayer. *Am Heart J* 2006;151(4):934–42.

32. Ziegler J. Spirituality returns to the fold in medical practice. *J Natl Cancer Inst* 1998; 90(17):1255–7.

Chapter 7

1. Modified from MM Hudson, A Hester. *After Completion of Therapy (ACT) Clinic.* Memphis, TN: St. Jude Children's Research Hospital. Portions adapted from *CCSS Newsletter,* Fall 1999 and Winter 2001.

2. Eliminating the suffering and death due to cancer. Special Issue, *JNCI Bulletin* 2006; 3(40).

3. Horning SJ, Adhikari A, Rizk N, Hoppe RT, Olshen RA. Effect of treatment for Hodgkin's disease on pulmonary function: results of a prospective study. *J Clin Oncol* 1994;12 (2):297–305.

4. Harle LK, Maggio M, Shahani S, et al. Endocrine complications of androgen-deprivation therapy in men with prostate cancer. *Clin Adv Hematol Oncol* 2006;4:687–96.

5. Brown BW, Brauner C, Minnotte MC. Noncancer deaths in white adult cancer patients. *J Natl Cancer Inst* 1993;85(12):979–87.

6. Hancock SL, Hoppe RT. Long-term complications of treatment and causes of mortality after Hodgkin's disease. *Semin Radiat Oncol* 1996;6(3):225–42.

7. Mauch P, Ng A, Aleman B, et al. Report from the Rockefeller Foundation sponsored International Workshop on Reducing Mortality and Improving Quality of Life in Long-Term Survivors of Hodgkin's Disease, July 9–16, 2003, Bellagio, Italy. *Eur J Haematol* 2005; 66(Suppl):68–76.

Chapter 8

1. Effect of chest x-rays on the risk of breast cancer among BRCA1/2 mutation carriers in the International BRCA1/2 Carrier Cohort Study: a report from the EMBRACE, GENEPSO, GEO-HEBON, and IBCCS Collaborators' Group. *J Clin Oncol* 2006;24(21):3361–6.

2. King MC, Marks JH, Mandell JB, New York Breast Cancer Study Group. Breast and ovarian cancer risks due to inherited mutations in BRCA1 and BRCA2. *Science* 2003;302 (5645):643–6.

3. McCance KL, Jones RE. Estrogen and insulin crosstalk: breast cancer risk implications. *Nurse Pract* 2003;28(5):12–23. Shi R, Yu H, McLarty J, Glass J. IGF-I and breast cancer: a meta-analysis. *Int J Cancer* 2004;111(3):418–23. Yu H, Rohan T. Role of the insulin-like growth factor family in cancer development and progression. *J Natl Cancer Inst* 2000;92(18):1472–89. Muti P. The role of endogenous hormones in the etiology and prevention of breast cancer: the epidemiological evidence. *Ann N Y Acad Sci* 2004;1028:273–82.

4. Lee AV, Jackson JG, Gooch JL, et al. Enhancement of insulin-like growth factor signaling in human breast cancer: estrogen regulation of insulin receptor substrate-1 expression in vitro and in vivo. *Mol Endocrinol* 1999 13(5):787–96.

5. Malin A, Dai Q, Yu H, et al. Evaluation of the synergistic effect of insulin resistance and insulin-like growth factors on the risk of breast carcinoma. *Cancer* 2004;100(4):694–700.

6. Hadsell DL, Bonnette SG. IGF and insulin action in the mammary gland: lessons from transgenic and knockout models. *J Mammary Gland Biol Neoplasia* 2000;5(1):19–30.

7. Yu H, Rohan T. Role of the insulin-like growth factor family in cancer development and progression. *J Natl Cancer Inst* 2000;92 (18):1472–89. Hankinson SE, Willett WC, Colditz GA, et al. Circulating concentrations of insulin-like growth factor–I and risk of breast cancer. *Lancet* 1998;351(9113):1393–6. Schernhammer ES, Holly JM, Pollak MN, Hankinson SE. Circulating levels of insulin-like growth factors, their binding proteins, and breast cancer risk. *Cancer Epidemiol Biomarkers Prev* 2005; 14(3):699–704.

8. Stoll BA. Biological mechanisms in breast cancer invasiveness: relevance to preventive interventions. *Eur J Cancer Prev* 2000;9(2):73–9.

9. McCance KL, Jones RE. Estrogen and insulin crosstalk: breast cancer risk implications. *Nurse Pract* 2003;28(5):12–23.

10. Gonullu G, Ersoy C, Ersoy A, et al. Relation between insulin resistance and serum concentrations of IL-6 and TNF-alpha in overweight or obese women with early stage breast cancer. *Cytokine* 2005;31(4):264–9.

11. Goodwin PJ, Ennis M, Pritchard KI, et al. Fasting insulin and outcome in early-stage breast cancer: results of a prospective cohort study. *J Clin Oncol* 2002;20(1):42–51.

12. Ford JM, Whittemore AS. Predicting and preventing hereditary colorectal cancer. *JAMA* 2006;296(12):1521–3.

13. Platz EA, Willett WC, Colditz GA, Rimm EB, Spiegelman D, Giovannucci E. Proportion of colon cancer risk that might be preventable in a cohort of middle-aged US men. *Cancer Causes Control* 2000;11(7):579–88. Danaei G, Vander Hoorn S, Lopez AD, Murray CJ, Ezzati M, Comparative Risk Assessment Collaborating Group (Cancers). Causes of cancer in the world: comparative risk assessment of nine behavioural and environmental risk factors.

Lancet 2005;366(9499):1784–93. Colditz GA, Sellers TA, Trapido E. Epidemiology: identifying the causes and preventability of cancer. *Nat Rev Cancer* 2006;6(1):75–83.

14. Watson P, Ashwathnarayan R, Lynch HT, Roy HK. Tobacco use and increased colorectal cancer risk in patients with hereditary nonpolyposis colorectal cancer (Lynch syndrome). *Arch Intern Med* 2004;164(22):2429–31.

15. van de Vijver MJ, He YD, van't Veer LJ, et al. A gene-expression signature as a predictor of survival in breast cancer. *N Engl J Med* 2002;347(25):1999–2009.

16. Hampton T. Breast and colon cancer genomes sequenced. *JAMA* 2006;296(15):1825–6.

17. Potti A, Mukherjee S, Petersen R, et al. A genomic strategy to refine prognosis in early-stage non–small-cell lung cancer. *N Engl J Med* 2006;355(6):570–80.

Chapter 9

1. Nessim S, Smith DS. Survivorship: obstacles and opportunities. In *Everyone's Guide to Cancer Therapy* 4th ed., eds. M Dollinger, EH Rosenbaum, SJ Mulvihill, M Tempero. Kansas City, MO: Andrews McMeel, 2002.

2. Hoffman B. Cancer survivors at work: a generation of progress. *CA Cancer J Clin* 2005; 55(5):271–80.

3. Short PF, Vasey JJ, Tunceli K. Employment pathways in a large cohort of adult cancer survivors. *Cancer* 2005;103(6):1292–301.

4. Wheatley GM, Cunnick WR, Wright BP, Van Keuren D. Proceedings: the employment of persons with a history of treatment for cancer. *Cancer* 1974;33(2):441–5.

5. Yabroff KR, Lawrence WF, Clauser S, Davis WW, Brown ML. Burden of illness in cancer survivors: findings from a population-based national sample. *J Natl Cancer Inst* 2004; 96 (17):1322–30.

6. Hewitt M, Rowland JH, Yancik R. Cancer survivors in the United States: age, health, and disability. *J Gerontol A Biol Sci Med Sci* 2003; 58(1):82–91.

7. Bradley CJ, Bednarek HL. Employment patterns of long-term cancer survivors. *Psycho-oncology* 2002;11(3):188–98.

8. Ferrell BR, Grant M, Dean GE, Funk B, Ly J. Bone tired: the experience of fatigue and its impact on quality of life. *Oncol Nurs Forum* 1996;23:1539–47.

9. Fobair P, Hoppe RT, Bloom J, Cox R, Varghese A, Spiegel D. Psychosocial problems among survivors of Hodgkin's disease. *J Clin Oncol* 1986;4(5):805–14.

10. Feldman F. *Work and Cancer Health Histories*. Atlanta, GA: American Cancer Society, 1982.

11. Yankelovich Clancy Shulman Inc. *Cerenex Survey on Cancer Patients in the Workplace: Breaking Down Discrimination Barriers*. Unpublished, 1992.

12. Bloom JR, Hoppe RT, Fobair P, Cox RS, Varghese A, Spiegel D. Effects of treatment on the work experiences of long-term survivors of Hodgkin's disease. *Journ Psychosoc Oncol* Special Issue: Clinical research issues in psychosocial oncology. 1988,6(3-4):65-80.

13. Fobair P, ed. *Work Patterns Among Long Term Survivors of Hodgkin's Disease*. New York: Praeger, 1988. Barofsky I, ed. *Work and Illness: The Cancer Patient*. New York: Praeger, 1989.

14. Americans with Disabilities Act of 1990. 42 U.S.C. 2000; 12101–13.

15. Federal Rehabilitation Act of 1973. 29 U.S.C. 2000; 701–96.

16. Family and Medical Leave Act of 1993. 29 U.S.C. 2000; 2611–2654.

17. Employment Retirement and Income Security Act of 1974. 29 U.S.C. 2000; 1001–91.

18. Hewitt MGS, Stovall E. *From Cancer Patient to Cancer Survivor*. Washington, DC: National Academies Press, 2006.

19. McCarthy EP, Ngo LH, Roetzheim RG, et al. Disparities in breast cancer treatment and survival for women with disabilities. *Ann Intern Med* 2006;145:637–45.

20. Harvey J. Cohen Center for the Study of Aging and Human Development, Duke University and Federal Administration Medical Center, Durham, NC 27710.

Chapter 10

1. Kushi LH, Byers T, Doyle C, et al. American Cancer Society 2006 Nutrition and Physical Activity Guidelines Advisory Committee. American Cancer Society guidelines on nutrition and physical activity for cancer prevention: reducing the risk of cancer with healthy food choices and physical activity. *CA Cancer J Clin* 2006;56(5):254–81.

2. Adams KF, Schatzkin A, Harris T, et al. Overweight, obesity, and mortality in a large prospective cohort of persons 50–71 years of age. *N Engl J Med* 2006;355:763–78.

3. National Institutes of Health. *The Practical Guide: Identification, Evaluation, and Treatment of Overweight and Obesity in Adults*. Report of the National Institutes of Health (NHI-BI) Obesity Education Initiative and NAASCO. Washington, DC: National Institutes of Health, 1998, www.nhlbi.nih.gov/guidelines/obesity/practgde.htm.

4. Romero-Corral A, Montori VM, Somers VK, et al. Association of bodyweight with total mortality and with cardiovascular events in coronary artery disease: a systematic review of cohort studies. *Lancet* 2006;368(9536):666-78.

5. Franzosi MG. Should we continue to use BMI as a cardiovascular risk factor? *Lancet* 2006;368(9536):624–5. Romero-Corral A, Montori VM, Somers VK, et al. Association of bodyweight with total mortality and with cardiovascular events in coronary artery disease: a systematic review of cohort studies. *Lancet* 2006;368(9536):666–78. Li TY, Rana JS, Manson JE, et al. Obesity as compared with physical activity in predicting risk of coronary heart disease in women. *Circulation* 2006;113(4):499–506.

6. Price GM, Uauy R, Breeze E, Bulpitt CJ, Fletcher AE. Weight, shape, and mortality risk in older persons: elevated waist-hip ratio, not high body mass index, is associated with a greater risk of death. *Am J Clin Nutr* 2006;84(2):449–60.

7. International Agency for Research on Cancer, Globocan, http://www-dep.iarc.fr (accessed April 20, 2007).

8. Key TJ, Allen NE, Spencer EA, Travis RC. The effect of diet on risk of cancer. *Lancet* 2002;360(9336):861–8.

9. Greenlee RT, Hill-Harmon MB, Murray T, Thun M. Cancer statistics, 2001. *CA Cancer J Clin* 2001;51(1):15-36. Key TJ, Allerri NE, Spencer EA. The effect of diet on risk of cancer. *Lancet* 2002;360:861–8.

10. King MC, Marks JH, Mandell JB, New York Breast Cancer Study Group. Breast and ovarian cancer risks due to inherited mutations in BRCA 1 and BRCA 2. *Science* 2003;302(5645):643–6.

11. Biddinger SB, Ludwig DS. The insulin-like growth factor axis: a potential link between glycemic index and cancer. *Am J Clin Nutr* 2005;82(2):277–8.

12. McGinnis JM, Foege WH. Actual causes of death in the United States. *JAMA* 1993;270(18):2207–12.

13. Ito Y, Gajalakshmi KC, Sasaki R, Suzuki K, Shanta V. A study on serum carotenoid levels in breast cancer patients of Indian women in Chennai (Madras), India. *J Epidemiol* 1999;9(5):306–14. Nkondjock A, Ghadirian P. Intake of specific carotenoids and essential fatty acids and breast cancer risk in Montreal, Canada. *Am J Clin Nutr* 2004;79(5):857–64. Kim MK, Park YG, Gong G, Ahn SH. Breast cancer, serum antioxidant vitamins, and p53 protein overexpression. *Nutr Cancer* 2002;43(2):159–66. Sato R, Helzlsouer KJ, Alberg AJ, Hoffman SC, Norkus EP, Comstock GW. Prospective study of carotenoids, tocopherols, and retinoid concentrations and the risk of breast cancer. *Cancer Epidemiol Biomarkers Prev* 2002;11(5):451–7. Ching S, Ingram D, Hahnel R, Beilby J, Rossi E. Serum levels of micronutrients, antioxidants and total antioxidant status predict risk of breast cancer in a case control study. *J Nutr* 2002;132(2):303–6. Toniolo P, Van Kappel AL, Akhmedkhanov A, et

al. Serum carotenoids and breast cancer. *Am J Epidemiol* 2001;153(12):1142–7.

14. Chidambaram N, Baradarajan A. Influence of selenium on glutathione and some associated enzymes in rats with mammary tumor induced by 7,12-dimethylbenz(a)-anthracene. *Mol Cell Biochem* 1996;156(2):101–7. El-Bayoumy K, Sinha R. Mechanisms of mammary cancer chemoprevention by organoselenium compounds. *Mutat Res* 2004;551(1–2):181–97.

15. Thompson LU, Chen JM, Li T, Strasser-Weippl K, Goss PE. Dietary flaxseed alters tumor biological markers in postmenopausal breast cancer. *Clin Cancer Res* 2005;11(10):3828–35. Chen J, Stavro PM, Thompson LU. Dietary flaxseed inhibits human breast cancer growth and metastasis and downregulates expression of insulin-like growth factor and epidermal growth factor receptor. *Nutr Cancer* 2002;43(2):187–92. Denis L, Morton MS, Griffiths K. Diet and its preventive role in prostatic disease. *Eur Urol* 1999;35(5–6):377–87. Demark-Wahnefried W, Price DT, Polascik TJ, et al. Pilot study of dietary fat restriction and flaxseed supplementation in men with prostate cancer before surgery: exploring the effects on hormonal levels, prostate-specific antigen, and histopathologic features. *Urology* 2001;58(1):47–52.

16. Aronson WJ, Tymchuk CN, Elashoff RM, et al. Decreased growth of human prostate LNCaP tumors in SCID mice fed a low-fat, soy protein diet with isoflavones. *Nutr Cancer* 1999;35(2):130–6. Jacobsen BK, Knutsen SF, Fraser GE. Does high soy milk intake reduce prostate cancer incidence? The Adventist Health Study (United States). *Cancer Causes Control* 1998;9(6):553–7. Kolonel LN, Hankin JH, Whittemore AS, et al. Vegetables, fruits, legumes and prostate cancer: a multi-ethnic case-control study. *Cancer Epidemiol Biomarkers Prev* 2000;9(8):795–804. Messina MJ. Emerging evidence on the role of soy in reducing prostate cancer risk. *Nutr Rev* 2003;61(4):117–31.

17. Allred CD, Allred KF, Ju YH, Goeppinger TS, Doerge DR, Helferich WG. Soy processing influences growth of estrogen-dependent breast cancer tumors. *Carcinogenesis* 2004;25(9):1649–57. Boyapati SM, Shu XO, Ruan ZX, et al. Soyfood intake and breast cancer survival: a followup of the Shanghai Breast Cancer Study. *Breast Cancer Res Treat* 2005;92(1):11–7.

18. Kumar NB, Cantor A, Allen K, Riccardi D, Cox CE. The specific role of isoflavones on estrogen metabolism in premenopausal women. *Cancer* 2002;94(4):1166–74. Xu X, Duncan AM, Merz BE, Kurzer MS. Effects of soy isoflavones on estrogen and phytoestrogen metabolism in premenopausal women. *Cancer Epidemiol Biomarkers Prev* 1998;7(12):1101–8.

19. Sartippour MR, Heber D, Henning S, et al. cDNA microarray analysis of endothelial cells in response to green tea reveals a suppressive phenotype. *Int J Oncol* 2004;25(1):193–202.

20. Kuriyama S, Shimazu T, Ohmori K, et al. Green tea consumption and mortality due to cardiovascular disease, cancer, and all causes in Japan: the Ohsaki study. *JAMA* 2006; 296(10):1255–65.

21. Bradlow HL, Sepkovic DW, Telang NT, Osborne MP. Multifunctional aspects of the action of indole-3-carbinol as an antitumor agent. *Ann NY Acad Sci* 1999;889:204–13. Fowke JH, Longcope C, Hebert JR. Brassica vegetable consumption shifts estrogen metabolism in healthy postmenopausal women. *Cancer Epidemiol Biomarkers Prev* 2000;9(8):773–9.

22. Mozaffarian D, Rimm EB. Fish intake, contaminants, and human health: evaluating the risks and the benefits. *JAMA* 2006;296(15):1885–99.

23. Cho E, Chen WY, Hunter DJ, et al. Red meat intake and risk of breast cancer among premenopausal women. *Arch Intern Med* 2006;166(20):2253–9.

24. Hughes-Fulford M. *Not All Fats Are Created Equal.* Report from UCSF Compre-

hensive Cancer Center, Volume 8.2, Summer 2006, p. 3.

25. Chajes V, Bougnoux P. Omega-6/omega-3 polyunsaturated fatty acid ratio and cancer. *World Rev Nutr Diet* 2003;92:133–51.

26. Ziegler RG, Hoover RN, Nomura AM, et al. Relative weight, weight change, height, and breast cancer risk in Asian-American women. *J Natl Cancer Inst* 1996;88(10):650–60.

27. Bermudez O. *Consumption of sweet drinks among American adults from the NHANES 1999–2000.* Experimental Biology 2005, San Diego, Abstract 839.5.

28. Galli F, Stabile AM, Betti M, et al. The effect of alpha- and gamma-tocopherol and their carboxyethyl hydroxychroman metabolites on prostate cancer cell proliferation. *Arch Biochem Biophys* 2004;423(1):97–102.

29. Deneo-Pellegrini H, De Stefani E, Ronco A, Mendilaharsu M. Foods, nutrients and prostate cancer: a case-control study in Uruguay. *Br J Cancer* 1999;80(3–4):591–7. Heinonen OP, Albanes D, Virtamo J, et al. Prostate cancer and supplementation with alpha-tocopherol and beta-carotene: incidence and mortality in a controlled trial. *J Natl Cancer Inst* 1998; 90(6):440–6. Helzlsouer KJ, Huang HY, Alberg AJ, et al. Association between alpha-tocopherol, gamma-tocopherol, selenium, and subsequent prostate cancer. *J Natl Cancer Inst* 2000;92 (24):2018–23. Huang HY, Alberg AJ, Norkus EP, Hoffman SC, Comstock GW, Helzlsouer KJ. Prospective study of antioxidant micronutrients in the blood and the risk of developing prostate cancer. *Am J Epidemiol* 2003; 157(4):335–44.

30. Garland CF, Garland FC, Gorham ED, et al. The role of vitamin D in cancer prevention. *Am J Public Health* 2006;96(2):252–61. Holick MF. The role of vitamin D for bone health and fracture prevention. *Curr Osteoporos Rep* 2006;4(3):96–102. Holick MF. Defects in the synthesis and metabolism of vitamin D. *Exp Clin Endocrinol Diabetes* 1995;103(4):219–27. Peterlik M, Cross HS. Dysfunction of the vitamin D endocrine system as common cause for multiple malignant and other chronic diseases. *Anticancer Res* 2006;26(4A):2581–8.

31. Doyle C, Kushi LH, Byers T, et al.; American Cancer Society 2006 Nutrition, Physical Activity, and Cancer Survivorship Committee. Nutrition and physical activity during and after cancer treatment: an American Cancer Society Guide for informed choices. *CA Cancer J Clin* 2006;56(6):323–53.

32. Grant WB. An estimate of premature cancer mortality in the U.S. due to inadequate doses of solar ultraviolet-B radiation. *Cancer* 2002;94(6):1867–75.

33. Kushi LH, Byers T, Doyle C, et al.; American Cancer Society 2006 Nutrition and Physical Activity Guidelines Advisory Committee. American Cancer Society guidelines on nutrition and physical activity for cancer prevention: reducing the risk of cancer with healthy food choices and physical activity. *CA Cancer J Clin* 2006;56(5):254–81.

34. Vainio H, Bianchini F. *Weight Control and Physical Activity,* Vol. 6. Lyon, France: International Agency for Cancer Research Press, 2002.

35. Halabi S, Small EJ, Vogelzang NJ. Elevated body mass index predicts for longer overall survival duration in men with metastatic hormone-refractory prostate cancer. *J Clin Oncol* 2005;23(10):2434-5; author's reply p. 2435. A comment on Amling CL, Riffenburgh RH, et al. Pathologic variables and recurrence rates as related to obesity and race in men with prostate cancer undergoing radical prostatectomy. *J Clin Oncol* 2004;22(3):439-45.

Chapter 11

1. Kushi LH, Byers T, Doyle C, et al.; American Cancer Society 2006 Nutrition and Physical Activity Guidelines Advisory Committee. American Cancer Society guidelines on nutrition and physical activity for cancer prevention: reducing the risk of cancer with healthy food choices and physical activity. *CA Cancer J Clin* 2006;56(5):254–81.

2. Holmes MD, Chen WY, Feskanich D, Kroenke CH, Colditz GA. Physical activity and survival after breast cancer diagnosis. *JAMA* 2005;293(20):2479–86.

3. Curry S, Byers T, Hewitt M, eds. *Fulfilling the Potential of Cancer Prevention and Early Detection.* Washington, DC: National Academies Press, 2003.

4. McTiernan A. Obesity and cancer: the risks, science, and potential management strategies. *Oncology (Williston Park)* 2005;19(7):871–81; discussion 881–2, 885–6.

5. Rosner GL, Hargis JB, Hollis DR, et al. Relationship between toxicity and obesity in women receiving adjuvant chemotherapy for breast cancer: results from cancer and leukemia group B study 8541. *J Clin Oncol* 1996;14(11):3000–8.

6. Amling CL. Relationship between obesity and prostate cancer. *Curr Opin Urol* 2005; 15(3):167–71.

7. Lippman SM, Levin B. Cancer prevention: strong science and real medicine. *J Clin Oncol* 2005;23(2):249–53.

8. Thorpe KE, Florence CS, Howard DH, Joski P. The rising prevalence of treated disease: effects on private health insurance spending. *Health Aff (Millwood)* 2005, Jan–Jun:W5-317–25.

9. Colliver V. *Zooming Obesity Rate Has Price Tag.* New Bern, NC: Health Management Associates of New Bern, NC Study for California Health Services, 2005.

10. Adams KF, Schatzkin A, Harris TB, et al. Overweight, obesity, and mortality in a large prospective cohort of persons 50 to 71 years old. *N Engl J Med* 2006;355(8):763–78.

11. Wing RR, Tate DF, Gorin AA, Raynor HA, Fava JL. A self-regulation program for maintenance of weight loss. *N Engl J Med* 2006;355:1563–71.

12. National Institutes of Health. Childhood obesity. *Word on Health,* June 2002: http://www.nih.gov/news/WordonHealth/jun2002/childhoodobesity.htm (accessed on April 11, 2007).

13. Tominaga S, Kuroishi T. *Epidemiology and Prevention of Breast Cancer in the 21st Century.* Nagoya, Japan: Aichi Cancer Center Research Institute.

14. Chlebowski RT, Aiello E, McTiernan A. Weight loss in breast cancer patient management. *J Clin Oncol* 2002;20(4):1128–43.

15. Prentice R, Thompson D, Clifford C, Gorbach S, Goldin B, Byar D. Dietary fat reduction and plasma estradiol concentration in healthy postmenopausal women. The Women's Health Trial Study Group. *J Natl Cancer Inst* 1990;82(2):129–34. Wu AH, Pike MC, Stram DO. Meta-analysis: dietary fat intake, serum estrogen levels, and the risk of breast cancer. *J Natl Cancer Inst* 1999;91(6): 529–34.

16. Chlebowski RT, Aiello E, McTiernan A. Weight loss in breast cancer patient management. *J Clin Oncol* 2002;20(4):1128–43.

17. Demark-Wahnefried W, Peterson B, McBride C, Lipkus I, Clipp E. Current health behaviors and readiness to pursue life-style changes among men and women diagnosed with early stage prostate and breast carcinomas. *Cancer* 2000;88(3):674–84.

18. Newman VA, Thomson CA, Rock CL, et al, Women's Healthy Eating and Living (WHEL) Study Group. Achieving substantial changes in eating behavior among women previously treated for breast cancer: an overview of the intervention. *J Am Diet Assoc* 2005;105(3):382–91. Pierce JP, Faerber S, Wright FA, et al. A randomized trial of the effect of a plant-based dietary pattern on additional breast cancer events and survival: the Women's Healthy Eating and Living (WHEL) Study. *Control Clin Trials* 2002;23(6): 728–56.

19. Ligibel JA, Chlebowski RT, Goodwin PJ. *The Effect of Lifestyle Factors on Breast Cancer Prognosis.* American Society of Clinical Oncology 2006 Educational Book, pp. 16–20, and ASCO oral presentation, Atlanta, Georgia, June 4, 2006.

20. Michael YL, Kawachi I, Berkman LF, Holmes MD, Colditz GA. The persistent impact of breast carcinoma on functional health status: prospective evidence from the Nurses' Health Study. *Cancer* 2000;89(11):2176–86.

21. Eliassen AH, Colditz GA, Rosner B, Willett WC, Hankinson SE. Adult weight change and risk of postmenopausal breast cancer. *JAMA* 2006;296(2):193–201.

22. Eng SM, Gammon MD, Terry MB, et al. Body size changes in relation to postmenopausal breast cancer among women on Long Island, New York. *Am J Epidemiol* 2005;162 (3):229–37.

23. McTiernan A. Obesity and cancer: the risks, science, and potential management strategies. *Oncology (Williston Park)* 2005;19 (7):871–81. Dignam JJ, Wieand K, Johnson KA, Raich P, Anderson SJ, Somkin C, Wickerham DL. Effects of obesity and race on prognosis in lymph node–negative, estrogen receptor–negative breast cancer. *Breast Cancer Res Treat* 2006;97(3):245–54. Whiteman MK, Hillis SD, Curtis KM, McDonald JA, Wingo PA, Marchbanks PA. Body mass and mortality after breast cancer diagnosis. *Cancer Epidemiol Biomarkers Prev* 2005;14(8):2009–14. Berclaz G, Li S, Price KN, et al. Body mass index as a prognostic feature in operable breast cancer: the International Breast Cancer Study Group experience. *Ann Oncol* 2004;15(6): 875–84. Kroenke CH, Chen WY, Rosner B, Holmes MD. Weight, weight gain, and survival after breast cancer diagnosis. *J Clin Oncol* 2005;23(7):1370–8. Ryu SY, Kim CB, Nam CM, et al. Is body mass index the prognostic factor in breast cancer? A meta-analysis. *J Korean Med Sci* 2001;16(5):610–14. Loi S, Milne RL, Friedlander ML, et al. Obesity and outcomes in premenopausal and postmenopausal breast cancer. *Cancer Epidemiol Biomarkers Prev* 2005; 14(7):1686–91.

24. Pollak M, Costantino J, Polychronakos C, et al. Effect of tamoxifen on serum insulin-like growth factor I levels in stage I breast cancer patients. *J Natl Cancer Inst* 1990;82 (21):1693–7. McTiernan A. Obesity and cancer: the risks, science, and potential management strategies. *Oncology (Williston Park)* 2005;19 (7):871–81.

25. Thomson CA, Giuliano AR, Shaw JW, et al. Diet and biomarkers of oxidative damage in women previously treated for breast cancer. *Nutr Cancer* 2005;51(2):146–54.

26. Slavin JL. Mechanisms for the impact of whole grain foods on cancer risk. *J Am Coll Nutr* 2000;19(3 Suppl):300S–307S. Stoll BA. Can supplementary dietary fibre suppress breast cancer growth? *Br J Cancer* 1996;73(5): 557–9. Rock CL, Flatt SW, Thomson CA, et al. Effects of a high-fiber, low-fat diet intervention on serum concentrations of reproductive steroid hormones in women with a history of breast cancer. *J Clin Oncol* 2004; 22(12):2379–87.

27. Michels KB, Holmberg L, Bergkvist L, Ljung H, Bruce A, Wolk A. Dietary antioxidant vitamins, retinol, and breast cancer incidence in a cohort of Swedish women. *Int J Cancer* 2001;91(4):563–7.

28. Ziegler RG, Hoover RN, Nomura AM, et al. Relative weight, weight change, height, and breast cancer risk in Asian-American women. *J Natl Cancer Inst* 1996;88(10):650–60.

29. Byers T. Overweight and mortality among baby boomers: now we're getting personal. *N Engl J Med* 2006;355(8):758–60.

30. King MC, Marks JH, Mandell JB, New York Breast Cancer Study Group. Breast and ovarian cancer risks due to inherited mutations in BRCA1 and BRCA2. *Science* 2003; 302(5645):643–6.

31. Kauff ND, Satagopan JM, Robson ME, et al. Risk-reducing salpingo-oophorectomy in women with a BRCA1 or BRCA2 mutation. *N Engl J Med* 2002;346(21):1609–15.

32. Moyad MA. The use of complementary/preventive medicine to prevent prostate cancer recurrence/progression following definitive therapy: part I—lifestyle changes. *Curr Opin Urol* 2003;13(2):137–45.

33. Moyad MA. Promoting general health during androgen deprivation therapy (ADT): a rapid 10-step review for your patients. *Urol Oncol* 2005;23(1):56–64.

34. Wei IT, Gross M, Jaffe CA, et al. Androgen-deprivation therapy for prostate cancer results in significant loss of bone density. *Urology* 1999;54:607–11.

35. Braga-Basaria M, Dob AS, Muller DC, et al. Metabolic syndrome in men with prostate cancer undergoing long-term androgen-deprivation therapy. *J Clin Oncol* 2006;24:3979–83.

36. Veierod MB, Laake P, Thelle DS. Dietary fat intake and risk of prostate cancer: a prospective study of 25,708 Norwegian men. *Int J Cancer* 1997;73(5):634–8.

37. Calle EE, Rodriguez C, Walker-Thurmond K, Thun MJ. Overweight, obesity, and mortality from cancer in a prospectively studied cohort of U.S. adults. *N Engl J Med* 2003;348(17):1625–38.

38. Amling CL, Riffenburgh RH, Sun L, Moul JW, Lance RS, Kusuda L. Pathologic variables and recurrence rates as related to obesity and race in men with prostate cancer undergoing radical prostatectomy. *J Clin Oncol* 2004;22(3):439–45. Freedland SJ, Aronson WJ, Kane CJ, Presti JC Jr, Amling CL. Impact of obesity on biochemical control after radical prostatectomy for clinically localized prostate cancer: a report by the Shared Equal Access Regional Cancer Hospital Database Study Group. *J Clin Oncol* 2004;22(3):446–53.

39. Amling CL. Relationship between obesity and prostate cancer. *Curr Opin Urol* 2005;15(3):167–71.

40. Amling CL, Riffenburgh RH, Sun L, et al. Pathologic variables and recurrence rates as related to obesity and race in men with prostate cancer undergoing radical prostatectomy. *J Clin Oncol* 2004;22(3):439–45.

41. Pasquali R, Casimirri F, Cantobelli S, et al. Effect of obesity and body fat distribution on sex hormones and insulin in men. *Metabolism* 1991;40(1):101–4. Gann PH, Hennekens CH, Ma J, Longcope C, Stampfer MJ. Prospective study of sex hormone levels and risk of prostate cancer. *J Natl Cancer Inst* 1996;88(16):1118–26.

42. Smith MR. Changes in fat and lean body mass during androgen-deprivation therapy for prostate cancer. *Urology* 2004;63(4):742–5. Nowicki M, Bryc W, Kokot F. Hormonal regulation of appetite and body mass in patients with advanced prostate cancer treated with combined androgen blockade. *J Endocrinol Invest* 2001;24(1):31–6. Smith MR. Osteoporosis and other adverse body composition changes during androgen deprivation therapy for prostate cancer. *Cancer Metastasis Rev* 2002;21(2):159–66. Basaria S, Lieb J II, Tang AM, et al. Long-term effects of androgen deprivation therapy in prostate cancer patients. *Clin Endocrinol (Oxf)* 2002;56(6):779–86. Berruti A, Dogliotti L, Terrone C, et al. Changes in bone mineral density, lean body mass and fat content as measured by dual energy x-ray absorptiometry in patients with prostate cancer without apparent bone metastases given androgen deprivation therapy. *J Urol* 2002;167(6):2361–7.

43. Wei IT, Gross M, Jaffe CA, et al. Androgen-deprivation therapy for prostate cancer results in significant loss of bone density. *Urology* 1999;54:607–11.

44. Moyad MA, Carroll PR. Lifestyle recommendations to prevent prostate cancer, part II: time to redirect our attention? *Urol Clin North Am* 2004;31(2):301–11. Moyad MA. The use of complementary/preventive medicine to prevent prostate cancer recurrence/progression following definitive therapy: part I—lifestyle changes. *Curr Opin Urol* 2003;13(2):137–45.

45. Wolk A, Larsson SC, Johansson JE, Ekman P. Long-term fatty fish consumption and renal cell carcinoma incidence in women. *JAMA* 2006;296(11):1371–6.

Chapter 12

1. Mustian KM, Griggs JJ, Morrow GR, et al. Exercise and side effects among 749 patients during and after treatment for cancer: a University of Rochester Cancer Center Community Clinical Oncology Program Study. *Support Care Cancer* 2006;14(7):732–41.

2. Demark-Wahnfried W, Clipp EC, Morey MC. *Lifestyle Intervention Development Study to Improve Physical Function in Older Adults with Cancer: Outcomes from Project LEAD*. Durham, NC: School of Nursing, Department of Surgery, Older Americans Independence Center, Duke University Medical Center.

3. Erikson, J. New evidence that exercise improves cancer survival fuels interest in large randomized study. *Oncology Times* 2006;28 (17):8.

4. Centers for Disease Control and Prevention. CDC's National Physical Activity Initiative, www.cdc.gov/nccdphp/sgr/pdf/npal.pdf.

5. Meyerhardt JA, Giovannucci EL, Holmes MD, Chan AT, Chan JA. Physical activity and survival after colorectal cancer diagnosis. *J Clin Oncol* 2006;24(22):3527–34.

6. Mustian KM, Katula JA, Gill DL, Roscoe JA, Lang D, Murphy K. Tai chi chuan, health-related quality of life and self-esteem: a randomized trial with breast cancer survivors. *Support Care Cancer* 2004;12(12):871–6.

7. Mustain KM, Gillies L, Williams J, et al. *A Pilot Study on the Influence of Tai Chi Chuan (TCC) on the Immune Function and Association with Cardiorespiratory Fitness Among Breast Cancer Survivors,* poster presentation at the MASCC Meeting, Toronto, June 24, 2006.

8. Cohen L, Chandwani K, Thornton B, et al. G. Randomized trial of yoga in women with breast cancer undergoing radiation treatment. *J Clin Oncol* 2006 ASCO Annual Meeting Proceedings Part I. Vol. 24, No. 18S (June 20 Supplement), 2006: 8505.

9. Lee IM. Physical activity and cancer prevention: data from epidemiologic studies. *Med Sci Sports Exerc* 2003;35(11):1823–7.

10. Holmes MD, Chen WY, Feskanich D, Kroenke CH, Colditz GA. Physical activity and survival after breast cancer diagnosis. *JAMA* 2005;293(20):2479–86.

11. Nelson ME, Meredith CN, Dawson-Hughes B, Evans WJ. Hormone and bone mineral status in endurance-trained and sedentary postmenopausal women. *J Clin Endocrinol Metab* 1988;66(5):927–33.

12. Irwin ML, Crumley D, McTiernan A, Bernstein L, Baumgartner R. Physical activity levels before and after a diagnosis of breast carcinoma: the Health, Eating, Activity, and Lifestyle (HEAL) study. *Cancer* 2003;97(7): 1746–57.

13. Poniatowski BC, Mock V, Cohen G. Sleep disturbance, fatigue, and exercise in women receiving radiation therapy or chemotherapy for breast cancer. *Proc Am Soc Clin Oncol* 20:400a, 2001.

14. King MC, Marks JH, Mandell JB; New York Breast Cancer Study Group. Breast and ovarian cancer risks due to inherited mutations in BRCA1 and BRCA2. *Science* 2003; 302(5645):643–6.

15. Bardia A, Wang AH, Hartmann LC, et al. Abstract 1002 (page 32): physical activity and risk of postmenopausal breast cancer by hormone receptor status and histology: a large prospective cohort study with 18 years of follow up. Mayo Clinic College of Medicine, Rochester, Minnesota, from the proceedings of the Oral Abstract Presentation and Plenary Sessions from the 42nd Annual Meeting, American Society of Clinical Oncology, Atlanta, GA, 2006.

16. Brown BW, Brauner C, Minnotte MC. Noncancer deaths in white adult cancer patients. *J Natl Cancer Inst* 1993;85(12):979–87.

17. Torti DC, Matheson GO. Exercise and prostate cancer. *Sports Med* 2004;34(6):363–9.

18. Torti DC, Matheson GO. Exercise and prostate cancer. *Sports Med* 2004;34(6):363-9.

19. Giovannucci EL, Liu Y, Leitzmann MF, Stampfer MJ, Willett WC. A prospective study of physical activity and incident and fatal prostate cancer. *Arch Intern Med* 2005;165(9):1005–10.

20. Windsor PM, Nicol KF, Potter J. A randomized, controlled trial of aerobic exercise for treatment-related fatigue in men receiving radical external beam radiotherapy for localized prostate carcinoma. *Cancer* 2004;101(3):550–7.

21. Pierotti B, Altieri A, Talamini R, Montella M, Tavani A. Lifetime physical activity and prostate cancer risk. *Int J Cancer* 2005; 114(4):639–42. Jian L, Shen ZJ, Lee AH, Binns CW. Moderate physical activity and prostate cancer risk: a case-control study in China. *Eur J Epidemiol* 2005;20(2):155–60.

22. Bairati I, Larouche R, Meyer F, Moore L, Fradet Y. Lifetime occupational physical activity and incidental prostate cancer (Canada). *Cancer Causes Control* 2000;11(8):759–64.

23. Barnard RJ, Ngo TH, Leung PS, Aronson WJ, Golding LA. A low-fat diet and/or strenuous exercise alters the IGF axis in vivo and reduces prostate tumor cell growth in vitro. *Prostate* 2003;56(3):201–6.

24. Leung PS, Aronson WJ, Ngo TH, Golding LA, Barnard RJ. Exercise alters the IGF axis in vivo and increases p53 protein in prostate tumor cells in vitro. *J Appl Physiol* 2004;96(2):450–4.

25. Zeegers MP, Dirx MJ, van den Brandt PA. Physical activity and the risk of prostate cancer in the Netherlands cohort study, results after 9.3 years of follow-up. *Cancer Epidemiol Biomarkers Prev* 2005;14(6):1490-5.

26. Lee IM, Paffenbarger RS Jr, Hsieh C. Physical activity and risk of developing colorectal cancer among college alumni. *J Natl Cancer Inst* 1991;83(18):1324–9. Severson RK, Nomura AM, Grove JS, Stemmermann GN. A prospective analysis of physical activity and cancer. *Am J Epidemiol* 1989;130(3):522–9.

27. Sandhu MS, Dunger DB, Giovannucci EL. Insulin, insulin-like growth factor–I (IGF-I), IGF binding proteins, their biologic interactions, and colorectal cancer. *J Natl Cancer Inst* 2002;94(13):972–80.

28. Meyerhardt JA, Giovannucci EL, Holmes MD, Chan AT, Chan JA. Physical activity and survival after colorectal cancer diagnosis. *J Clin Oncol* 2006;24(22):3527–34.

29. Meyerhardt JA, Heseltine D, Niedzwiecki D, Hollis D, Saltz LB. Impact of physical activity on cancer recurrence and survival in patients with stage III colon cancer: findings from CALGB 89803. *J Clin Oncol* 2006;24(22):3535–41.

30. Haydon AM, Macinnis RJ, English DR, Morris H, Giles GG. Physical activity, insulin-like growth factor 1, insulin-like growth factor binding protein 3, and survival from colorectal cancer. *Gut* 2006;55(5):689–94.

Chapter 13

1. Brody J. Personal health: women and alcohol—heart benefit versus cancer risk. *New York Times,* Sept. 15, 1993, p. C13.

2. Chen WY, Willett WC, Rosner B, Colditz GA. Moderate alcohol consumption and breast cancer risk. *J Clin Oncol,* 2005 ASCO Annual Meeting Proceedings, Part I of II, 23(16S) (June 1 Supplement), 2005:515. Horn-Ross PL, Canchola AJ, West DW, Stewart SL. Patterns of alcohol consumption and breast cancer risk in the California Teachers Study cohort. *Cancer Epidemiol Biomarkers Prev* 2004;13(3):405–11. Tjonneland A, Christensen J, Thomsen BL, Olsen A, Stripp C. Lifetime alcohol consumption and postmenopausal breast cancer rate in Denmark: a prospective cohort study. *J Nutr* 2004;134(1):173–8. Hamajima N, Hirose K, Tajima K Collaborative Group on Hormonal Factors in Breast Cancer. Alcohol, tobacco and breast cancer: collaborative reanalysis of individual data from 53 epidemiological studies, including 58,515 women with breast cancer and 95,067 women without the disease. *Br J Cancer* 2002;87(11):1234–45. Petri AL, Tjonneland A, Gamborg M, Johansen D, Hoidrup S. Alcohol intake, type of beverage, and risk of breast cancer in pre- and postmenopausal women. *Alcohol Clin Exp Res* 2004; 28(7):1084–90. Key TJ, Schatzkin A, Willett

WC, Allen NE, Spencer EA. Diet, nutrition and the prevention of cancer. *Public Health Nutr* 2004;7(1A):187–200. Terry MB, Zhang FF, Kabat G, Britton JA, Teitelbaum SL. Lifetime alcohol intake and breast cancer risk. *Ann Epidemiol* 2006;16(3):230–40.

3. Key TJ, Schatzkin A, Willett WC, Allen NE, Spencer EA, Travis RC. Diet, nutrition and the prevention of cancer. *Public Health Nutr* 2004;7(1A):187–200.

4. Terry MB, Zhang FF, Kabat G, Britton JA, Teitelbaum SL, Neugut AI. Lifetime alcohol intake and breast cancer risk. *Ann Epidemiol* 2006;16(3):230–40.

5. Schatzkin A, Longnecker MP. Alcohol and breast cancer. Where are we now and where do we go from here? *Cancer* 1994;74(3 Suppl):1101–10.

6. Chen WY, Willett WC, Rosner B, Colditz GA. Moderate alcohol consumption and breast cancer risk. *J Clin Oncol,* 2005 ASCO Annual Meeting Proceedings, Part I of II, 23 (16S) (June 1 Supplement), 2005:515.

7. Chen WY, Willett WC, Rosner B, Colditz GA. Moderate alcohol consumption and breast cancer risk. *J Clin Oncol,* 2005 ASCO Annual Meeting Proceedings, Part I of II, 23(16S) (June 1 Supplement), 2005:515. Petri AL, Tjonneland A, Gamborg M, Johansen D, Hoidrup S. Alcohol intake, type of beverage, and risk of breast cancer in pre- and postmenopausal women. *Alcohol Clin Exp Res* 2004;28 (7):1084–90. Enger SM, Ross RK, Paganini-Hill A, Longnecker MP, Bernstein L. Alcohol consumption and breast cancer oestrogen and progesterone receptor status. *Br J Cancer* 1999;79(7–8):1308–14.

8. Sellers TA, Vierkant RA, Cerhan JR, Gapstur SM, Vachon CM. Interaction of dietary folate intake, alcohol, and risk of hormone receptor–defined breast cancer in a prospective study of postmenopausal women. *Cancer Epidemiol Biomarkers Prev* 2002;11(10 Pt 1): 1104–7.

9. Volkow ND, Wang GJ, Begleiter H, et al. High levels of dopamine D2 receptors in unaffected members of alcoholic families: possible protective factors. *Arch Gen Psychiatry* 2006;63(9):999–1008. McGue, M. The behavioral genetics of alcoholism. *Curr Dir in Psychol Sci* 1999;8(4):109–115.

10. Kranzler HR. Evidence-based treatments for alcohol dependence: new results and new questions. *JAMA* 2006;295(17):2075–6. Grant BF, Dawson DA, Stinson FS, Chou SP, Dufour MC. The 12-month prevalence and trends in *DSM-IV* alcohol abuse and dependence: United States, 1991–1992 and 2001–2002. *Drug Alcohol Depend* 2004;74(3):223–34.

11. Anton RF, O'Malley SS, Ciraulo DA, Cisler RA, Couper D COMBINE Study Research Group. Combined pharmacotherapies and behavioral interventions for alcohol dependence: the COMBINE study—a randomized controlled trial. *JAMA* 2006;295(17): 2003–17.

Chapter 14

1. Berrettini WH, Lerman CE. Pharmacotherapy and pharmacogenetics of nicotine dependence. *Am J Psychiatry* 2005;162(8):1441–51.

2. www.nih.gov/news/pr/jun2006/od-14.htm.

3. Johnson BA. New weapon to curb smoking: no more excuses to delay treatment. *Arch Intern Med* 2006;166(15):1547–50.

4. Tom Glynn, senior director, International Tobacco, American Cancer Society.

5. Hughes J, Stead L, Lancaster T. Antidepressants for smoking cessation. *Cochrane Database Syst Rev.* 2004;4:CD000031.

6. Oncken C, Gonzales D, Nides M, Rennard S, Watsky E, Billing CB. Efficacy and safety of the novel selective nicotinic acetylcholine receptor partial agonist, varenicline, for smoking cessation. *Arch Intern Med* 2006; 166(15):1571–7.

7. Etter JF. Cytisine for smoking cessation: a literature review and a meta-analysis. *Arch Intern Med* 2006;166(15):1553–9.

Chapter 15

1. Classen C, Butler LD, Koopman C, Miller E, DiMiceli S. Supportive-expressive group therapy and distress in patients with metastatic breast cancer: a randomized clinical intervention trial. *Arch Gen Psychiatry* 2001;58(5):494–501. Spiegel D. Health caring. Psychosocial support for patients with cancer. *Cancer* 1994; 74(4 Suppl):1453–7. Spiegel D. A 43-year-old woman coping with cancer. *JAMA* 1999;282 (4):371–8. Spiegel D, Bloom JR, Yalom I. Group support for patients with metastatic cancer. A randomized outcome study. *Arch Gen Psychiatry* 1981;38(5):527–33. Spiegel, D. *Living Beyond Limits: New Help and Hope for Facing Life-Threatening Illness*. New York: Times Books/Random House, 1993.

Chapter 16

1. Lieberman B. Nutrition action health letter. *Center for Science in the Public Interest;* 34 (2):1–8.

2. Grodstein F, Manson JE, Stampfer MJ. Hormone therapy and coronary heart disease: the role of time since menopause and age at hormone initiation. *J Womens Health (Larchmt)* 2006;15(1):35–44.

Chapter 17

1. Twiss JJ, Waltman N, Ott CD, Gross GJ, Lindsey AM, Moore TE. Bone mineral density in postmenopausal breast cancer survivors. *J Am Acad Nurse Pract* 2001;13(6):276–84.

2. Fisher B, Dignam J, Bryant J, DeCillis A, Wickerham DL. Five versus more than five years of tamoxifen therapy for breast cancer patients with negative lymph nodes and estrogen receptor–positive tumors. *J Natl Cancer Inst* 1996;88(21):1529–42.

3. Avenell A, Gillespie WJ, Gillespie LD, O'Connell DL. Vitamin D and vitamin D analogues for preventing fractures associated with involutional and post-menopausal osteoporosis. *Cochrane Database Syst Rev* 2005;3: CD000227.

4. Fisher B, Costantino JP, Wickerham DL, Redmond CK, Kavanah M. Tamoxifen for prevention of breast cancer: report of the National Surgical Adjuvant Breast and Bowel Project P-1 Study. *J Natl Cancer Inst* 1998;90(18): 1371–88.

5. Love RR, Mazess RB, Barden HS, Epstein S, Newcomb PA, Jordan VC. Effects of tamoxifen on bone mineral density in postmenopausal women with breast cancer. *N Engl J Med* 1992;326(13):852–6.

6. Stefanick ML. Risk–benefit profiles of raloxifene for women. *N Engl J Med* 2006;355 (2):190–2.

7. Hortobagyi, GM. Clinical issues and therapeutic advances. *MD Anderson Breast Medical Oncology,* May 2006.

8. Twiss JJ, Waltman N, Ott CD, Gross GJ, Lindsey AM, Moore TE. Bone mineral density in postmenopausal breast cancer survivors. *J Am Acad Nurse Pract* 2001;13(6):276–84.

9. Lan C, Lai JS, Chen SY. Tai chi chuan: an ancient wisdom on exercise and health promotion. *Sports Med* 2002;32(4):217–24.

10. Adapted from Freeman G. *Prevent Falls, Know Your Elderly Patients.* Oakland, CA: National Lymphedema Network. www.Lymphnet.org.

11. Adapted from *Treating Patients Age 65 and Older: A Guide for California Physicians.* [This material is valid March 1, 2006–March 1, 2009.] Sponsored by Thomson American Health Consultants. Atlanta, GA: Thomson American Health Consultants, 2006.

12. Avidan AY, Fries BE, James ML, Szafara KL, Wright GT, Chervin RD. Insomnia and hypnotic use, recorded in the minimum data set, as predictors of falls and hip fractures in Michigan nursing homes. *J Am Geriatr Soc* 2005;53(6):955–62.

13. Fisher B, Dignam J, Bryant J, DeCillis A, Wickerham DL. Five versus more than five years of tamoxifen therapy for breast cancer

patients with negative lymph nodes and estrogen receptor–positive tumors. *J Natl Cancer Inst* 1996;88(21):1529–42.

14. Fisher B, Costantino JP, Wickerham DL, Redmond CK, Kavanah M. Tamoxifen for prevention of breast cancer: report of the National Surgical Adjuvant Breast and Bowel Project P-1 Study. *J Natl Cancer Inst* 1998;90(18): 1371–88.

15. Love RR, Mazess RB, Barden HS, Epstein S, Newcomb PA, Jordan VC. Effects of tamoxifen on bone mineral density in postmenopausal women with breast cancer. *N Engl J Med* 1992;326(13):852–6.

16. Eliminating the Suffering and Death Due to Cancer. Special Issue, *JNCI Bulletin,* 2006; 3(40).

17. Stefanick ML. Risk–benefit profiles of raloxifene for women. *N Engl J Med* 2006;355 (2):190–2.

18. Wei JT, Gross M, Jaffe CA, et al. Androgen-deprivation therapy for prostate cancer results in significant loss of bone density. *Urology* 1999;54:607–11.

19. Holmes-Walker DJ, Woo H, Gurney H, Do VT, Chipps DR. Maintaining bone health in patients with prostate cancer. *Med J Aust* 2006;184(4):176–9.

Chapter 18

1. Nathan DM, Cleary PA, Backlund JY, et al, Diabetes Control and Complications Trial/ Epidemiology of Diabetes Interventions and Complications (DCCT/EDIC) Study Research Group. Intensive diabetes treatment and cardiovascular disease in patients with type 1 diabetes. *N Engl J Med* 2005;353(25):2643–53. Writing Team for the Diabetes Control and Complications Trial/Epidemiology of Diabetes Interventions and Complications Research Group. Sustained effect of intensive treatment of type 1 diabetes mellitus on development and progression of diabetic nephropathy: the Epidemiology of Diabetes Interventions and Complications (EDIC) study. *JAMA* 2003;290 (16):2159–67.

Chapter 19

1. American Cancer Society. *What Are the Key Statistics About Nonmelanoma Skin Cancer?* Atlanta, GA: Author, 2006.

2. American Cancer Society. *What Are the Key Statistics About Melanoma?* Atlanta, GA: Author, 2006.

Chapter 20

1. Aziz NM, Rowland JH. Trends and advances in cancer survivorship research: challenge and opportunity. *Semin Radiat Oncol* 2003;13(3):248–66. Slatkin N. Cancer-related pain and its pharmacologic management in the patient with bone metastasis. *J Support Oncol* 2006;4(2 Suppl 1):15–21.

2. Koopman C, Butler LD, Classen C, et al. Traumatic stress symptoms among women with recently diagnosed primary breast cancer. *J Trauma Stress* 2002;15(4):277–87. Han WT, Collie K, Koopman C, et al. Breast cancer and problems with medical interactions: relationships with traumatic stress, emotional self-efficacy, and social support. *Psychooncology* 2005;14(4):318–30.

Chapter 21

1. "Chemotherapy related cardiac toxicity," based on oral presentation at ASCO, June 2006, Atlanta, GA.

2. Dr. Yuer from M. D. Anderson Cancer Center, based on oral report at ASCO, June 2006, Atlanta, GA.

Chapter 23

1. Monk JP, Phillips G, Waite R, Kuhn J, Schaaf LJ, Otterson GA. Assessment of tumor necrosis factor alpha blockade as an interven-

tion to improve tolerability of dose-intensive chemotherapy in cancer patients. *J Clin Oncol* 2006;24(12):1852–9.

2. Bradbury J. Taking fatigue out of cancer. *Lancet Oncol* 2006;7(6):457. Collado-Hidalgo A, Bower JE, Ganz PA, Cole SW, Irwin MR. Inflammatory biomarkers for persistent fatigue in breast cancer survivors. *Clin Cancer Res* 2006;12(9):2759–66.

3. Morrow GR, Ryan J, Kohli S, et al. Modafinil (Provigil) for persistent post-treatment fatigue: an open label study of 82 women with breast cancer. Abstracts of the 18th MASCC International Symposium, Toronto, Canada, June 22–24, 2006. *Supportive Care in Cancer* 2006;14:583-687. Abstract no. 11-070.

4. Servaes P, Verhagen S, Bleijenberg G. Determinants of chronic fatigue in disease-free breast cancer patients: a cross-sectional study. *Ann Oncol* 2002;13(4):589–98.

Chapter 25

1. This chapter is adapted from *Everyone's Guide to Supportive Cancer Care* and *Everyone's Guide to Cancer Therapy.*

2. Dahn JR, Penedo FJ, Molton I, Lopez L, Schneiderman N, Antoni MH. Physical activity and sexual functioning after radiotherapy for prostate cancer beneficial effects for patients undergoing external beam radiotherapy. *Urology* 2005;65(5):953–8.

3. Casper RF, Yen SS. Neuroendocrinology of menopausal flushes: an hypothesis of flush mechanism. *Clin Endocrinol (Oxf)* 1985;22: 293–312.

4. McLeod DC. Gynecomastia. *N Engl J Med* 1993;328:490.

5. The Women's Health Initiative studied the effects of menopausal hormone use in women 50–80 years of age and provided no guidance as to hormone use in women with premature ovarian failure.

Chapter 26

1. Nieman CL, Kazer R, Brannigan RE, Zoloth LS, Chase-Lansdale PL. Cancer survivors and infertility: a review of a new problem and novel answers. *J Support Oncol* 2006;4(4):171–8.

2. Dr. Charles Shapiro, ASCO presentation, June 2006, Atlanta, GA.

3. Byrne J, Fears TR, Gail MH, Pee D, Connelly RR, Austin DF. Early menopause in long-term survivors of cancer during adolescence. *Am J Obstet Gynecol* 1992;166(3):788–93.

4. Critchley HO, Wallace WH, Shalet SM, Mamtora H, Higginson J. Abdominal irradiation in childhood: the potential for pregnancy. *Br J Obstet Gynaecol* 1992;99(5):392–4.

5. Holmes GE. Long-term survival in childhood and adolescent cancer. Five-center study: U.S.A. *Ann NY Acad Sci* 1997;824:180–9.

6. Audrins P, Holden CA, McLachlan RI, Kovacs GT. Semen storage for special purposes at Monash IVF from 1977 to 1997. *Fertil Steril* 1999;72(1):179–81.

7. Tournaye H, Goossens E, Verheyen G, Frederickx V, De Block G. Preserving the reproductive potential of men and boys with cancer: current concepts and future prospects. *Hum Reprod Update* 2004;10(6):525–32.

8. Bisharah M, Tulandi T. Laparoscopic preservation of ovarian function: an underused procedure. *Am J Obstet Gynecol* 2003;188(2): 367–70.

9. Alkhouri N, Patrizio P, Abraham J. Pregnancy after breast cancer. *Community Oncol* 2007;4(5):331–48

Chapter 27

1. Adapted from Dollinger M, Rosenbaum E, Mulvahill S, Tempero M. *Everyone's Guide to Cancer Therapy,* 5th ed. Kansas City, MO: Andrews McMeel, 2007.

Chapter 28

1. Adapted from *Treating Patients Age 65 and Older: A Guide for California Physicians.* [This

material is valid March 1, 2006–March 1, 2009.] Sponsored by AHC Media LLC. Atlanta, GA: AHC Media LLC, 2006.

2. Avidan AY, Fries BE, James ML, Szafara KL, Wright GT, Chervin RD. Insomnia and hypnotic use, recorded in the minimum data set, as predictors of falls and hip fractures in Michigan nursing homes. *J Am Geriatr Soc* 2005;53(6):955–62.

3. Lan C, Lai JS, Chen SY. Tai chi chuan: an ancient wisdom on exercise and health promotion. *Sports Med* 2002;32(4):217–24.

4. Adapted from Freeman G. *Prevent Falls, Know Your Elderly Patients*. Oakland, CA: National Lymphedema Network. www.Lymphnet.org.

Chapter 29

1. Kissin MW, Querci della Rovere G, Easton D, Westbury G. Risk of lymphoedema following the treatment of breast cancer. *Br J Surg* 1986;73(7):580–4. Armer J, Fu MR, Wainstock JM, Zagar E, Jacobs LK. Lymphedema following breast cancer treatment, including sentinel lymph node biopsy. *Lymphology* 2004;37(2):73–91.

2. Wilke LG, McCall LM, Posther KE, et al. Surgical complications associated with sentinel lymph node biopsy: results from a prospective international cooperative group trial. *Ann Surg Oncol* 2006;13(4):491–500.

3. National Lymphedema Network, www.Lymphnet.org.

4. Ahmed RL, Thomas W, Yee D, Schmitz KH. Randomized controlled trial of weight training and lymphedema in breast cancer survivors. *J Clin Oncol* 2006;24(18):2765–72.

Chapter 30

1. Adapted from Iqbal Y. "Patients' fears help keep incontinence in the closet." *Am Coll Physicians Obs* March 2006. www.acponline.org/journals/news/march06/incontinence.htm.

2. Hendrix SL, Cochrane BB, Nygaard IE, et al. Effects of estrogen with and without progestin on urinary incontinence. *JAMA* 2005;293(8):935–48.

Chapter 31

1. Gawande A. On washing hands. *N Engl J Med* 2004;350(13):1283–6.

2. Aiello AE, Marshall B, Levy SB, Della-Latta P, Larson E. Relationship between triclosan and susceptibilities of bacteria isolated from hands in the community. *Antimicrob Agents Chemother* 2004;48(8):2973–9.

3. Bosch FX, de Sanjose S. Human papillomavirus and cervical cancer: burden and assessment of causality. *J Natl Cancer Inst Monogr* 2003;31:3–13.

4. Koutsky L. Epidemiology of genital human papillomavirus infection. *Am J Med* 1997;102(5A):3–8.

5. CDC. *HPV Vaccine Questions and Answers*, August 2006. www.cdc.gov/std/hpv/hpv-vaccine.pdf (accessed Nov. 20, 2006). CDC. *HPV and HPV Vaccine: Information for Healthcare Providers,* revised August 2006. www.cdc.gov/std/hpv/hpv-vacc-hcp-3-pages.pdf (accessed Nov. 20, 2006).

6. Bistrian BR, Sherman M, Blackburn GL, Marshall R, Shaw C. Cellular immunity in adult marasmus. *Arch Intern Med* 1977;137(10):1408–11.

7. Wilson MM, Vaswani S, Liu D, Morley JE, Miller DK. Prevalence and causes of undernutrition in medical outpatients. *Am J Med* 1998;104(1):56–63F.

Chapter 32

1. Adapted from "Creative Expression" in *Everyone's Guide to Cancer Supportive Care.*

Summary and Review

1. Ferrell BR, Grant M, Dean GE, Funk BLYJ. Bone tired: the experience of fatigue and its impact on quality of life. *Oncol Nurs Forum* 1996;23:1539–47.

2. Radimer KL, Ballard-Barbash R, Miller JS, et al. Weight change and the risk of late-onset breast cancer in the original Framingham cohort. *Nutr Cancer* 2004;49(1):7–13.

3. Demark-Wahnefried W, Aziz NM, Rowland JH, Pinto BM. Riding the crest of the teachable moment: promoting long-term health after the diagnosis of cancer. *J Clin Oncol* 2005;23(24):5814–30.

4. *Fruits and Vegetables,* Vol. 8. Lyon, France: International Agency for Research on Cancer, World Health Organization, 2003.

5. He K, Hu FB, Colditz GA, Manson JE, Willett WC, Liu S. Changes in intake of fruits and vegetables in relation to risk of obesity and weight gain among middle-aged women. *Int J Obes Relat Metab Disord* 2004;28(12): 1569–74.

6. Kushi LH, Byers T, Doyle C, et al, American Cancer Society 2006 Nutrition and Physical Activity Guidelines Advisory Committee. American Cancer Society guidelines on nutrition and physical activity for cancer prevention: reducing the risk of cancer with healthy food choices and physical activity. *CA Cancer J Clin* 2006;56(5):254–81.

7. *Healthy Youth: An Investment in Our Nation's Future.* Atlanta, GA: Centers for Disease Control and Prevention, National Center for Chronic Disease Prevention and Health Promotion, 2003. www.cdc.gov/healthyyouth.

8. Curry S, Byers T, Hewitt M, eds. *Fulfilling the Potential of Cancer Prevention and Early Detection.* Washington, DC: National Academies Press, 2003.

9. Mustian K, Williams J, Moynihan J, et al. A pilot study of the influence of Tai Chi Chuan on immune function and associations with cardiorespiratory fitness among breast cancer survivors. Abstracts of the 18th MASCC International Symposium, Toronto, Canada, June 22–24, 2006. *Supportive Care in Cancer* 2006;14:583–687. Abstract no. 10-064.

10. Poniatowski BC, Mock V, Cohen D. Sleep disturbance, fatigue, and exercise in women receiving radiation therapy or chemotherapy for breast cancer. *Proc Am Soc Clin Oncol* 20:400A, 2001.

11. Kushi LH, Byers T, Doyle C, et al, American Cancer Society 2006 Nutrition and Physical Activity Guidelines Advisory Committee. American Cancer Society guidelines on nutrition and physical activity for cancer prevention: reducing the risk of cancer with healthy food choices and physical activity. *CA Cancer J Clin* 2006;56(5):254–81.

Appendix B: Bibliography of Selected Cancer Survivorship Resources

Gail Sorrough, M.L.I.S., and Gloria Won, M.L.I.S., medical librarians at the H. M. Fishbon Memorial Library, UCSF Medical Center at Mount Zion

Cancer Survivorship: Selected Resources

This bibliography consists of selected key works on cancer survivorship that have been published since 2000. The increasing number of cancer survivors has triggered an increase in published works about survivorship. By the time this list is published, there will no doubt be newer editions of many of these titles and many more new articles and books available.

Personal testimonies about surviving cancer abound; many are beautifully written, inspirational, and filled with good advice. They have not been included in this list in part because there are so many, and it was decided that choosing among them would be best left to the individual reader.

Places to Look for the Latest Professional Literature

PubMed — www.pubmed.gov

PubMed is a bibliographic database produced by the U.S. National Library of Medicine (NLM) that provides access to professional biomedical and some selected health-related lay journals. Coverage includes all aspects of medicine, medical research, nursing and nursing research, integrative medicine, and allied health. It is the largest, most comprehensive biomedical database in the world (more than 16 million citations and growing). Use by a novice searcher is facilitated by a powerful search engine interface and an excellent online tutorial. We also suggest consulting a medical librarian for assistance with precision searching to achieve optimal results. PubMed is freely available to anyone anywhere via the Internet. The NLM has also negotiated free access to full text of many journals that are indexed in PubMed.

Places to Look for the Latest Lay Literature

National Cancer Institute Office of Cancer Survivorship (OCS) — dccps.nci.nih.gov/ocs

The OCS provides information to patients, their families, healthcare providers, advocates, and the research community. OCS has an extensive Web site with current information on survivorship issues. One of the most useful sections on their Web site is "Post Treatment Resources: Follow-Up Medical Care After Cancer Treatment." Here you can find published fact sheets, tips, and access to adult and pediatric guidelines for follow-up care from selected organizations.

The National Coalition for Cancer Survivorship (NCCS) — www.canceradvocacy.org

The NCCS, founded in 1986, is the oldest survivor-led cancer advocacy organization in the country, with a mission to address the full spectrum of survivorship issues of living with, through, and beyond cancer. NCCS pursues systemic changes at the federal level to influence how the government researches cancer and regulates, finances, and delivers cancer care. NCCS publishes educational materials and develops online networks and tools on various aspects of survivorship.

Centers for Disease Control and Prevention (CDC) "Cancer Survivorship" — www.cdc.gov/cancer/survivorship

The CDC works with national, state, and local partners to create and implement successful strategies to help the millions of people in the United States who live with, through, and beyond cancer. Materials are available for patients, physicians, and public health professionals. These materials may be downloaded and printed or ordered through CDC's Cancer Resource Library at www.cdc.gov/cancer/dcpc/library/index.htm.

General Texts

Cancer Nursing: Principles AND Practice. Connie Henke Yarbro, Margaret Hansen Frogge, and Michelle Goodman, eds. 6th ed. Sudbury, MA: Jones & Bartlett Publishers, 2005. Part VII, "Dimensions of Cancer Survivorship," pp. 1663–1726.

The Cancer Survivor's Guide: The Essential Handbook to Life After Cancer. Michael Feuerstein and Patricia Findley. New York: Marlowe & Co., 2006.

Choices: The Most Complete Sourcebook for Cancer Information. Marion E. Morra and Eve Potts. 4th ed. New York: HarperCollins, 2003.

The Complete Revised and Updated Cancer Survival Guide: Everything You Must Know and Where to Go for State-of-the-Art Treatment of the 25 Most Common Forms of Cancer. Peter Teeley and Philip Bashe. New York: Broadway, 2005.

A Guide to Survivorship for Women with Ovarian Cancer. F. J. Montz, Robert E. Bristow, and Paula J. Anastasia. Baltimore: Johns Hopkins University Press, 2005.

Living Through Breast Cancer. Carolyn M. Kaelin and Francesca Coltera. New York: McGraw-Hill, 2005.

Living Well with Cancer: A Nurse Tells You Everything You Need to Know About Managing the Side Effects of Your Treatment. Katen Moore and Libby Schmais. New York: Perigee, 2002.

Managing the Side Effects of Chemotherapy and Radiation Therapy. Marylin J. Dodd. San Francisco: UCSF Nursing Press, 2001.

Oncology: An Evidence-Based Approach. Alfred E. Chang, Patricia A. Ganz, Daniel F. Hayes, et al., eds. New York: Springer, 2006. Section 8, "Cancer Survivorship," pp. 1753–1958.

Survivors of Childhood and Adolescent Cancer: A Multidisciplinary Approach. 2nd ed. Cindy L. Schwartz. Berlin: Springer, 2005.

Alternative and Complementary Medicine

American Cancer Society's Complete Guide to Complementary and Alternative Cancer Methods. 2nd ed. Atlanta, GA: American Cancer Society, 2006.

American Cancer Society's Guide to Complementary and Alternative Cancer Methods Handbook. Atlanta, GA: American Cancer Society, 2002.

Breast Cancer: Beyond Convention—The World's Foremost Authorities on Complementary and Alternative Medicine Offer Advice on Healing. Mary Tagliaferri, Isaac Cohen, and Debu Tripathy, eds. Foreword by Dean Ornish. New York: Atria, 2002.

Complementary Cancer Therapies: Combining Traditional and Alternative Approaches for the Best Possible Outcome. Dan Labriola. Roseville, CA: Prima Publishing, 2000.

Complementary and Integrative Medicine in Cancer Care and Prevention: Foundations and Evidence-Based Interventions. Marc S. Micozzi. New York: Springer, 2006.

The Complete Natural Medicine Guide to Breast Cancer: A Practical Manual for Understanding, Prevention and Care. Sat Dharam Kaur. Toronto: Robert Rose Inc., 2003.

Comprehensive Cancer Care: Integrating Alternative, Complementary, and Conventional Therapies. James S. Gordon and Sharon R. Curtin. Cambridge, MA: Perseus Books Group, 2000.

Healing Outside the Margins: The Survivor's Guide to Integrative Cancer Care. Carole O'Toole with Carolyn B. Hendricks, M.D., medical advisor. Washington, DC: Lifeline Press, 2002.

Integrated Cancer Care: Holistic, Complementary, and Creative Approaches. Jennifer Barraclough, ed. New York: Oxford University Press, 2001.

Government Publications

Childhood Cancer Survivorship: Improving Care and Quality of Life. National Cancer Policy Board and the Institute of Medicine. Maria Hewitt, Susan L. Weiner, and Joseph V. Simone, eds. Washington, DC: National Academies Press, 2003. Also available online: www.nap.edu/catalog/10767.html#toc.

From Cancer Patient to Cancer Survivor: Lost in Transition. Committee on Cancer Survivorship: Improving Care and Quality of Life, National Cancer Policy Board; Maria Hewitt, Sheldon Greenfield, and Ellen Stovall, eds. Washington, DC: National Academies Press, 2006. Also available online: www.nap.edu/catalog/11468.html.

Living Beyond Cancer: Finding a New Balance; President's Cancer Panel 2003–2004 Annual Report. Suzanne H. Rueben. Washington, DC: U.S. Department of Health and Human Services, 2004. Also available online: deainfo.nci.nih.gov/advisory/pcp/pcp03-04rpt/Survivorship.pdf.

A National Action Plan for Cancer Survivorship: Advancing Public Health Strategies. Centers for Disease Control and Prevention (U.S.); National Center for Chronic Disease Prevention and Health Promotion (U.S.); Lance Armstrong Foundation. Austin, TX: Lance Armstrong Foundation, 2004. Also available online: www.cdc.gov/cancer/survivorship/pdf/plan.pdf.

Nutrition and Health

American Cancer Society's Healthy Eating Cookbook. 3rd ed. Atlanta, GA: American Cancer Society, 2005.

Cancer Fitness: Exercise Programs for Patients and Survivors. Anna L. Schwartz. Foreword by Lance Armstrong. New York: Simon & Schuster, 2004.

Eat, Drink, and Be Healthy: the Harvard Medical School Guide to Healthy Eating. Walter C. Willett, et al. New York, NY: Free Press, 2005.

Eating Well, Staying Well During and After Cancer. Abby S. Bloch, Barrie Cassileth, Michelle Holmes, and Cynthia Thomson, eds. Atlanta, GA: American Cancer Society, 2004.

Exercise and Cancer Recovery. Carole M. Schneider, Carolyn A. Dennehy, and Susan D. Carter. Champaign, IL: Human Kinetics Publishers, 2003.

The FORCE Program: The Proven Way to Fight Cancer Through Physical Activity and Exercise. Jeffrey Berman, Fran Fleegler, John Hanc, and Nancy Brinker. New York: Ballantine Books, 2003.

Healthy Eating for Life to Prevent and Treat Cancer. Physicians Committee for Responsible Medicine. New York: Wiley, 2002.

One Bite at a Time: Nourishing Recipes for People with Cancer, Survivors, and Their Caregivers. Rebecca Katz, Marsha Tomassi, and Mat Edelson. Berkeley, CA: Celestial Arts Publishing Company, 2004.

Staying Alive! Cookbook for Cancer Free Living: Real Survivors . . . Real Recipes . . . Real Results.

Sally Errey and Trevor Simpson. Vancouver: Belissimo Books, 2004.

The Strang Cancer Prevention Center Cookbook: A Complete Nutrition and Lifestyle Plan to Dramatically Lower Your Cancer Risk. Laura J. Pensiero, Michael P. Osborne, and Susan Oliveria. New York: McGraw-Hill, 2004.

Survivor's Guide to Reversing Cancer: A Journey from Cancer to Cure. Gerald H. Smith. Langhorne, PA: International Center for Nutritional Research, 2004.

Planning for the Future

Be Prepared: The Complete Financial, Legal, and Practical Guide to Living with a Life-Challenging Condition. David S. Landay. New York: St. Martin's Press, 2000.

A Cancer Survivor's Almanac: Charting Your Journey. Barbara Hoffman, ed. 3rd ed. National Coalition for Cancer Survivorship, 2004.

Financial assistance from national organizations for cancer survivors. J. Levy. *Cancer Pract* 2002;10(1):48–52.

What Cancer Survivors Need to Know About Health Insurance. Kimberly J. Calder and Karen Pollitz. 5th ed. Silver Spring, MD: National Coalition for Cancer Survivorship, 2003.

Working It Out: Your Employment Rights as a Cancer Survivor. Barbara Hoffman. 7th ed. Silver Spring, MD: National Coalition for Cancer Survivorship, 2003.

Psycho-Oncology

After Breast Cancer: A Common-Sense Guide to Life After Treatment. Hester Hill Schnipper and Lowell E. Schnipper. New York: Bantam Books, 2003.

Battling Prostate Cancer: Getting from "Why Me" to "What Next." Marvin A. McMickle. Valley Forge, PA: Judson Press, 2004.

Cancer and the Family Caregiver: Distress and Coping. Ora Gilbar and Hasida Ben-Zur. Springfield, IL: Charles C Thomas, 2002.

Living Under the Sword: Psychosocial Aspects of Recurrent and Progressive Life-Threatening Illness. Austin H. Kutscher. Lanham, MD: Scarecrow Press, 2004.

Meeting Psychosocial Needs of Women with Breast Cancer. Maria Elizabeth Hewitt, Roger Herdman, and Jimmie C. Holland, with a contribution by the National Cancer Policy Board (U.S.) Staff. Washington, DC: National Academies Press, 2004. Also available online: www.nap.edu/catalog/10909.html.

Staying Alive: Life-Changing Strategies for Surviving Cancer—Restoring the Body, Mending the Mind, Strengthening the Spirit. Brenda Hunter. Colorado Springs, CO: WaterBrook Press, 2004.

Supportive and Palliative Care

American Cancer Society's Guide to Pain Control: Understanding and Managing Cancer Pain. Atlanta, GA: American Cancer Society, 2004.

Cancer Pain: Assessment and Management. Eduardo Bruera and Russell Portenoy, eds. New York: Cambridge University Press, 2003.

The Complete Guide to Relieving Cancer Pain and Suffering. Richard B. Patt and Susan S. Lang. New York: Oxford University Press, 2004.

Fatigue in Cancer. Jo Armes, Meinir Krishnasamy, and Irene Higginson, eds. New York: Oxford University Press, 2004.

Handbook of Cancer-Related Fatigue. Roberto Patarca-Montero. New York: Haworth Medical Press, 2004.

Lymphedema: Understanding and Managing Lymphedema After Cancer Treatment. Atlanta, GA: American Cancer Society, 2006.

Principles and Practice of Palliative Care and Supportive Oncology, 2nd ed. Ann M. Berger, Russell K. Ortenoy, and David E. Weissman, eds. Philadelphia, PA: Lippincott Williams & Wilkins, 2002. Chapter 74, "Long-Term Survivorship: Late Effects," by Noreen M. Aziz.

Journal Literature

Cancer survivorship in the adult: an annotated bibliography. Mitchell SA. *Am J Nurs* 2006; 106(3 Suppl):e1–e19.

Clinical practice guidelines for the care and treatment of breast cancer: follow-up after treatment for breast cancer (summary of 2005 update). Grunfeld E, Dhesy-Thind S, Levine M, Steering Committee on Clinical Practice Guidelines for the Care and Treatment of Breast Cancer. *CMAJ* 2005;172(10):1319–20.

Health care of young adult survivors of childhood cancer: a report from the Childhood Cancer Survivor Study. Oeffinger KC, Mertens AC, Hudson MM, et al. *Ann Fam Med* 2004;2(1):61–70.

Health status of adult long-term survivors of childhood cancer: a report from the Childhood Cancer Survivor Study. Hudson MM, Mertens AC, Yasui Y, et al. *JAMA* 2003;290 (12):1583–92.

Improving health care for adult survivors of childhood cancer: recommendations from a Delphi Panel of Health Policy Experts. Mertens AC, Cotter KL, Foster BM, et al. *Health Policy* 2004;69(2):169–78.

Intensive lifestyle changes may affect the progression of prostate cancer. Ornish D, Weidner G, Fair WR, et al. *J Urol* 2005;174 (3):1065–9; discussion 1069–70.

Limitations on physical performance and daily activities among long-term survivors of childhood cancer. Ness KK, Mertens AC, Hudson MM, et al. *Ann Intern Med* 2005;143(9): 639–47. Summary for patients on p. I30.

Long-term follow-up guidelines for survivors of childhood, adolescent, and young adult cancers. Children's Oncology Group, version 2.0, March 2006. http://www.survivorshipguidelines.org.

Long-term follow-up of people who have survived cancer during childhood. Skinner R, Wallace WH, Levitt GA UK Children's Cancer Study Group Late Effects Group. *Lancet Oncol* 2006;7(6):489–98.

Long-term outcomes of adult survivors of childhood cancer. Robison LL, Green DM, Hudson M, et al. *Cancer* 2005;104(11 Suppl): 2557–64.

Nutrition and Physical Activity During and After Cancer Treatment: An American Cancer Society Guide for Informed Choices. Doyle C, et al. *CA Cancer J Clin* 2006;56(6):323–53.

Riding the crest of the teachable moment: promoting long-term health after the diagnosis of cancer. Demark-Wahnefried W, Aziz NM, Rowland JH, Pinto BM. *J Clin Oncol* 2005;23(24):5814–30; comment, 5458–60.

The state of the science on nursing approaches to managing late and long-sequelae of cancer and cancer treatment. *Am J Nurs* 2006;106(3 Suppl):1–102.

Appendix C: Useful Web Addresses

Alexandra Andrews, Webmaster, cancersupportivecare.com, and Ernest H. Rosenbaum, M.D.

American Cancer Society – www.cancer.org

The American Cancer Society is the nationwide community-based voluntary health organization dedicated to eliminating cancer as a major health problem by preventing cancer, saving lives, and diminishing suffering from cancer through research, education, advocacy, and service. English and Spanish versions. Toll-free number: 1-800-ACS-2345 (hotline).

American Chronic Pain Association – www.theacpa.org

The American Chronic Pain Association offers education and support for people living with chronic pain.

American Hospice Foundation – www.americanhospice.org

The American Hospice Foundation opens new doors to hospice care through public education programs focused on strategically selected audiences such as employers, schools, insurance companies, and religious organizations.

American Institute for Cancer Research Online – www.aicr.org

The American Institute for Cancer Research is the nation's leading charity in the field of diet, nutrition, and cancer prevention.

American Pain Foundation – www.painfoundation.org

The American Pain Foundation is a nonprofit organization that provides information, advocacy, research, and support for people living with pain.

American Red Cross – www.redcross.org

The American Red Cross helps keep people safe every day, especially in emergencies.

American Society of Breast Disease – www.asbd.org

The American Society of Breast Disease advocates a multidisciplinary team approach to breast health management and to breast disease prevention, early detection, treatment, and research.

American Society of Clinical Oncology (ASCO) – www.asco.org

ASCO Online is an interactive resource for oncology professionals and cancer patients.

Association of Cancer Online Resources (ACOR) – www.acor.org

ACOR.org offers access to mailing lists that provide support, information, and community to everyone affected by cancer and related disorders.

Association of Oncology Social Work (AOSW) World Wide Web Site – www.aosw.org

Oncology social work is the primary professional discipline providing psychosocial services to patients, families, and caregivers facing the impact of cancer diagnosis and treatment.

R. A. Bloch Cancer Foundation, Inc. – www.blochcancer.org

Richard Bloch Cancer Foundation's Web site. More than 8 million Americans are alive today with a history of serious cancer because they didn't give up hope and fought their disease.

The Cancer Answer – www.thecanceranswer.org

"Cancer Answer Second Opinions," by Malin Dollinger, M.D., F.A.C.P., of *Everyone's Guide to Cancer Therapy,* clinical professor, University of Southern California.

CancerCare – www.cancercare.org 1-800-813-HOPE

CancerCare is a national nonprofit organization that provides free, professional support services for anyone affected by cancer.

Cancer Links – www.cancerlinks.com

A thoughtful source and guide to cancer information on the Web. Choose from hundreds of helpful and useful links worldwide, with more added daily for your cancer needs.

Cancerlynx: We Prowl the Net – www.cancerlynx.com

Cancer Lynx: We Prowl the Net advocates for cancer patients and their families. The site provides news information and very human stories about cancer.

Cancer Supportive Care – www.cancersupportivecare.com

Supportive care becomes the fifth dimension in therapy after a diagnosis of cancer. Cancer patients face an uncertain future with potential problems and fears related to medical situations, such as side effects from therapy and loss or exacerbation of physical and mental function. This Web site is designed to help you cope with the myriad challenges that accompany the diagnosis and treatment of cancer.

cancerTrials: A Service of the National Cancer Institute – www.cancer.gov/clinicaltrials

NCI's gateway to information on cancer clinical trials, including what they are and how they work, how to find ongoing trials, results from recent studies, and resources for cancer researchers conducting trials.

Candlelighters Childhood Cancer Foundation (CCCF) – www.candlelighters.org

CCCF was founded in 1970 by concerned parents of children with cancer. Today the organization has more than 50,000 members of the national office and more than 100,000 members across the country, including Candlelighters affiliate groups.

Centers for Disease Control and Prevention (CDC) – www.cdc.gov/cancer

CDC works with national, state, and local partners to create and implement successful strategies to help the millions of people in the United States who live with, through, and beyond cancer. Materials are available for patients, physicians, and public health professionals. These materials may be downloaded and printed or ordered through CDC's Cancer Resource Library at www.cdc.gov/cancer/dcpc/library/index.htm.

Children's Hospice International (CHI) – www.chionline.org

CHI is committed to the concept of care called hospice. It recognizes the right and need for children and their families to choose healthcare and support, whether in their own home, hospital, or hospice.

Colorectal Cancer Prevention: Chemoprevention Database – www.inra.fr/reseau-nacre/sci-memb/corpet/indexan.html

Database of agents and diets ranked by efficacy and a systematic review of experimental studies.

Comprehensive Cancer Information: National Cancer Institute – www.cancer.gov

Accurate, up-to-date, comprehensive cancer information from the U.S. government's principal agency for cancer research.

Coping with Cancer – www.copingmag.com

Coping with Cancer is America's consumer magazine for people whose lives have been touched by cancer, now in its twenty-first year of providing knowledge, hope, and inspiration. Its readers include cancer patients (survivors) and their families, caregivers, healthcare teams, and support group leaders.

Diseases, Disorders and Related Topics – micf.mic.ki.se/Diseases

The library at Karolinska Institutet has for years collected links to free medical Web resources. The result is an extensive directory of quality-controlled links to Web sites and information resources on the Net.

Fertile Hope – www.fertilehope.org

A nonprofit organization, Fertile Hope provides fertility resources for cancer patients and can be contacted on the Web, by phone at 212-202-3692 or 888-994-HOPE, or by mail at P.O. Box 624, New York, NY 10014.

Food and Drug Administration Home Page – www.fda.gov

The FDA is the nation's foremost consumer protection agency.

healthfinder – www.healthfinder.gov

Your free guide to reliable health information, developed by the U.S. Department of Health and Human Services.

Health Library – healthlibrary.stanford.edu

The Health Library is a free public consumer health information source. The Health Library is a community service of Stanford Hospital and Clinics.

Hospice Foundation of America – www.hospicefoundation.org

Hospice Foundation of America is a not-for-profit organization that provides leadership in the development and application of hospice and its philosophy of care.

Institute of Medicine (IOM) – www.iom.edu

The Institute of Medicine is a nonprofit organization providing science-based information on biomedical science, medicine, and health.

International Federation of Red Cross and Red Crescent Societies – www.ifrc.org

The International Federation of Red Cross and Red Crescent Societies is the world's largest humanitarian organization, providing assistance without regard to nationality, race, religious beliefs, class, or political opinions.

International Union Against Cancer – www.uicc.org

The International Union Against Cancer is the only international nongovernment organization dedicated uniquely to the global control of cancer.

Leukemia & Lymphoma Society – www.leukemia-lymphoma.org

The Leukemia & Lymphoma Society is the world's largest voluntary health organization dedicated to funding blood cancer research, education, and patient services.

Look Good . . . Feel Better Cosmetic Program – www.lookgoodfeelbetter.org

The Look Good . . . Feel Better Cosmetic Program is a free national public service program designed to teach women and teens with cancer practical techniques that help restore their appearance during treatments. For more information, or to find out about programs in your area, call your local office of the American Cancer Society or the Look Good . . . Feel Better toll-free number (1-800-395-LOOK) or visit the Web site.

Medicare.gov: The Official U.S. Government Site for People with Medicare – www.medicare.gov

Medicare.gov is a consumer beneficiary Web site that provides access to information about Medicare and Medicare health plans, contact information and publications, and information about healthcare fraud and abuse and nursing homes.

Multinational Association of Supportive Care in Cancer (MASCC) – www.mascc.org

The MASCC is an international, multidisciplinary organization with more than 1,000 members representing more than thirty countries and five continents. It operates in collaboration with the International Society for Oral Oncology.

National Cancer Survivors Day Internet Information Guide – www.ncsdf.org

A survivor is anyone living with a history of cancer. This includes newly diagnosed survivors and long-term survivors. For many, National Cancer Survivors Day marks another year of life, truly the very best reason to celebrate.

National Center for Complementary and Alternative Medicine (NCCAM) – www.nccam.nih.gov

The NCCAM explores complementary and alternative healing practices in the context of rigorous science, trains researchers, and provides authoritative information to the public and professionals.

National Coalition for Cancer Survivorship (NCCS) – www.canceradvocacy.org

The NCCS is the oldest survivor-led cancer advocacy organization in the country and a highly respected authentic voice at the federal level, advocating for high-quality cancer care for all Americans and empowering cancer survivors. Includes a Spanish version.

National Institutes of Health (NIH) – www.nih.gov

The NIH is one of the world's foremost medical research centers. An agency of the U.S. Department of Health and Human Services, the NIH is the federal focal point for health research. The NIH Web site offers health information for the public and medical professionals. It includes extensive information on funding opportunities and links to the many institutes and centers that make up the NIH, such as the National Cancer Institute and the National Library of Medicine.

National Library of Medicine – ww.nlm.nih.gov

The National Library of Medicine, on the campus of the National Institutes of Health in Bethesda, Maryland, is the world's largest medical library. It collects materials in all major areas of the health sciences and to a lesser degree in such areas as chemistry, physics, botany, and zoology. The collections stand at 5 million items: books, journals, technical reports, manuscripts, microfilms, photographs, and images. Housed in the library is one of the world's finest medical history collections of old (pre-1914) and rare medical texts, manuscripts, and incunabula.

OncoLink: A University of Pennsylvania Cancer Center Resource – www.oncolink.com

OncoLink provides in-depth information about cancer.

Oncology Nursing Society (ONS) Online – www.ons.org

The official Web service of the Oncology Nursing Society.

Osher Center for Integrative Medicine – www.osher.ucsf.edu

The mission of the Osher Center for Integrative Medicine is to search for the most effective treatments by combining conventional and alternative approaches that address all aspects of health and wellness: biological, psychological, social, and spiritual. They are working to transform healthcare by conducting rigorous research on the medical outcomes of complementary and alternative healing practices; educating medical students, health professionals, and the public about these practices; and creating new models of clinical care.

San Antonio Breast Cancer Symposium – www.sabcs.org

This is an international scientific symposium for interaction and exchange between basic scientists and clinicians in breast cancer.

University of California San Francisco (UCSF) Medical Center – www.ucsfhealth.org

UCSF Medical Center and UCSF Children's Hospital are recognized throughout the world as leaders in healthcare, known for innovative medicine, advanced technology, and compassionate care. For almost a century, they have offered unparalleled medical treatment.

Index

References to graphics and sidebars are in *italics*.

E

J

P